DISORDERED THINKING AND THE RORSCHACH

DISORDERED THINKING
AND THE RORSCHACH

Theory, Research, and Differential Diagnosis

James H. Kleiger

THE ANALYTIC PRESS

1999   Hillsdale, NJ   London

Published by The Analytic Press, Inc.
101 West Street, Hillsdale, NJ 07642
www.analyticpress.com

Text designed and typeset by CompuDesign, Charlottesville, VA.
Index by Leonard S. Rosenbaum.

Library of Congress Cataloging-in-Publication Data

Kleiger, James H., 1952–
    Disordered thinking and the Rorschach : theory, research, and
differential diagnosis / James H. Kleiger.
        p.   cm.
    Includes bibliographical references and index.
    ISBN 0-88163-232-5
    1. Rorschach Test—Interpretation.   2. Psychoses—Diagnosis.
3. Diagnosis, Differential.   I. Title.
    [DNLM: 1. Psychotic Disorders—diagnosis. 2. Thinking.
3. Rorschach Test.   4. Psychoanalytic Theory.   5. Diagnosis,
Differential. WM 200 K63d 1999]
RC473.R6K54   1999
616.89'075—dc21
DNLM/DLC
for Library of Congress   99-11816
                                                                CIP

Printed in the United States of America

10   9   8   7   6   5   4   3   2   1

For M.J., my special rose

CONTENTS

PART 4 DIFFERENTIAL DIAGNOSIS OF
RORSCHACH THOUGHT DISORDER

ACKNOWLEDGMENTS

Writing a book about the Rorschach assessment of thought disorder was a daunting task. It was at times exhilarating and fascinating, and at other times frustrating and tiresome; but without the major contributions of a broad community of others, it would have been clearly impossible. How can one approach a subject like this without standing on the shoulders of intellectual heroes who have made monumental contributions to the field of Rorschach assessment? Thus, it is fitting to begin by acknowledging the seminal Rorschach contributions of such figures as Hermann Rorschach, David Rapaport, Robert Holt, Roy Schafer, Phil Holzman, Irv Weiner, John Exner, Sidney Blatt, and Paul Lerner. This is not to mention other historic figures, such as Beck, Klopfer, Piotrowski, Hertz, and Schachtel, who helped establish the empirical, theoretical, and conceptual foundations of the Rorschach. Each has contributed something directly or indirectly to my Rorschach education and in turn to the writing of this book. Were it not for their substantive endowments to the field, I would no doubt be occupying my time and energies in some other direction.

The circle of influence tightens when I think of four colleagues who have been of immeasurable help with my education about thought disorder and the Rorschach. This work would have also not been possible without their consultation and tutelage. I mention here Bob Athey, the master in conceptualizing thought disorder; Debbie Levy, who originally piqued my interest in studying thought disorder and has always been generous with her time and information; and Don Colson, who gave me the opportunity to join him and Athey in a project to develop an alternative method for scoring thought disorder on the Rorschach. Although the project did not survive, our friendship has, as well Don's thoughtful contributions to my understanding of thought disorder. Finally, I hold Marty Leichtman directly responsible for this book. Without his role as a teacher, role model, colleague, and cheerleader, I would have never undertaken a project such as this.

More peripheral, but no less important, has been the community of Rorschach peers and kindred spirits who have taught me through their own contributions to the literature and through correspondence in recent times and over the years. I include my evil twin Don Viglione, Marvin Acklin, Reid Meloy, Charles Peterson, Bruce Smith, Jed Yaloff, and Marvin Podd.

I could not fail to mention my esteem for my teachers and colleagues at Menninger who have guided me over the years through an apprenticeship that connects me to the likes of Rapaport, Holt, Schafer, Mayman, and Appelbaum. I thank Jon Allen, Sid Frieswyk, Lisa Lewis, Mary Jo Peebles-Kleiger, Sharon Nathan, Lui Leichtman, Len Horwitz, Bill Smith, Mel Berg, Arnie Schneider, Meredith Titus, Fred Shectman, and Mary Cerney for their patient mentoring, support, and friendship. They continue to embody the finest traditions and values of the Menninger psychologist.

Marty Leichtman could not have put me in touch with a better editor than John Kerr. I have valued John's expert advice that goes far beyond editoral assistance. Not only has he provided crucial input into the style and substance of my manuscript, but he was always extremely generous with his encouragement and support. This book would have remained a figment of my imagination without his help. I am also grateful to Melanie Livergood for her assistance in preparing this manuscript and to the staff librarians at Menninger for their cheerful assistance over the years and their patience with my frequent tardiness in returning books to the library.

Irv Rosen listened to me too often to remember as I ruminated about writing this book. What he offered was a space to explore much more than my musings about the content of the book or my experience as I embarked on the project. I am grateful to him for lessons about patience and persistence, about necessary losses, self acceptance, and integrity.

My family offered steady encouragement and showed great interest in trying to understand what the heck I was devoting my free time to. In particular, I'd like to thank my mother, father, sister, and Uncle Bert. My immediate family deserves no less than a purple heart for enduring several years of living with a temperamental writer, chest high in books and papers. Nicky and Katie are my pride and joy and each day with them sustains me. Thanks, guys, for your suggestions for a title to this book. At the core of this experience is, of course, Mary Jo, my teacher, my love, and my fellow traveler, who has perhaps endured most of the privation associated with her husband's stubborn preoccupation.

Finally, I would be remiss if I did not acknowledge the countless patients who have endured the anxiety, tedium, and shame that can sometimes result from our noble efforts to study them with the Rorschach. For over twenty years they have been my tutors. For all they have given to me, I hope that I can continue giving something forward.

INTRODUCTION

For three quarters of a century, the Rorschach Test has captured the interest and imagination of several generations of psychodiagnosticians and researchers interested in the nature of personality functioning. Like all psychodiagnostic instruments, the Rorschach's popularity has periodically ebbed and flowed; however, it has proven to be a remarkably durable technique that continues to occupy a prominent place in graduate school curricula and the clinical practice of psychology.

Many fine books have been written about the the nature of the test and the response process. Rorschach scholars have differed on whether the Rorschach is best regarded as a "test," a "method," or a "technique"; whether it is a test of perception, cognitive-perceptual problem solving, or representation. Many have written about the methods of administration and scoring, the interpretative significance of key variables, and their experimental, psychometric, and experiential foundations. Others have devoted themselves to elucidating pertinent developmental issues or elaborating the theoretical underpinnings of the Rorschach. In addition to focusing on these issues, most texts address the subject of verbalization, or more specifically, pathological forms of verbalizing a response.

Rapaport (Rapaport, Gill, and Schafer, 1968) originally viewed verbalization as a component of the fifth major scoring category (along with frequency and organization) and the fourth major interpretative dimension (in addition to the quantitative and qualitative wealth of the record and the form level) of the Rorschach protocol. Perhaps more than anyone, Rapaport and his colleagues tried to discover the meaning of different forms of pathological reasoning and verbalization expressed in the response. Long interested in the structure and pathology of thinking, Rapaport sought to penetrate the scoring categories and capture the psychological rationale and diagnostic significance of the major categories of disturbed thinking and verbalization on the Rorschach.

Rapaport laid the groundwork for subsequent writers who attempted to extend the meaning of thought disorder scoring on the Rorschach. Some sought to broaden the interpretative scope of thought disorder scores (Athey, 1974, 1986; Blatt and Ritzler, 1974; Kleiger and Peebles-Kleiger, 1993); others have tried to refine the psychometric characteristics of these scoring categories (Exner, Weiner, and Schuyler, 1976; Exner and Weiner, 1982, 1995); and still others have labored to identify the differential diagnostic implications of thought disorder scores among various clinical groups (Shenton, Solovay, and Holzman, 1987; Solovay, Shenton, and Holzman, 1987). Viewed separately, each of these contributions has increased our understanding of thought disorder on the Rorschach. Taken together, they add significant depth and breadth to the study of disordered thinking in general.

Reviewing and integrating these various approaches is the mission of this book. Whereas other texts have addressed thought disorder as one among many salient variables, I wish to focus solely on thought disorder, the various ways in which it is scored, the conceptual and empirical underpinnings of these scores, and their normative and diagnostic implications. More specifically, I am interested in deconstructing various scoring categories in order to ascertain the psychological experience that underlies the scores. The premise of this book is that Rorschach thought disorder scores can provide a basis for making inferences about a broad range of experience.

I believe that serious-minded students and clinicians alike, despite the de-skilling climate of managed care, remain vitally interested in careful and comprehensive diagnostic work aimed at plumbing the depth of personality organization and mental experience. Many practitioners are not satisfied with a formula approach to interpreting test data and prefer, instead, an approach that allows them to "get inside" the scores and puzzle over the psychological meaning of different scoring categories and response patterns. I also believe that many clinicians hunger for a deeper understanding about the phenomena underlying the scoring categories on the test. As a serious study of Rorschach methods for assessing and conceptualizing thought disorder, I hope that this book will also contribute something to the understanding of the psychology of disordered thinking.

The book itself is rooted in the tradition of careful and comprehensive psychodiagnostic work that originated at the Menninger Foundation in the 1940s. Passed from one generation of psychologists to another in the form of a painstaking apprenticeship, the method of inference making from instruments like the Rorschach continues to focus on the unique experience of the individual taking the test. Although not tied to any specific scoring or theoretical tradition, my interest in the conceptual underpinnings of thought disorder scoring categories is influenced by the approaches of Rapaport, Holt, Holzman, Athey, Mayman, Lerner, Levy, and Leichtman, all of whom have had at one time or another an affiliation with the Menninger tradition. However, thoughtful diagnostic work was never the sole purview of Menninger. The scholarly work of others such as Weiner, Exner, and Blatt also contributed significantly to the ideas about which I have written. An integrationist at heart, I have attempted to pull together the best ideas of all of those who have attempted to make a serious study of the Rorschach assessment of thought disorder.

The book is organized in four parts. Part 1 examines the conceptual definitions of the phenomenon of thought disorder and the history of Rorschach approaches to measuring disordered thinking. Part 2 reviews a range of popular and less well-known thought disorder scoring systems. In Part 3, I have organized thought disorder scores into several conceptual frameworks, beginning with Pine's (1990) pluralistic psychoanalytic model (Drive, Ego, Object, and Self) and progressing to a detailed study of the meaning of each of the major scoring categories. Part 4 involves the differential diagnostic implication of the scoring categories and a review of the relationship between thought disorder and creativity. In the final chapter, I attempt to formulate some conclusions about the salient issues related to scoring and conceptualizing thought disorder on the Rorschach.

It must be stressed from the outset that as an in-depth study of one particular aspect of the total Rorschach experience, this book artificially focuses exclusively on thought disorder to the exclusion of other variables pertaining to formal scoring categories, thematic content, and patient-examiner interaction, not to mention data available from other testing instruments. Such a narrow focus falls short of the standard of adequate practice and is not intended to be a model for diagnostic work. Clearly, in practice, sound clinical inferences are based on converging lines of evidence from independent sources of data. No credible text would advocate using only one test, let alone only one score from that test. Therefore, it is assumed that clinicians will always weigh their inferences carefully and evaluate them in light of the data from other components of the overall evaluation. My effort to cast thought disorder scoring into bold relief will, I hope, encourage readers to consider the multiple meanings and implications of these scores as they view them in the context of the entire diagnostic picture.

PART

1

INTRODUCTION TO THOUGHT DISORDER AND THE RORSCHACH

The subject of thought disorder and the Rorschach test create a natural harmony. Not only do they share a number of similar concepts, but they also have overlapping historical roots. Beginning with a conceptual review of past and current theories and controversial issues regarding the nature of thought disorder, I will then turn to the subject of measurement and describe how the Rorschach has always been regarded as an ideal method for measuring and studying thought disorder. In chapter 2, I examine the role that the Rorschach has played over the last 75 years as a major method for assessing and studying disordered thinking.

CHAPTER

1

CONCEPTUALIZING

DISORDERED THOUGHT

Mrs. A eyed me suspiciously as I handed her Card III of the Rorschach. From the outset, she had expressed her reluctance to look at the inkblots, repeatedly asking about the purpose of the test and the nature of the blots. Gingerly accepting the card, she responded promptly: "Oh, this is two people with insectoid heads, ripping the scalp off some fat guy in the middle so they can drop a red wig into his brain. He has to be really fat because it would take two people to do something like that." Without so much as a breath, she added, "This isn't so bad. These blots are interesting."

Although taken by surprise by the sudden emergence of this strikingly primitive and bizarre response, I had to agree with her sentiments: these blots *are* interesting. Moreover, I began to wonder about the meaning of this unusual, rather unforgettable response. Beyond the obvious indication that her thinking was disturbed and that this regressive shift in her thought processes and reality testing was associated with primitive aggressive fantasies, I was not quite satisfied that my inferences had gone far enough. I could play more with the thematic content of the response and infer a self-other paradigm characterized by sado-masochistic themes or a feeble and vulnerable sense of self. Likewise, I could concentrate on the formal aspects of the response and conclude that Mrs. A's reasoning was severely strained, and that she had the capacity to become delusional. However, I felt that these inferences, while useful as possible starting points, were static and did not go far enough in helping me understand what her strained logic, idiosyncratic use of language, primitive content, and unrealistic combinations might actually mean about how she experienced the world. Put simply, I was left wondering more about the meaning of the psychological processes underlying this bizarre response.

Apart from the circular conclusion that thought disorder scores tell us that a person has a "thought disorder" or "impaired reasoning," what do they actually mean in terms of how an individual perceives the world, interacts with others, or feels about him or herself? Is it possible to derive more than static, one-dimensional inferences from Rorschach thought disorder scores? This is the question that inspired this book— how to go about deepening our understanding of different manifestations of thought disorder using the Rorschach. In particular, I am interested in exploring the conceptual meaning of different types of thought disorder, not only in terms of their differential diagnostic implications (and associated treatment considerations) but, more interestingly, in terms of what different forms of thought disorder can tell us about the psychological/phenomenological experience of the respondent.

Although there are many ways to measure and understand thought disorder, the Rorschach Test seems particularly well suited to this endeavor. With its lengthy history in the field of psychodiagnostic assessment, the Rorschach has been widely used as a research and clinical instrument for assessing and studying varieties of disordered thinking. In the last century, researchers pioneered a variety of Rorschach-based systems for scoring and interpreting manifestations of thought disorder. This book is a tribute to the work of these individuals and an attempt to synthesize and extend their contributions.

However, before attempting to explore the meanings of traditional thought disorder scoring on the Rorschach, it is important to begin at a more basic starting point. What is "thought disorder" anyway? How might we define, conceptualize, and measure it?

What Is Thought Disorder?

Accurate assessment of complex clinical phenomena rests on the clarity of the concepts that we seek to measure. Without agreement about the nature and scope of the clinical entity under question, assessment efforts can be confusing and contradictory as different approaches yield different findings about concepts that are inherently unrelated. Regardless of what kind of instrumentation is used, the clinical assessment of thought disorder must begin with a clarification of the meaning of the concept.

"Thought disorder" is a widely used and often misunderstood term with a history of controversy regarding scope of definition, underlying mechanisms, and diagnostic specificity. Following the presentation of a comprehensive working definition of disordered thinking, various controversies regarding the conceptual nature and the measurement of thought disorder can be addressed. A brief examination of these issues will set the stage for a review of pioneering efforts to use the Rorschach to evaluate and understand thought disorder.

THE NATURE OF THOUGHT DISORDER

Definition of Thought Disorder

More than 80 years ago, Emil Kraepelin (1896) and Eugen Bleuler (1911) identified disturbances in thinking as an important feature in dementia praecox (Kraepelin's term) or schizophrenia (Bleuler's term). Kraepelin described the deterioration in intellectual processes as an incoherent ordering of ideas which, instead of flowing in a linear manner, become "derailed" from their appropriate course. Kraepelin cared about thought disorder because it helped him isolate diagnostic groups with differing prognoses.

Bleuler made formal thought disorder the cornerstone of his theory for understanding the clinical phenomena of schizophrenia. He cared about thought disorder because it offered a path to understanding the central defect in a syndrome (the group of schizophrenias) otherwise marked by different, varied, and florid symptomatology. Bleuler thought that if he could identify and measure the central defect of the syndrome, he might be able to home in on the underlying cause and possibly discover a treatment. According to Bleuler's theory, the key to understanding schizophrenia lay in the pathological nature of the patient's thinking, specifically the disturbed associations among thoughts and feelings that are split from one another. He termed this splitting process "loosening of associations," which he viewed as the primary symptom of schizophrenia and the basis for all the clinical phenomena that follow.

Although by today's standards Bleuler's associationist approach provides an outdated and restricted explanation of thought disorder, it held sway in psychiatric circles up until the mid-1970s. For example, The Comprehensive Textbook of Psychiatry/II (Freeman, Kaplan, and Saddock, 1976) defined formal thought process disorder in terms of "irrelevance and incoherence of the patient's verbal productions. It ranges from simple blocking and mild circumstantiality to total loosening of associations, as in word salad" (p. 1333).

Even today, many psychiatric clinicians retain a one-dimensional view of thought disorder by equating it with the concept of "looseness of associations." The following DSM IV (American Psychiatric Association, 1994), definition of schizophrenic thought disorder is characterized by this narrow associationist approach, which tends to ignore the complexity and varied nature of disordered thinking.

> Disorganized thinking ("formal thought disorder," "loosening of associations") has been argued by some (Bleuler, in particular) to be the single most important feature of schizophrenia. . . . The person may "slip off track" from one topic to another ("derailment" or "loose associations"); answers to questions may be obliquely related or completely unrelated ("tangentiality") [p. 276].

Other attempts to conceptualize thought disorder go beyond the singularity of associational psychology. Fish (1962), for example, defined thought disorder as a disturbance of conceptual thinking in the absence of serious brain disease and in the presence of adequate intelligence. Harrow and Quinlan (1985) provided another simple definition by stating that thought disorder describes a variety of diverse types of verbalization and thinking that are labeled by others as bizarre and idiosyncratic. One cannot argue with this defintion; however, it does not take us very far. Harrow and Quinlan's definition amounts to stating that "crazy people say crazy things" without beginning to consider what it is about "crazy" thinking—and there are many things, not one thing—that makes it seem "crazy" to others. Used in this limited way, "thought disorder" is an empty concept. It may satisfy the professional's need for a more dignified term than "crazy," but offers no starting point for either a more precise taxonomy of different kinds of crazy presentations or a starting point for an analytic inquiry into what the various causes and implications of these presentations may be.

A more comprehensive definition of thought disorder would be one that encompasses a broader perspective that includes not only traditional concepts such as impaired pace and flow of associations, but also such factors as errors in syntax, word usage, syllogistic reasoning, inappropriate levels of abstracting, failure to maintain conceptual boundaries, and a breakdown in the discrimination of internal perceptions from external ones. Such a definition comes closer to capturing the multidimensional nature of disturbances in thought organization. Defined in this broad manner, disordered thinking has been conceptualized and elaborated in a variety of ways, some of which have led to confusion and sparked disagreement and controversy over the decades.

Unraveling the Conceptual Tangles of Thought Disorder

What are other ways in which disorders of thinking may be characterized, studied, and understood? The study of thought disorder covers broad conceptual territory, with clear historical roots, controversial issues and dialectical positions, and links to related fields of linguistics and the neurosciences. I believe that it is useful to understand something about the background of the concept, the arguments that have cropped up along the way, and the different perspectives from which thought disorder can be studied and applied. The following review is not intended to be exhaustive but highlights a number of important vantage points along the conceptual pathway.

THOUGHT DISORDER OR SPEECH DISORDER. Psychiatric researchers and psycholinguists have disagreed about the conceptual and terminogical nature of thought disorder. The term "thought disorder" has been widely accepted among psychiatric researchers who view language and speech as representative of thought (Harrow and Quinlan, 1985; Lanin-Kettering and Harrow, 1985; Holzman, Shenton, and Solovay, 1986). Holzman, probably the clearest spokesman for this group, has asserted that language is a transparent medium through which thought is expressed. According to Holzman, since deviant verbal productions of psychotic patients reveal disturbed thought processes, the peculiarities in psychotic communication should be labeled "thought disorders" and not speech or language disorders. Harrow and Quinlan (1985) acknowledged that speech and thought are not necessarily isomorphic with one another and that bizarre communication may, in some cases, be a product of impaired expression of reasonable ideas. However, like Holzman, they believed that their research supported the conclusion that faulty language or speech is generally a result of strange thinking and, hence they, too, favor the term "thought disorder." Andreasen (Andreasen, Hoffman, and Grove, 1985) also retained the term "thought disorder" in her research; however, she was more troubled by the "conceptual entangling of thought and language" (p. 202). Despite her use of the traditional terminology, Andreasen favored scrapping the term "thought disorder" and substituting terms such as "communication disorders," "dysphasia," or "dyslogia" (Andreasen, 1982).

Linguists have typically challenged the assumptions of psychiatric researchers and disputed the empirical basis for equating speech with thought. Chaika (1990), who introduced the term "speech disorder," accused psychiatric researchers of circular reasoning in claiming that disturbed thinking necessarily underlies disturbed speech. She said that there is no empirical evidence that demonstrates that disordered thinking always produces disordered speech. Although thought is expressed through language, it is a logical fallacy, according to Chaika, to conclude that language is a direct expression of thought. Chaika's view, echoed by others (Harvey and Neale, 1983), is that language, speech, and thought cannot be equated, and that all that we can study are observable disturbances in speech. Making inferences about the nature of underlying thought processes, based on the quality of an individual's verbal productions, is unwarranted.

Both Holzman and Chaika agreed that thought disorder and language or speech disturbances can occur independently. Holzman used this finding to argue that since language and speech disorders are separate entities (clinically distinct from psychotic thought disorders), it is reasonable to conclude that the verbal anomalies of psychotic patients result directly from disordered thinking. Conversely, Chaika viewed the independence of thought and language/speech as the basis for concluding that thought is not equivalent with and cannot always be inferred from speech. Chaika reminded us that psychotic thought disorder is not necessarily accompanied by any of the florid speech disorders, nor do any of these automatically indicate disordered thinking.

Regardless of whom one chooses to believe, it is clear that thought and speech are independent and can coexist in a variety of ways. People can either say things strangely, they can say strange things, or they can do both. In other words, people can express logical ideas in the form of bizarre speech, bizarre ideas in the form of coherent speech, or bizarre ideas through the medium of bizarre and deviant speech.

Harvey and Neale (1983) criticized the term "thought disorder," which they felt was confounded with disturbances in speech and language, and recommended that traditional terminology be replaced with two new categories, one called "discourse failure" and the other, "deviant cognitive processes that relate to discourse failures." Andreasen's (1982) terms "dysphasia" and "dyslogia" seem to capture this same division between deviant speech and deviant ideas. This bifurcated view of thought disorder is also suggestive of the distinction traditionally made between thought disorders of form versus thought disorders of content.

Part of the difficulty may be that, by virtue of training and interests, psychiatric researchers and linguists place emphasis on different areas of functioning. Holzman, for example, is a psychologist and psychoanalyst interested primarily in studying underlying thought processes, while Chaika is a linguist chiefly interested in the pragmatic analysis of verbal discourse. Chaika is more concerned with the form of deviant speech, such as disturbances in syntax, semantics, and coherence, while Holzman is concerned as much with the content as with the form. Furthermore, Chaika looks at the formal qualities of deviant speech and entertains a range of possible causative explanations, whereas Holzman assumes that deviant verbalizations and strange ideas reflect disturbed thinking. In essence, Holzman's approach is consistent with psychiatric and psychodiagnostic methodology, in which one assumes that inferences about underlying psychological structures and organization can be made on the basis of observable behavior. By contrast, Chaika challenges these assumptions and questions the validity of inferring the nature of that which is not available for direct observation.

Despite Chaika's cogent arguments, there are a number of reasons that Rorschach clinicians will choose to retain the traditional term "thought disorder" to describe deviant verbal productions of psychotic patients. First, "thought disorder" is the traditional term used in clinical diagnostic and treatment settings to describe the deviant verbal productions and peculiar ideas of psychotic patients. Introducing new terminology, such as "speech disorder," "dysphasia," or "dyslogia," may clear up confusion for some; but it would undoubtedly contribute to a further muddying of the water in a more general sense, as clinicians and researchers would now have multiple terms to argue about and use in contradictory ways. Relatedly, all of the major Rorschach thought disorder systems have retained the traditional terminology, making for a shared conceptual language. Even non-Rorschach thought disorder researchers such as Andreasen, who has been quite critical of the term "thought disorder," has elected to continue using this term. Secondly, psychodiagnosticians spend as much, if not more time, evaluating the nature of patients' fallacious reasoning and peculiar ideas (often expressed in the context of normal and coherent speech) as they do evaluating the formal qualities of their deviant or bizarre speech. It is unclear how the term "speech disorder" would apply to the kinds of problems in logical reasoning that psychologists encounter on testing. Further, using the term "dysphasia" to describe deviant speech and "dyslogia" to describe strained logic seems somewhat cumbersome. Although intended to increase clarity and precision in clinical thinking, these new terms may actually invite more confusion. To make the distinction between dysphasia and dyslogia, psychologists can instead employ the traditional concepts of disorders in the "form" versus "content" of thought. These more recognizable terms can then be subsumed under the broader heading of either "thought disorder" or "disordered thinking."

Thus, for the purposes of this book the traditional terminology will be used. Although the terms "thought disorder" or "disordered thinking" are surely flawed and surrounded by a degree of conceptual unclarity, they are the best terms we have to communicate our understanding of commonly encountered clinical phenomena in psychotic patients.

SPECIFICITY: DISENTANGLING THOUGHT DISORDER FROM SCHIZOPHRENIA.
From a historical perspective, the psychiatric and psychodiagnostic
study of thought disorder has been inseparable from the evaluation
and diagnosis of schizophrenia. Up to the mid-1970s, the centrality
and specificity of thought disorder to schizophrenia was largely
unquestioned (a fact that will be echoed repeatedly throughout this
book). Until relatively recently, the work of the Andreasen group
(Andreasen and Powers, 1974; Andreasen, 1979a, b) and the Harrow
group (Harrow and Quinlan, 1977; Harrow et al., 1980, 1982;
Rattenbury et al., 1983) demonstrated convincingly that disordered
thinking is as prominent in manic psychosis as it is in schizophrenia.
Harrow and Quinlan (1985) found that not only do high levels of
thought disorder occur in both manic and schizophrenic patients but
that there is no difference in the extent of thought disorder between
the two groups. This is an issue that will be examined in more detail
in later chapters.

Having established that disordered thinking is not specific to schizophrenia and that it is associated with manic psychosis as well, Marengo
and Harrow (1985) wondered whether thought disorder is simply a general function of psychosis as opposed to being a manifestation of any
particular diagnostic syndrome. They found that even though psychotic
patients were more thought disordered than nonpsychotic patients,
severely disordered thinking was not just a basic function of psychosis
but occured significantly more frequently among manic and schizophrenic patients than it did in other psychotic conditions. They observed
that the frequency of thought disorder occurred most frequently in
mania, followed in descending order by schizophrenia, schizoaffective
disorders, other psychotic conditions, nonpsychotic disorders, and
depression. Thus, while severe thought disorder is not specific to and
pathognomonic of one diagnostic entity in particular, it is more frequently observed in mania and schizophrenia (both in acutely psychotic
and nonpsychotic manic patients alike) than in other types of psychotic
and nonpsychotic disorders.

Holzman's group further refined the specificity issue by demonstrating that schizophrenia, mania, and schizoaffective conditions can
be distinguished by qualitative aspects of their disordered thinking
(Shenton et al., 1987; Solovay et al., 1987). Although they found certain types of thought disorder were nonspecific and occurred in each
psychotic group, they discovered that each psychotic condition had a
distinctive thought disorder "signature," characterized by different
patterns of disordered thinking, that could play an important role in
differential diagnosis.

Over the last two decades, additional studies have documented the presence of thought disorder, previously associated exclusively with schizophrenia (and later, mania), in a greater variety of patient groups. Psychological test findings demonstrated a range of thought disorder phenomena in borderlines (Singer, 1977; Kwawer et al., 1980; Carr and Goldstein, 1981; Armstrong, Silberg, and Parente, 1986; Edell, 1987) and eating disordered patients (Small et al., 1988). Other studies have established the presence of varieties of disordered thinking in depression (Ianizito, Cadoret, and Pugh, 1974; Silberman, Weingartner, and Post, 1983; Carter, 1986); in schizoid personality disorders (Wolff, 1991); among the nonschizophrenic relatives of schizophrenic individuals (Shenton et al., 1989); and, occasionally, in normal subjects (McConaghy and Clancy, 1968).

POSITIVE OR NEGATIVE THOUGHT DISORDER. Like most of the controversies surrounding the concept of thought disorder, the distinction between positive and negative symptoms is an outgrowth of research on schizophrenia. First used by Hughlings-Jackson (1931), the terms "positive" and "negative symptoms" describe two qualitatively distinct types of schizophrenic thought disorder symptomatology. Positive thought disorder includes examples of flagrantly apparent bizarreness in speech and logic and may manifest itself in unusual ideas, delusions, and hallucinations. Most of the Schneiderian first rank symptoms, such as thought broadcasting, thought withdrawal, and thought insertion (Schneider, 1959), reflect forms of positive thought disorder, which are highly related to schizophrenia. However, as we have already seen, the presence of positive thought disorder, or what Harrow and Quinlan (1985) called "bizarre-idiosyncratic thinking," may be sensitive but not specific to schizophrenia.

Negative thought disorder is usually conceived of as a deficit condition or absence of normal functioning. Based on their review of the literature, Lewine and Sommers (1985) divided the negative signs and symptoms into four domains including affect-arousal, perception-cognition, physical, and interpersonal. Generally recognized features include blunted affect, anhedonia, apathy, poverty of speech and thought content, social withdrawal, slowed speech, and psychomotor retardation. Unlike positive thought disorder, negative symptoms are generally regarded as specific to a subtype of schizophrenia (Andreasen, 1982) and associated with poor outcome (Astrup and Noreik, 1966; Pogue-Geile and Harrow, 1984). Some have referred to this subtype as "Type II" schizophrenia (as compared to "Type I" or the positive thought disordered form of the syndrome). Type II is said to be characterized by negative symptoms, neurological abnormalities, impaired cognition, and poor response to treatment (Crow, 1980).

Lewine and Sommers raised questions about a number of traditional assumptions regarding the conceptual nature of negative symptoms. In particular, they took issue with the automatic tendency to equate negative symptoms with a deficit state. Koistinen (1995) highlighted other problems associated with studies of positive and negative symptoms. For example, the patients diagnosed as schizophrenic in these studies often cannot be easily separated into pure culture groups with only negative or positive symptoms. Gur et al. (1991) found that the largest group of patients in their study was classified as having both positive and negative symptoms with a much smaller number falling specifically into one group or the other. A number of others have begun to question whether the positive-negative dichotomy is an oversimplification which fails to capture the complexity of forms of schizophrenic (and nonschizophrenic) thought disorder (Arndt, Alliger, and Andreasen, 1991; Van Der Does et al., 1993).

SINGLE COMPONENT OR MULTIPLE FACTORS. The early history of thought disorder research was characterized by a proliferation of theories which attempted to account for all schizophrenic thought disorder phenomena on the basis of a central explanatory mechanism or defect. In their seminal study of disordered thinking in schizophrenia, Chapman and Chapman (1973) provided a detailed review and critique of these theories, most of which were stimulated by Bleuler's (1911) belief in a single underlying psychological defect in schizophrenia. For Bleuler this defect was the breaking of associative threads between ideas that could account for all the symptoms of schizophrenia. Vigotsky (1934) and Goldstein (Goldstein and Scheerer, 1941) moved away from associationist theories and focused instead on schizophrenic patients' inability to think abstractly and tendency to think concretely. Cameron (1938) rejected the notion that schizophrenics were overly literal and concrete and paid attention to their failure to maintain conceptual boundaries and tendency to engage in overinclusive thinking. Von Domarus (1944) and Arieti (1955, 1974) emphasized the primacy of illogical reasoning in schizophrenic thought disorder. They used the terms "paralogical" (von Domarus, 1944) and "paleological" thinking (Arieti, 1955) to describe classical errors in syllogistic reasoning in which two things are identified on the basis of common predicates as opposed to similar subjects. Chapman and Chapman (1973) reviewed a number of other single component theories including their own theory which they called "excessive yielding to normal biases." According to the Chapmans, the intrusive associations in schizophrenic speech are not arbitrary but are common associates which are then substituted for more appropriate responses.

Harrow and Quinlan (1985) empirically evaluated the centrality and validity of a number of these classic single component theories. Like the

Chapmans, Harrow and Quinlan did not find empirical support for the primacy of any one of the theories in the samples of schizophrenic patients they studied. Moreover, both groups of researchers found that not all types of thought disorder (as represented by different theories) are equally important. Especially if examined at different phases of the disorder, such as the acute phase, partial remission, and chronic phases, several of the classic types of thought disorder studied by the central defect theorists are less important. For example, some of the types of disordered thinking that were hypothesized as central to schizophrenia were found more frequently during the acute phase of the illness and others were associated more with chronicity. Looseness, conceptual overinclusiveness, errors in reasoning, and boundary problems were all observed to occur more frequently in acute stages of schizophrenia. Conversely, an inability to think abstractly and excessively concrete thinking were more prominent among chronic schizophrenic patients and were associated with impoverished thinking associated with negative symptomatology.

In general Harrow and Quinlan concluded that looseness, overinclusiveness, and fallacious logic occur more readily in acute schizophrenia; but as time passes, there is usually a reduction in each type and the total composite of bizarre-idiosyncratic thinking. They proposed a model in which disordered thinking is not a consequence of a single factor or defect but of several factors which may often interact. One key factor involves something they termed "impaired perspective" which reflects a failure in one's ability to judge critically the social appropriateness of one's verbal productions. According to Harrow and Quinlan, thought disordered individuals fail to discern whether or not they will sound bizarre or comprehensible to others. Harrow and Quinlan also consider the intermingling of material from idiosyncratic experiences and preoccupations into one's verbalizations to be another critical underlying aspect of thought disorder. The final underlying aspect of thought pathology is a general "confusion-disorganization" factor that occurs in the acute phase of any psychotic condition.

One other approach to categorizing thought pathology and thinking in general was presented by Weiner (1966) and later elaborated by Johnston and Holzman (1979). According to Weiner, thought processes chiefly consist of concept formation, cognitive focusing, and logical reasoning. Concept formation implies the ability to interpret experience at appropriate levels of abstraction and reflects the continuum of concreteness on one end and overinclusion on the other. Cognitive focusing involves scanning, establishing, and maintaining a focus on relevant stimuli, and ignoring irrelevant details. Stimulus overinclusion (Shield, Harrow, and Tucker, 1974) is a term which describes an individual's tendency to be distracted by a wide range of irrelevant stimuli. The intrusion of idiosyncratic thoughts and loose associations that reflect a deviation from the task at hand are also subsumed under the heading of problems in maintaining a focus. Finally, problems in reasoning reflect difficulties in drawing logical inferences about the relationships between things, people, events, and so on. Illogical conclusions can be formed on the basis of syllogistic errors (von Domarus, 1944; Arieti, 1967), the tendency to establish meaning on the basis of minimal evidence, or the collapse of appropriate conceptual boundaries between incompatible ideas or objects. Weiner's framework will be presented in more detail in chapter 12 when we review the conceptual meaning of different thought disorder scores on the Rorschach.

DICHOTOMOUS OR CONTINUOUS VARIABLE. Classical researchers in the field of thought disorder presented theories that viewed thought pathology as the product of a single underlying defect that was dichotomous in nature. In other words, thought disorder was seen as a unitary phenomenon which was either present or absent. Thinking was either normal or bizarre; there was no conception that thinking may exist along a continuum from normal to pathological. However, just as theories regarding the specificity and unitary nature of thought disorder gave way to more complex and holistic conceptual understanding, so too did the belief that disordered thinking is dichotomous in nature.

Contemporary researchers and practitioners agree that disordered thinking fits along a continuum extending to normal, nondisturbed thinking (Harrow and Quinlan, 1977, 1985; Johnston and Holzman, 1979; Andreasen and Grove, 1986; Holzman et al., 1986). The distinction between milder forms of thought pathology and more severe levels of disordered thinking is widely accepted. Harrow and Quinlan (1977) demonstrated that mild levels of thought disorder occur quite frequently in many acutely disturbed schizophrenic and nonschizophrenic individuals alike, but that the most severe levels of thought disorder occur less frequently among all patients except for acutely disturbed schizophrenic patients. Marengo and Harrow (1985) later showed that acutely disturbed psychotic and nonpsychotic manic patients may exhibit similarly high levels of severe thought disorder as schizophrenic patients and significantly greater levels of severe thought disorder than either other psychotic or nonpsychotic patients. Even within the same diagnostic group or individual per se, there is variability in the level or degree of thought disorder between individuals and within the same individual depending on the phase of illness (Harrow and Quinlan, 1977).

Because pathological thought processes occur along a continuum of severity, as opposed to occupying a discrete realm of functioning, Harrow and Quinlan (1977) proposed that the term "disordered thinking" be substituted for the term "thought disorder." They argued that the term "thought disorder" is misleading in that it implies a distinct and unique entity dichotomous with normal thinking.

I find the term "disordered thinking" consistent with the concept of action language (Schafer, 1976; Harty, 1986) and one that helps avoid reification of constructs by remaining closer to the raw data of observable behavior. The observable behavior most relevant to the study of disordered thinking in this book is a range of verbalizations that convey the bizarre and idiosyncratic structure and content of Rorschach responses. In the scoring systems we will study, these responses are coded into scores which reflect gradations in the degree of disturbed thinking, from mild to more severe. The concept of a continuum of functioning is, thus, inherent in all extant Rorschach approaches for assessing thought disorder. For this reason, the term "disturbed or disordered thinking" is preferred to the more static term "thought disorder."

NEUROPSYCHOLOGICAL OR PSYCHOLOGICAL DEFICIT. Traditionally studied as a psychological construct, researchers have increasingly sought to understand disordered thinking from a cognitive neuroscience perspective. Actually, both Bleuler (1911) and Kraepelin (1896) paved the way for later efforts to conceptualize thought disorder neuropsychologically. Both highlighted the attentional deficits in schizophrenia. As a result, the domain of attention early captured the interest of neuroscientists seeking to understand the cognitive and neurological substrata of thought disorder. Most of these efforts focused more narrowly on schizophrenic thought disorder as opposed to the manifestations of disordered thinking in other clinical syndromes. McGhie and Chapman (1961) studied disorders of attention and perception in schizophrenia and stressed the importance of integrating and stabilizing sensory data to reduce the chaotic flow of information that reaches consciousness. Venables (1960) put forth the concept of "flooding" by sensory overload in schizophrenia.

More recently, Nuechterlein and Dawson (1984) postulated that impairments in attention and information processing were the underlying cause of thought disorder in schizophrenia. Using tests that require sustained attention and information processing (a span of apprehension test and a special version of the Continuous Performance Test), Nuechterlein's group subsequently examined both the stability of information processing performance across time and the relationship between attentional variables and thought disorder (Nuechterlein et al., 1986). Comparing the performances of schizophrenic and manic patients, the researchers concluded that attentional impairment may be more of a "trait" variable for schizophrenic subjects than it is for manic ones.

Through a series of investigations, Braff and his colleagues have demonstrated that schizophrenic patients exhibit abnormal information processing when compared to nonpatient controls (Braff and Saccuzzo,

1981; Braff and Geyer, 1990; Braff, Saccuzzo, and Geyer, 1991; Braff, Grillon, and Geyer, 1992). When information processing deficits occur, sensory registration may be impaired, resulting in problems in higher order cognitive operations. When attention and information processing functions are impaired, schizophrenic subjects may experience increased distractibility in response to a flooding by excessive and poorly inhibited internal and external stimuli, leading to cognitive fragmentation and markedly disordered thinking.

Cutting edge research is being conducted to examine the correlation between thought disorder, neuropsychological measures, and neuroanatomical brain structures (Spitzer, 1997; Nestor et al., 1998). These researchers are attempting to understand thought disorder (primarily in schizophrenia) by studying components of verbal memory as they relate to information processing. In particular, the concepts of (1) "working memory," an auditory and visuospatial subsystem for the storage of transient information, (2) a "central executive" subsystem (which coordinates the processing of material in both of these subsystems and the accessing of long-term storage), and (3) "semantic associative memory" have been employed to conceptualize schizophrenic thought disturbances. Goldman-Rakic (1992) suggested that because of a prefrontally-based deficit in working memory, schizophrenic patients may lose their train of thought, fail to perceive causal relationships, and be unable to regulate their behavior by internal schemata and ideas. Other studies suggested that thought disorder in schizophrenia may be related to left temporal lobe abnormalities in semantic processing (Shenton et al., 1992). Nestor and his colleagues (Nestor et al., 1993) also suggested that a dysfunctional semantic system may underlie disordered forms of thinking in schizophrenia as a result of temporal lobe pathology.

It is certain that neuroscientists will push their investigations of disordered cognitive processes into the realm of nonschizophrenic syndromes. Increasingly we can expect neuropsychological studies of thought disturbances in affective, trauma-based, characterological, and anxiety-related disorders.

ASSESSING DISORDERED THINKING

Controversies, Problems, and Challenges

Measuring disordered thinking is beset with a number of controversies, potential problems, and challenges. As we have already seen, making inferences about an intangible variable such as thinking from overt speech is controversial and has led to questions about the validity of the construct of "thought disorder." Because the construct itself is called into question, instruments which purport to measure disordered thinking, instead of disordered speech, for example, are vulnerable to the criticism that they lack sufficient construct validity to justify claims of their effectiveness as diagnostic tools. Nonetheless, despite, this potential criticism, the construct of "thought disorder" (versus speech or language disorder) has gained ascendancy in the fields of psychopathology and psychodiagnostic testing and continues to be an accepted variable that clinicians and researchers seek to measure with instruments and techniques of all sorts.

Another difficulty that hinders assessment efforts is the lack of universal agreement on what constitutes disordered thought. As we have seen above, there may now be general agreement that disordered thinking exists along a continuum of severity and reflects a number of different anomalies in thinking. However, there is no absolute standard for classifying these anomalies of thought. Furthermore, different researchers tend to employ different techniques to assess different types of disturbed thinking. Although there may be overlap in many of the variables studied by different assessment techniques, comparison between the various techniques is often difficult. Different assessment methods may employ different names for similar variables or use the same name for essentially different types of disordered thinking.

Achieving sufficiently high interrater reliability or clinical sensitivity with the instruments is a challenge since many of the rating or scoring systems themselves are quite intricate, difficult to learn, and subject to interpretation. Research on the most prominent scales and scoring systems demonstrates that significantly high interrater reliablity is possible; however, learning some of these rating systems usually requires more than familiarizing oneself with the manuals. Often consultation with the researchers, who pioneered the rating scales or scoring systems, is necessary in order to use the instruments competently. For example, serious researchers interested in using the Thought Disorder Index or TDI (Johnston and Holzman, 1979) are encouraged to attend an intensive workshop with the Cambridge group who originated the TDI in order to calibrate their sensitivities and scoring thresholds with this original group of researchers.

Many of the categories of disordered thinking are not independent of one another and occur together in more severely disturbed cases. Scoring the presence and discerning the meaning of one particular type of thought disturbance may be obscured by the presence of several other types. Just as the simultaneous mixing of several different colors together can produce an impenetrable blackness, the concurrence of multiple types of disordered thought in one sample of speech or Rorschach response makes for a similar kind of obscurity in scoring and interpretation. Should all examples of disordered thinking in a given sample (e.g., a single response) be scored or just the predominent process? If one scores each subtype separately, how does one make sense of the contribution of each subtype in the presence of others? Can each be understood separately, or does the simultaneous presence of several subtypes of disordered thinking simply suggest severe confusion and disorganization characteristic of an acute disturbance? On the other hand, since some subtypes of disordered thinking have more specificity to certain types of disorders than others, the coincidence of these subtypes with other subtypes may have special diagnostic significance.

The impact of phase of illness, medication, and context must be taken into consideration when assessing disordered thinking. The degree to which an individual's thinking is disorganized will depend on whether he or she is in an acute phase, or in a partial or complete remission from the active disturbance. Valid measurement of disordered thinking also requires one to evaluate the subject's motivation, attitude, and the context in which the idiosyncratic thinking is revealed. Is the subject aware of the bizarreness of his or her speech or ideas; and if so, what is his or her attitude toward it? Is idiosyncratic thought used to shock, control, or entertain? As Johnston and Holzman (1979) pointed out, the presence of odd and difficult-to-understand material does not constitute immediate grounds for inferring the incursion of a psychotic process.

Finally, disordered thinking can be assessed by a variety of instruments ranging from formal psychological tests to structured interview techniques specifically designed to measure disordered thought. Although some of these better known instruments have achieved convergent validity with one another, there are few comparative studies and none that have established the superiority of one method over others.

What follows is a brief review of the categories of instruments used to measure disordered thinking. Here I will focus primarily on the non-Rorschach methods that have acheived credible results as diagnostic tools, as well as some of those that have been less successful in assessing bizarre and idiosyncratic thinking.

Methods and Procedures

Chapman and Chapman (1973) reviewed five methods of measuring thought disorder in schizophrenic patients including: (1) clinical description of spontaneous verbalizations; (2) clinical interpretation of verbalizations made to standardized stimuli; (3) classification of verbalizations into predetermined categories; (4) standardized tests with standardized scoring of verbalizations; (5) multiple choice techniques. These methods

differ from one another in the degree to which the examiner (1) speci-
fies the stimulus situation, (2) restricts the number of possible responses
that an individual can give, and (3) limits the scoring categories for these
responses. Koistinen (1995) divided assessment techniques into two
broad categories, those using structured interview techniques and those
based on psychological testing instruments. Structured interviews can
serve as standardized stimuli for responses which are then either interpreted clinically (without any prescribed scoring schema) or scored
according to rigorous scoring or rating specifications. However, semistructured or unstructured interviews can also be used as a basis for rating specific categories of thought disorder according to clearly defined
criteria. Psychological tests, on the other hand, always involve standardized stimuli which are most often associated with predetermined
response categories scored according to specific criteria. Interview techniques, used together with rating scales, and formal psychological
assessment instruments are the most common procedures for measuring
disordered thinking. Examples of these two widely used categories of
measurement will be reviewed below.

INTERVIEWS WITH RATING SCALES. Structured and unstructured interview techniques are usually accompanied by rating scales which attempt
to categorize degrees of severity of different types of thought disorder.
Johnston and Holzman (1979) mentioned several thought disorder rating scales that have been based on interview techniques over the last 25
years. Among these are Bellak's thought process rating scale (Bellak,
1969); Cancero's rating scale for thought disorder (Cancero, 1969); and
Grinker and Holzman's Schizophrenia State Inventory (Grinker and
Holzman, 1973). The Psychotic Inpatient Profile (PIP) (Lorr and Vest,
1969; Knight and Blaney, 1977; Knight et al., 1986) is another rating
scale designed to quantify verbal and nonverbal behavior of psychiatric
inpatients.

Perhaps the best contemporary example of rating scales based on
interview and observational data is Andreasen's Scale for the Assessment
of Thought, Language, and Communication (TLC) (Andreasen, 1978).
The scale consists of definitions and directions for rating the severity on
a 0–3 or 0–4 scale of 18 subtypes of formal thought disorder. Subjects
are ordinarily given a standard interview approximately 45 minutes in
length. The interview was designed to avoid focusing on the subject's
psychopathology and generally begins by asking the subjects to talk
about themselves uninterrupted for about five minutes. Following this
initial unstructured monologue, the examiner asks specific questions
regarding a variety of topics such as family life, politics, and religion.

Remember that Andreasen objected to the global term "thought disorder" and favors, instead, subdividing this concept into three categories

including "communication," "language," and "thought disorders." Like Harrow and Quinlan (1985), she believed that many subtypes of communication disorders result when the speaker fails to follow conventional rules that are used to make it easier for listeners to understand what is being said. Among these communication disorders, Andreasen lists poverty of speech content, pressured speech, distractible speech, tangentialiality, derailment or looseness, stilted speech, echolalia, self-reference, circumstantiality, loss of goal directedness, perseveration, and blocking. She reserves the term "language disorders" for those pathological instances in which the speaker violates syntactical and semantic conventions which guide language usage. Andreasen includes word approximations, neologisms, incoherence, and clanging among her language disorder category. Finally, she does not entirely eliminate the concept of "thought disorder," which she continues to use for those situations in which thinking by itself appears to be deviant. Poverty of speech, in which thought does not seem to occur, and illogical processes of forming conclusions or making inferences are examples of Andreasen's thought disorder category.

The TLC disorders defined by Andreasen are not all associated with a similar level of pathology. Some are suggestive of more severe psychopathology than others. These most severe TLC signs are grouped together and comprise the first 11 items of the scale. The remaining four items are generally indicative of less psychopathology. Andreasen provides a simple quantitative method to obtain a global rating of TLC disorder, which includes assigning greater weights to the more pathological subtypes.

The interrater reliabilities of each of the subtypes defined by Andreasen have been shown to be sufficiently high to make the TLC Scale a useful instrument for research and the clinical assessment of disordered thinking, speech, and language. Andreasen's research (Andreasen, 1979; Andreasen and Grove, 1986) has demonstrated both quantative and qualitative differences in TLC scores between different groups of psychotic patients.

PSYCHOLOGICAL TESTS. Psychological tests used to assess a wide range of psychological phenomena have been used by clinicians and researchers to assess disordered thinking. Tests such as the MMPI and MCMI offer the advantages of timeliness and ease of administration; however, they provide, at best, crude measures of deviant thinking. The unfortunate zeitgeist of equating thought disorder with schizophrenia led researchers to construct a variety of special indexes for the MMPI in order to diagnose or discriminate schizophrenia from neurotic conditions (Peterson, 1954; Taulbee and Sisson, 1957; Meehl and Dahlstrom, 1960; Heinrichs, 1964; Goldberg, 1965). More recently, Butcher and colleagues (Butcher et al., 1989) developed the MMPI 2 Content Scales, which included a Bizarre Mentation category. This special content scale, like Wiggins's Psychoticism Scale (Wiggins, 1966), was designed to measure patients' reports of strange thoughts and psychotic experiences. Researchers at Indiana University (Levitt, 1989) devised a scale that includes all MMPI items for which an endorsement indicates the existence of hallucinatory or delusional experience.

A variety of other self-administered paper and pencil tests have been used to assess aspects of schizophrenic functioning. The Psychosis Proneness Scales (Chapman, Chapman, and Miller, 1982), the Rust Inventory of Schizotypal Cognitions (Rust, 1987), the Venables Scale (Venables et al., 1990), and the Schizotypal Personality Questionnaire (Raine, 1991) were all developed to assess different core features of vulnerablity to schizophrenia or schizotypy (Meehl, 1962).

The Whitaker Index of Schizophrenic Thinking (WIST) (Whitaker, 1973) is a brief paper and pencil test designed to assess the presence of schizophrenic thought disorder. Although creatively constructed, the WIST was constructed before it was generally accepted that disordered thinking is both multidimensional in nature and not specific to schizophrenia. Based on a single defect theory that viewed thought disorder as a product of varying degrees of associational disturbances, the WIST seems somewhat antiquated by today's standards and to be of limited utility except for use as a screening device.

In general, self-report inventories cannot provide a detailed assessment of the nature of thought processes. Even attempting to diagnose generic psychosis with the MMPI or any other personality inventory is always a difficult task which is usually accompanied by an unacceptably high percentage of false positives and false negatives. True and false or multiple choice questions, if read carefully, understood correctly, and answered truthfully, might be sensitive to some unusual ideas and experiences; however, without a sample of verbal behavior, it is difficult to judge anything about the severity or quality of subtypes of disordered thinking or communication.

Researchers and clinicians have used other psychodiagnostic instruments which measure concept formation and verbal reasoning to assess disordered thinking. Object Sorting Tests (Vigotsky, 1934; Goldstein, 1939; Goldstein and Scheerer, 1941; Hanfmann and Kasanin, 1942) and the Proverbs Test (Benjamin, 1944; Gorham, 1956) have been used to measure concreteness and overinclusion, two of the early concepts which were viewed as central deficits in schizophrenic thought disorder. Marengo et al. (1986) constructed a comprehensive measure of bizarre-idiosyncratic thinking based on two brief verbal tests, the Gorham Proverbs Test (Gorham, 1956) and the Comprehension subtest of the

WAIS (Wechsler, 1955). This has proven to be a reliable technique that provides a measure of the presence, severity, and type of disordered thinking. The composite thought disorder index, based on the scoring of separate responses to items on both tests, has been used in a number of studies that have established the construct validity of this scale.

The Rorschach is one of the most widely used vehicles for assessing disordered thinking in clinical and research settings. The Rorschach may be considered a clinical diagnostic technique when it is used, in a loosely standardized manner, as a structured interview to elicit responses for clinical interpretation. On the other hand, it functions as a test when it is administered in a standardized manner and dimensions of the patient's responses are scored according to specific criteria. Although generally classified as a "projective" test, using the Rorschach to study disordered thinking does not really depend on the projective hypothesis, which holds that a subject projects idiosyncratic conflicts and other aspects of his or her internal world onto the ambiguous inkblot stimuli. Likewise, one does not need to make symbolic interpretations of response content to make inferences about underlying thought processes. On the contrary, Rorschach responses, as samples of verbal behavior, remain closely tied to actual phenomena that the investigator studying disordered thinking is trying to measure. Rorschach responses reflect consistent properties of an individual's style of perceiving, thinking, and communicating and as such, can provide a basis for making representational inferences (Weiner, 1977) about how an individual perceives, thinks, and communicates in other settings that are unstructured, open-ended, and not clearly defined.

Since the Rorschach was developed more than 70 years ago (Rorschach, 1921), researchers and clinicians have devoted enormous attention to identifying signs of schizophrenia and other forms of serious psychopathology. Although early psychodiagnostic studies with the Rorschach mirrored general psychiatric diagnostic trends which assumed an isomorphic relationship between schizophrenia and disordered thinking, Rorschach clinicians and researchers have gradually developed more sophisticated ways of conceptualizing and measuring thought pathology with the Rorschach. Chapters 2 and 3 provide a more in depth exploration of the evolution of past and contemporary Rorschach methods to assess disordered thinking.

CHAPTER

2

THE RORSCHACH ASSESSMENT
OF DISORDERED THINKING

Trends in the Rorschach assessment of disordered thinking have mirrored broader psychiatric trends in the diagnostic conceptualizing of thought disorder. Like their psychiatric counterparts, early Rorschach contributors did not consider thought disorder separately from schizophrenia. Much as early theorists viewed disordered thinking as a unitary and pathognomonic symptom of schizophrenia, pioneers in the field of Rorschach testing focused exclusively on the test's ability to identify diagnostic signs of schizophrenia. Only after the concept of thought disorder was liberated from schizophrenia, did Rorschach researchers turn their interest to using the instrument to identify different forms of disordered thinking in a variety of psychopathological conditions.

The development of different Rorschach approaches to assess disordered thinking can be ordered chronologically and also organized according to several broad methodological trends in Rorschach research. Weiner (1977) traced the evolution of four different methods or approaches to Rorschach validation and application, beginning with the "empirical sign" approach, the "cluster and configuration" approach, the "global impression" approach, and the "conceptual" approach. In this chapter, I trace the development of Rorschach approaches to assess disordered thinking as it evolved through three of Weiner's methodological epochs, the empirical-sign, the cluster-configuration, and the conceptual approaches. In many respects, each approach defines a different chronological period in Rorschach thought disorder research.

1920S–1940S: EMPIRICAL-SIGN APPROACH FOR ASSESSING SCHIZOPHRENIA

As Weiner (1977) pointed out, the empirical-sign approach originated with the work of Hermann Rorschach. Rorschach's approach to comparing inkblot responses from schizophrenic and other psychiatric groups with normal individuals set the stage for a generation of researchers to embark on similar attempts to compare dimensions of Rorschach responses between schizophrenic patients and other diagnostic groups.

Hermann Rorschach's Experiment

Rorschach conceived of his inkblot procedure as a test of perception. As such, he considered deviant response processes in terms of perceptual anomalies, as opposed to disturbed linguistic or ideational phenomena. Without using the term "thought disorder" or the like, Rorschach (1921) introduced three types of perceptual anomalies, which became forerunners of the major thought disorder scoring categories in all Rorschach scoring systems that followed.

When discussing the "mode of apperception," or location scores, Rorschach presented several atypical ways that subjects could deliver whole responses. In comparing his various patient samples, he noticed that certain test scores or "signs" appeared most often in psychotic records. He used the term "confabulated whole answer" (to which he gave the symbol DW) to describe how "a single detail, more or less clearly perceived, is used as the basis for the interpretation of the whole picture, giving very little consideration to other parts of the picture" (1921, p. 37). Rorschach gave as an example of a confabulated whole answer "A crab" on Card I, when it was based solely on the small claw-like figures in the center top portion of the blot. He went on to state that the accuracy of form of such "DW" responses, as he labeled them, would be poor.

Rorschach contrasted imaginative subjects with confabulating ones. He found that imaginative subjects could produce an integrated response without distortion of the individual elements of the blot, while confabulators took two elements of the blot and combined them in such a way that the rest of the inkblot, and the relative position of the parts that are used, were ignored. In further contrasting imaginative and confabulating subjects, Rorschach indicated that imaginative subjects gave responses with more complex associations than did confabulators. It is clear that for Rorschach, confabulation reflected a kind of stimulus-boundedness, in which the subject simply *perceived* the inkblot, albeit in an idiosyncratic and distorted manner, and then reported what he or she saw, whereas the imaginative subject *interpreted* it. Among his patient samples, Rorschach found confabulated whole responses in the records of "unintelligent normals," "morons," epileptics, organics, and schizophrenics.

Rorschach also discussed several kinds of "combinatory" responses in which the subject interpreted details separately and then combined them into a whole response. He termed one special type of combinatory response the "confabulatory-combined whole answer" which he described as "amalgamations of confabulation and combination in which the forms are vaguely seen and the individual objects interpreted are combined without any real consideration for their relative positions in the picture" (p. 38). Rorschach gave as his initial example of this type of response, the Card VIII response of "Two bears climbing from a rock, over an iceberg, onto a tree trunk" (p. 38). Although he acknowledged that this was an accurately perceived response, he concluded that the "position of the objects in the picture is neglected" (p. 38). Rorschach did not elaborate on this statement and thus left the meaning of what he had in mind somewhat unclear. It appears, however, as if he were introducing a precursor to another type of combinatory response which Rapaport later termed "fabulized combination" (Rapaport et al., 1968). Rorschach observed that confabuatory-combined responses occurred more often in "confabulating morons, Korsakoff cases, and delirious patients [who] are able to invent whole stories in this way" (p. 38). Schizophrenic and manic patients, on the other hand, produced fewer of these kinds of deviant whole responses.

Only Rorschach's "contaminated whole response" was found solely in schizophrenic patients, making it the first pathognomic diagnostic sign of schizophrenia. Instead of attempting to describe the "contamination" response, Rorschach simply defined the process of contamination by giving his now famous example of a Card IV response, "The liver of a respectable statesman" (p. 38). He said that Card IV is frequently seen as a "degenerated organ" or a man sitting on some sort of a stool. "The schizophrenic interprets the figure twice, once as a liver and once as a man, and then contaminates the two with each other, at the same time tossing in the associated ideas 'respectable' and 'statesman'" (p. 38). Rorschach concluded that schizophrenic patients gave many responses in which confabulation, combination, and contamination are intermingled in one response.

Rorschach also noted that schizophrenic patients may be influenced by factors other than the standard perceptual characteristics of the inkblot or the usual determinants of the response such as form, color, or movement. For example, he observed how schizophrenic individuals may base their responses on absurd features such as the number or position of the elements in the inkblot. Both of these response categories reflected a process in which idiosyncratic meaning was assigned based on concrete aspects of the inkblot. Thus, Rorschach added a fourth category, which he referred to as a "position response," to his rudimentary thought disorder scoring system.

For the third edition of Rorschach's text, Bohm (1958) produced a table which listed what he felt were three pathognomonic signs of schizophrenia. The first of these was Rorschach's position response (Po), which Bohm believed was found in other patients but most frequently among schizophrenics. The second sign was the juxtaposition of acceptable responses with ones that were absurd and extremely poor in form quality. Bohm's third schizophrenia sign was the contaminated whole response which, like Rorschach, he believed occurred *only* among schizophrenic patients. Klopfer and Kelley (1942) attributed several other signs to Rorschach's list of schizophrenia signs, including perseveration, abstract and personal references, and description of the card and compared these to the lists of other prominent Rorschach investigators who followed Rorschach.

Since Rorschach viewed the inkblots as a test of perception and his three primary "thought disorder" scores as deviations in the perceptual mode of approach to the inkblot, he paid less attention to bizarre verbalizations or the pathological thinking that these verbalizations might represent. Despite his reference to absurd and abstract responses, none of his scoring concepts could adequately capture some very peculiar sounding responses that he encountered in his patients. His sample Rorschach records from severely psychotic patients contain numerous examples of bizarre ideas and verbalizations, which are not captured by his confabulation, confabulatory-combination, or contamination scores. For example, he presented responses from one hebephrenic patient who saw on Card V, "[The] Head of an animal which has never existed" and on Card IX, "Feces like those made by dwarfs which are sold at fairs" (p. 160). Neither of these peculiar responses received the location score of DW for a confabulation, nor did they merit the scores of confabulatory-combination, contamination, or position. All Rorschach could say about these bizarre responses was that the patient's "associative series were interrupted by typically schizophrenic 'leaps' in his thinking" (p. 161).

Thus, in developing a method of assessing personality based chiefly on perceptual processes and anomalies, Rorschach was unable systematically to track and account for the linguistic, associative-ideational, and representational peculiarities that often occurred in the response processes of his sickest patients. It was then left to Rapaport, some twenty years later, to develop a more comprehensive system which provided a way of coding and understanding these nonperceptual aspects of deviant responses (Rapaport et al., 1968).

Skalweit's Investigation of Schizophrenia

In their review of the Rorschach assessment of dementia praecox, Klopfer and Kelley (1942) pointed out how after the publication of *Psychodiagnostik* (1921), Rorschach investigators virtually ignored the subject of schizophrenia until Skalweit (1935) presented his monograph on schizophrenia and the Rorschach. Skalweit attempted to investigate the nature of schizophrenia in order to determine whether it was a discrete disease entity that changed the entire personality or simply an exaggeration of those personality patterns already present within the individual. By studying roughly 23 schizophrenic patients longitudinally, he concluded that schizophrenia was a disease process that infiltrates and significantly alters basic personality functioning. To illustrate how schizophrenia fundamentally changed personality, Skalweit demonstrated how the "Erleipnestypus" (M:SUMC, which is the ratio of the sum of human movement responses [M] to the weighted sum of color responses [FC = .5, CF = 1.0, C = 1.5]) of schizophrenic individuals changed from introversive to extratensive.

The primary signs Skalweit associated with schizophrenia included (1) a "confused mode of approach" to interpreting the inkblots (the sequence of location used in responding to the inkblots; whether one begins with whole, conventional detail, or unusual detail responses first), (2) a high percentage of original responses with (3) poor form level, (4) a decrease in the number of human movement responses (M), together with (5) an increase in the number of color responses (typically C, CF, and Color naming as well).

Skaleit's approach was comparatively crude but marked the first real attempt, following Rorschach, to apply the Rorschach Test to the psychodiagnosis of schizophrenia. However, there is a surprising absence of any of Rorschach's rudimentary thought disorder scores among Skalweit's schizophrenia signs. Instead, Skalweit's study was generally determinant-based, that is, concerned with the formal aspects of the blot, like color, which determined the response. Little, if any, attention was paid to the more idiosyncratic aspects of the response itself.

Sign Approaches of Rickers-Ovsiankina, Beck, and Klopfer and Kelley

The sign approach to the Rorschach diagnosis of schizophrenia reached its zenith in the late 1930s and 40s in the work of Rickers-Ovsiankina (1938), Beck (1938), and Klopfer and Kelley (1942). Rickers-Ovsiankina studied the Rorschach records of different subtypes of schizophrenic patients, while Beck made an exhaustive study of the personality structure in schizophrenia by analyzing records from 81 schizophrenic and

64 normal control subjects. Finally, Klopfer and Kelley provided the most comprehensive comparative analysis of the different Rorschach sign approaches of the day, adding their own set of signs to the comparison as well. In their analysis, they compared the diagnostic signs from Rorschach's original work (1921) to those from Rickers-Ovsiankina's study contrasting schizophrenic patients and normals (1938) and those from Beck's book *Personality Structure and Schizophrenia* published in the same year (1938). Klopfer and Kelley also constructed their own list of 20 Rorschach signs empirically associated with schizophrenia.

All investigators agreed that the following signs were diagnostic of schizophrenia: (1) a confused mode of approach, (2) the presence of confabulatory whole responses (DW), (3) low F+%, (4) low P%, (5) extreme variability in the form level of responses, (6) blocking or card rejections, (7) position responses, (8) abstract and personal responses, (9) perseveration, (10) original responses of poor or variable form level, and (11) description of the card as an inkblot or design. Klopfer and Kelley believed that this last sign was typical of schizophrenic thinking which showed a poverty and inflexibility of thought. They also found that the two most discriminating factors were poor form level and the low percentage of popular responses in schizophrenic subjects. All investigators also agreed that form level variability was a key feature in schizophrenic records, with good quality responses juxtaposed with extremely poor form quality responses. In terms of core "thought disorder" scores, all researchers listed confabulatory wholes, position responses, perseveration, and abstract and personal reference responses among their schizophrenia signs.

Only Rorschach considered any of these signs to be unquestionably pathognomic of schizophrenia. According to Rorschach, these were contamination, position responses, and extreme variability in form level. Klopfer and Kelley were somewhat more conservative, finding only contamination and position responses to be "usually pathognomic," while Beck and Rickers-Ovsiankina did not believe that any of the signs were absolutely indicative of schizophrenia. Somewhat surprisingly, Rickers-Ovsiankina did not find the contamination response even to be diagnostically associated with schizophrenia.

Both Beck and Rickers-Ovsiankina's studies exemplified the essence of the problematic nature of the empirical sign approach. As Weiner (1977) pointed out, these investigators derived Rorschach schizophrenia signs from a comparison between schizophrenic and "normal" subjects. This type of comparison is generally not diagnostically useful because it does not simulate the kind of differential diagnostic task one encounters in clinical practice. Additionally, the global category of schizophrenia used in these studies did not adequately address the variability within the syndrome. (Rickers-Ovsiankina did, however, attempt to address this problem by subdividing her samples of schizophrenic patients in order to achieve a greater degree of homogeneity.) Finally, both Beck and Rickers-Ovsiankina's diagnostic signs were based on a single comparison study without regard for the "shrinkage" that occurs in empirical studies of this type. As Weiner (1977) pointed out, shrinkage occurs when any test score that is identified by inspection to differentiate among known groups with some degree of accuracy will generally demonstrate less accuracy when reexamined with another sample. Likewise, any newly identified list of differentiating scores will include some that hold up better than others.

Klopfer and Kelley issued an important caveat to those engaged in empirical analyses of the Rorschachs of schizophrenic patients. Their cautionary statements regarding the limitations of the empirical sign methodology seem to have anticipated Weiner's critique some 25 years later. In particular, Klopfer and Kelley warned that schizophrenia is a heterogeneous syndrome and that there is no single Rorschach personality picture typical of schizophrenia as a whole. Thus they recommended that researchers subdivide schizophrenic patients into more homogeneous subtypes instead of lumping these patients together and then comparing them to control groups. Similarly they pointed out that the psychiatric classification of the day for diagnosing schizophrenia was notoriously poor. As a result of these factors, Klopfer and Kelley believed that it would be hard for any method of assessment to show a typical or prototypical Rorschach pattern for schizophrenia. Almost portending Weiner's conceptual approach, Klopfer and Kelley stated that the diagnoses were made only indirectly by inference from the personality picture constructed out of the Rorschach data.

Klopfer and Kelley attempted to provide theoretical explanations for some of their signs. Most notably, they believed that the lack of human movement responses among schizophrenic patients reflected the lack of differentiated inner life and that the low F+% the failure of these patients' ability to exert control over their fantasy lives. Klopfer and Kelley also tried to provide an explanation for the regression seen in schizophrenic patients in terms of their greater number of contaminations, positions responses, perseverations, F– responses, pure C's, and animal content percentage, all of which were found in children's records. Finally, Klopfer and Kelley looked fleetingly at qualitative aspects of the patient's verbalizations including condensation of words, sentences, and phrases. Additionally, they pointed out how the schizophrenic patient may lose distance from the card and respond to it as if it represented reality.

None of these approaches looked specifically at thinking or isolated thinking as a subject of study. While predating the direct study of thought disorder per se, Klopfer and Kelley began to shift away from focusing only on perceptual aspects of the response process and started to look more closely at the specific nature of the schizophrenic patient's disturbed thinking and language.

Rapaport's Contributions

Unlike Beck and Klopfer, Rapaport's interest in the Rorschach occurred comparatively late in his brief career and seemed to wane in the years following his seminal Rorschach contributions (Rapaport et al., 1968). A leading figure in American Ego Psychology, Rapaport drifted away from psychodiagnostic research and clinical use of the Rorschach and, instead, immersed himself in the more abstract realm of interpreting and systematizing psychoanalytic metapsychology. However, the legacy of his brief years of active involvement in the Rorschach and other psychodiagnostic instruments left an indelible mark on the field of psychological testing in general and the assessment of disordered thinking in particular. Holt described Rapaport's work in the area of conceptualizing and measuring forms of disturbed thought processes on the Rorschach as his "most distinctive and original contribution to Rorschach testing" (Holt et al., 1968, p. 424). Many would agree that Rapaport's contributions in this area are second only to those of Rorschach himself.

Rapaport had a passionate interest in deciphering the nature of thought and in understanding how thinking progresses from drive-dominated ideation to socialized and logical thought processes. In particular, he was concerned with how pathology gains expression in formal aspects of thought processes. Rapaport's interest in understanding the organization and pathological expressions of thought led to a shift away from a strict focus on the perceptual characteristics of the Rorschach and paved the way for the analysis of verbalization. Verbalization, for Rapaport, revealed the organizing principles of thinking and held the key to understanding thought pathology. Unlike previous investigators who saw the Rorschach as a more direct route to diagnosing schizophrenia, Rapaport zeroed in on deviant thinking per se and made this the subject of intense scientific scrutiny. However, like most researchers of his day, Rapaport believed that severe thought pathology was specific to schizophrenia.

From his work with Merton Gill and Roy Schafer, Rapaport began to use the term "thought disorder." Prior to his formal introduction of this term in his book *Organization and Pathology in Thought* (1951), this now familiar term had not appeared frequently in Rorschach literature on schizophrenia. Thus, Rapaport's work marked the first time that the Rorschach was used to assess disordered thinking as a separate component or function of the mental apparatus. In their analysis of Rorschach verbalization, Rapaport and his colleagues introduced a fifth category to Rorschach scoring, which set the standard for almost every subsequent Rorschach system for scoring and conceptualizing thought disorder.

Prior to his interest in systematizing deviant verbalizations, most Rorschach investigators focused only on the content of verbalizations that could lend themselves to symbolic interpretation. However, Rapaport noted that "what has been lacking thus far was a psychological rationale to systematize the conspicuous verbalizations and to attempt to explain the deviant ones" (Rapaport et al., 1968, p. 425). Thus, Rapaport believed that deviant verbalizations, like other response dimensions, lent themselves to objective and systematic scoring and diagnostic evaluation. In this regard, he and his colleagues identified 25 different types of pathological verbalizations. Schafer (1954) later stated that these scores enabled clinicians to classify examples of formal thought disorder on the Rorschach. The names chosen for these variants were selected by Rapaport and his two colleagues based both on the previous Rorschach literature and on their own experience and concepts. Some of the names given such as "confabulation" were already in use, but Rapaport and his colleagues modified and extended their meaning and significance.

Further details of the Rapaport system will be taken up in the next chapter. Suffice it to say, Rapaport's work was widely and harshly criticized because of the methodological flaws in his research and statistical analyses. Some of these errors were glaring and led critics to dismiss the nature of Rapaport's contributions to the Rorschach assessment of disordered thinking. As Goldfried, Stricker, and Weiner (1971) pointed out, the basic method involved elements of a sign approach; however, I believe that it is inaccurate to characterize the Rapaport system as simply an empirical sign approach. In terms of identifying Rorschach variables that were used as differential diagnostic markers, the Rapaport system was certainly consistent with an empirical sign approach. However, the scoring of deviant verbalizations, like the scoring of other response dimensions, had rich theoretical underpinnings. Rapaport took care in crafting a complex conceptual rationale for all of his scoring dimensions.

What is most notable about the Rapaport system of assessing thought disorder is how it gave rise to all modern approaches to assessing disordered thinking with the Rorschach (see Figure 2.1). Compared to the rest of Rapaport's system, the thought disorder scoring has proven to be not only his "most distinctive" but his most enduring contribution.

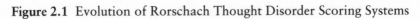

Figure 2.1 Evolution of Rorschach Thought Disorder Scoring Systems

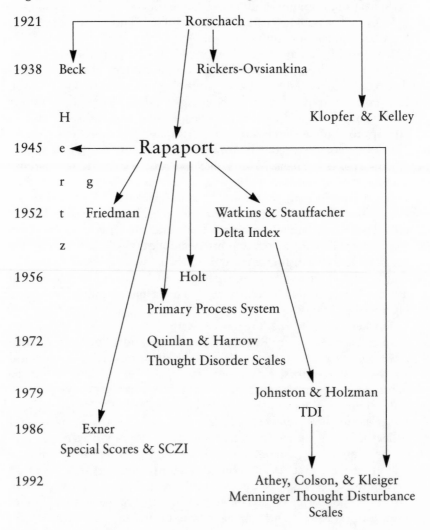

1950S: CLUSTER AND CONFIGURAL APPROACHES TO ASSESSING THOUGHT DISORDER

During the 1950s, researchers developed more sophisticated methods to achieve diagnostic sensitivity with the Rorschach. Perhaps in response to Klopfer and Kelley's (1942) caveat regarding the limitations of the empirical sign approaches of Beck and Rickers-Ovsiankina and of the methodological difficulties of the Rapaport study, a new generation of researchers began to combine Rorschach scores into clusters and configurations that could provide more powerful diagnostic tools for making reliable and valid inferences about the presence of schizophrenia. Instead of deriving a list of arbitrary signs that could be independent of one another, the individual elements of the cluster-configural approaches were often differentially weighted and added together to form a collective diagnostic index.

Four examples of cluster-configural approaches to diagnosing schizophrenic thought disorder include Piotrowski's Alpha Index (Piotrowski and Lewis,1950; Piotrowski and Berg, 1955), Watkins and Stauffacher's Delta Index (1952), the Thiesen Patterns (1952), and Weiner's Schizophrenia Signs (1960).

Piotrowski's Alpha Index

Piotrowski constructed his Alpha Index to identify mild, incipient and pseudoneurotic forms of schizophrenia (Piotrowski and Lewis, 1950; Piotrowski and Berg, 1955). The index was based on Rorschach indicators of energy capacity, energy control, overcontrol, underactivity, and underproductivity. The following five signs were assigned different weights depending on their value: (1) W (scored the traditional way including both DW and WS responses), (2) Sum C (scored the traditional way with 1.5 given for each C, 1.0 for each CF, and 0.5 for each FC response), (3) Sum c (diffuse shading scored with 1.5 given for each c response, 1.0 for each Fc response, and 0.5 for each subordinate c response), (4) C' Shock (scored if Card IV or V was rejected or if the reaction time to Card IV was longer than that of any other card, or if the reaction time to Card IV was excessively long), and (5) F+%. The index only applied when W was greater than 7 and Sum c was greater than Sum C.[1]

---

1. Readers unfamiliar with some of these scoring symbols are referred to Exner (1969) for basic scoring information regarding Piotrowski's Rorschach system.

The Alpha Index provided a global measure of psychotic functioning although Piotrowski believed that its clinical signs could distinguish preschizophrenic from manic depressive psychosis.[2] An Alpha Index of 3 or greater suggested that the patient was functioning at a neurotic level.

In their review of Rorschach indices for assessing schizophrenia, Goldfried et al. (1971), concluded that the Alpha Index could be useful in arriving at a diagnosis of schizophrenia but not in ruling it out. They pointed out that the index sacrificed a low number of false positives for a high number of false negatives and that when useful, it only applied to a small number of patients who met its requirements. One can also see that the index was not based on the subject's verbalizations and thus did not attempt to isolate either deviant verbalizations or their hypothesized underlying processes as major diagnostic indicators of schizophrenia. Somewhat surprisingly, Piotrowski ignored specific thought disorder scores when constructing his index. Instead, like earlier investigations which employed the empirical-sign approach, Piotrowski's Alpha Index focused on more traditional scoring determinants which reflected other aspects of personality functioning.

Thiesen Patterns

Like 1938, 1952 was a prodigious year for Rorschach research on diagnostic indices for schizophrenia. Thiesen (1952) identified five different patterns to diagnose schizophrenic patients. By comparing 60 schizophrenics against Beck's (1949) normal control group, Thiesen examined combinations of 20 major Rorschach variables and developed five patterns that differentiated the schizophrenic group from the normals at the .01 level of significance. Thiesen's five patterns were: (1) three or more anatomy responses and four or more sex responses, (2) F+% greater than or equal to 69 and Z score greater than 8.0, (3) no FC or M responses and A% less than or equal to 40, (4) F% less than or equal to 69, A% less than or equal to 40 and 5 populars, and (5) DW greater than or equal to 1 and no FC responses. The presence of just one of these patterns was thought to be diagnostic of schizophrenia. However, the absence of any pattern does not establish the presence of normalcy.

---

2. To arrive at an Alpha score, weighted scores from −2 to 4 were assigned to different levels of W, Sum C, Sum c minus Sum C, the presence or absence of c' shock, and the sign F+% <70. The reader is directed to Goldfried et al. (1971, p. 292) for a complete list of the weights assigned to different scores.

Like Piotrowski's Alpha Index, Thiesen's Patterns were curiously devoid of any of Rorschach's or Rapaport's core thought disorder scores. By today's standards, it is difficult to see how any of Thiesen's Patterns could be suggestive of, much less specific to, schizophrenia. Finally, attempts at cross validation have not supported Thiesen's original findings.

Weiner Signs

Weiner developed two sets of Rorschach schizophrenia signs based on empirical grounds and post facto theoretical rational. In his original derivation study, Weiner (1961) found that his schizophrenic patients could be distinguished from normal controls by the following three signs: (1) at least one to two CF responses, (2) sum C = 1.5–3.0, and (3) the presence of CF or C responses without C' responses. The presence of pure C responses formed the fourth sign when pure C was greater than or equal to one. Weiner called this series of signs the Color Stress Index, which he reasoned reflected inefficient defensive functioning characteristic of schizophrenia. He scored this index as positive when two of the first three conditions were met or when at least one pure C response was present in a patient's record.

Weiner's second index, which he termed Deviant Tempo (1962) consisted of the following four conditions: (1) more responses to Card V than IV; (2) more responses to Card V than VI; (3) more responses to Card IX than VIII; (4) more responses to Card IX than X. According to Weiner, anyone of these conditions suggested the presence of schizophrenia. Weiner's theoretical rationale was that deviations in normal response tempo reflected the types of disturbances in rate and flow of associations.

Although Weiner's two indices yielded a surprising degree of accuracy when used together and suffered from a low incidence of false positives and only a modest level of false negatives, Weiner's research was plagued with the same kinds of difficulties that troubled research employing the empirical-sign approach. However, Weiner's experience with shrinkage and other such methodological difficulties eventually led him to become a strong proponent of the conceptual approach to conducting research and making diagnostic inferences with the Rorschach.

Watkins and Stauffacher's Delta Index

Watkins and Stauffacher (1952) developed the most comprehensive index of this time period for assessing disordered thinking. Unlike previous signs or indices, Watkins and Stauffacher's Index of Pathological

Thinking or Delta Index focused specifically on deviant qualities of thinking as opposed to a more heterogenous conglomeration of determinant scores. Based on the thought disorder categories and scoring criteria introduced by Rapaport, the Delta Index was intended to measure the intrusion of primary process thinking.

Watkins and Stauffacher took 15 of Rapaport's thought disorder scores and assigned severity weights of .25, .50, and 1.0 to each based on the authors' clinical experience. The presence and severity of thought pathology was rated in each response and summed for the total score which was then divided by the number of responses recorded in the protocol. Watkins and Stauffacher called the degreee of deviation the "Delta Index" which was expressed as a percentage score. At the scoring level, they defined Delta as representing a quantitative measure of what Rapaport called either a pathological increase or loss of distance from the inkblot. Interpretatively, Watkins and Stauffacher viewed Delta as a measure of the degree to which a patient's adaptation to reality was contaminated by archaic and primary process ideation.

The Delta Index was derived from the records of 25 normal, 25 neurotic, and 25 psychotic patients. Watkins and Stauffacher's interrater reliabilities varied greatly among the three groups from .04 for the normals, .47 for the neurotics, and .91 for the psychotic group. Despite this variability, a combined reliability score for all 75 records was .78. Watkins and Stauffacher found that with a cutoff point of 10% Delta, all the normals were correctly identified, 8% of the neurotics were false positives, and 48% of the psychotics were correctly identified. The authors concluded that a Delta of 5% or lower could correctly identify nonpsychiatric subjects and a score of 10% of higher was a positive criterion for schizophrenia.

Two later studies evaluated both the reliability and validity of the Delta Index and found similarly high reliability scores for the total Delta Index (Pope and Jensen, 1957; Powers and Hamlin, 1955). In contrast to a high reliability for the total score, both studies found a lower percentage of agreement for individual responses and categories. Powers and Hamlin found significant Delta Index differences among five groups of subjects, with their socially adjusted subjects scoring lower than the neurotics, who in turn scored lower than the schizophrenic group. However, they did not find significant differences between their groups of latent, catatonic, and paranoid schizophrenics. Pope and Jensen found significant reductions in Delta in all of their psychiatric patients at the conclusion of their hospital treatments.

Goldfried et al. (1971) suggested that the Delta Index was cumbersome and difficult to score reliably with nonpsychotic subjects. They also stated that the utility of the index was limited by the fact that different researchers recommended using different cutoff scores and made various modifications in the scoring categories. However, Goldfried et al. concluded that the index could do a reasonably good job identifying schizophrenic subjects.

Despite some of its problems and the limitations of the research methodology (e.g., comparing heterogenous schizophrenic subjects to normal ones), the Delta Index must be heralded as the first carefully constructed quantifiable scale focused exclusively on measuring thought pathology per se, as opposed to the more global dependent variable of schizophrenia. In focusing more narrowly on a specific psychological process versus a more global psychiatric diagnosis, Watkins and Stauffacher brought the Delta Index a degree closer to a more sophisticated conceptual approach to identifying schizophrenia with the Rorschach.

1950s–1960s: CONCEPTUAL APPROACHES TO ASSESSING THOUGHT DISORDER

Weiner (1977) outlined the basis for a conceptual approach to the Rorschach diagnosis of schizophrenia. He stated that earlier approaches to Rorschach research in general suffered from a lack of understanding of how the instrument was to be used. He reminded us that the basic purpose of the Rorschach is not to make a diagnosis or predict a type of behavior but to assess personality processes or psychological functions. These personality processes or functions should then form a bridge between the Rorschach data, on the one hand, and whatever conditions or diagnosis that one is interested in investigating, on the other. Weiner pointed out that the first step in using the Rorschach to aid in psychiatric diagnosis of a particular condition is to specify the personality characteristics or variables associated with the condition under question. Those variables can be established on the basis of both empirical and theoretical factors. Once these variables have been identified, one then looks for features of the Rorschach that have been shown to measure reliably such variables or processes. From this definition, one can see how the Delta Index, by focusing more narrowly on deviant thought processes, had the quality of a conceptual approach.

Several scoring systems have been developed on more conceptual bases. The approaches of Hertz (1938, 1942), Friedman (1952, 1953), and Holt (1956; Holt and Havel, 1960, 1977) will be presented. I review Holt's system in greater detail in the following chapter because it is still used as a tool in contemporary Rorschach research.

The Organizational and Developmental Scoring Systems of Hertz and Friedman

Scoring organizational and developmental quality of responses is almost as old as the Rorschach itself. These concepts were derived from Rorschach's observations of the different kinds of whole responses (W) that subjects could produce. Although Rorschach did not refer to organizational activity directly or in any systematic way, he was aware that there were different kinds of W responses depending on the degree of articulation, organization, and accurate integration of the separate components of the inkblot. Aside from the simple, global W response, Rorschach noticed that subjects could produce W responses that reflected complex synthetic abilities requiring significant effort to construct. Rorschach also noted that some W responses could be confabulated (DW) by faulty pars pro toto thinking or contaminated by superimposing one whole response onto another.

After Rorschach, other investigators began to study organizational activity that occurred in the response process (Beck, 1933; Vernon, 1933; Guirdham, 1935; Hertz, 1938, 1942; Ford, 1946; Janoff, 1951; Friedman, 1952, 1953). By studying combinatory whole responses in particular, researchers were able to make inferences about the extent to which subjects could link together ideas and perceptions together in realistic and appropriate manner. Rapaport et al. (1968) realized that combinatory activity in the inkblots reflected a subject's integrative and abstracting abilities, and they developed a number of qualitative scoring categories to reflect various types of combinatory responses. In particular, his category of fabulized combination responses represented an extreme example of how combinatory activity could go awry and lead to the attribution of absurd and unrealistic relationships between inherently incompatible ideas and percepts. Thus, evaluating the complexity and quality of combination responses on the Rorschach became another means of examining the nature of an individual's thought processes and reality testing.

Hertz began developing a scoring system to assess organizational activity or "g" in 1938. For Hertz, the g score was intended to take into account not only the locations used, but also the form quality, vagueness, and originality of the response, as well as the appropriateness of the relationships that were described in the combinatory activity. Original responses that reflected good form, adequate articulation and integration, and realistic and logical relationships were given the highest g weighting of 1.5 and the score g+ O, 1.5. If the final original response was actually a combinatory response, involving two or more separately scored responses of good form level and realistic integration,

Hertz would assign the score g O+ comb, 1.5. At the other extreme, if the combinatory response was original and involved unrealistic, absurd, or illogical relationships between blot elements, whether or not the form quality was acceptable, the score would have been g O- comb!, 0.5. Hertz placed the exclamation point after this score to indicate that it was highly suggestive of severe thought impairment.

Hertz's g has been shown to be a sensitive indicator of impaired thinking, primarily among schizophrenic subjects (Hertz and Paolino, 1960; Loehrke, 1952). Hertz and Paolino (1960) used the g score to evaluate the thought processes of two groups of delusional paranoid schizophrenic and neurotic patients and found that the schizophrenic groups showed significantly more evidence of unrealistic, distorted, and personalized thinking that involved incongruous and inappropriate relationships between elements of the blot. As such, they viewed the g O-combination scores as clear indications of thought disorder. Additionally, Hertz and Paolino found that the schizophrenic subjects gave more fabulized content, contaminations, autistic logic, fluidity, incompatible alternatives, non sequitor reasoning, reference relationships, and peculiarities in speech and language usage.

Interestingly, Hertz also collected data on the organizational scores of obsessive-compulsive and manic patients (Hertz, 1977). Unfortunately, she lost much of her original data and could only piece together general impressions about the organizational pathology characteristic of these other two patient groups. It is not surprising that patients with obsessional styles often demonstrated high sum g weighting as they strived to see as many relationships as they could among the elements in the inkblot. Hertz found that manic patients achieved either high or low sum g weightings. When high, the qualitiative analysis showed the predominance of sum g- scores, reflecting inferior organizational activity which involved poor form and illogical combinations and vague abstractions. When low, Hertz found the Rorschachs to be sparse, erratic, unconnected, or disorganized.

Hertz suggested that the qualitative differentiations of the g score reflected the quality and efficiency of an individual's analytic, synthetic, combinative, and integrative capacity. Furthermore, Hertz was quite clear in linking qualitative aspects of g scores to thought organization, and more particularly disordered thought. Accordingly, Hertz stated that when subjects obtain scores such as g O- and g O- comb!, their thinking is seriously illogical and may reflect excessive fantasizing of a delusional nature.

Friedman (1952, 1953) was less interested in assessing organizational capacity, per se, but more concerned with using the Rorschach to measure developmental level. Based on Werner's developmental theory (1948), which held that development unfolds from a state of global functioning towards increasing capacity for differentation and integration, Friedman created a developmental approach to the structural aspects of Rorschach scores. According to Werner's theory, development proceeds along several bipolar continua: syncretic-discrete; diffuse-articulated; labile-stable; and rigid-flexible. Syncretic and diffuse modes of functioning were thought to indicate overly general and vague approaches to perceiving and organizing information, which signaled developmental immaturity and were also thought to be characteristic of schizophrenic individuals who function at lower developmental levels.

Based on the earlier work of Beck and Rapaport, Friedman developed a simple scoring system that took into account the structural and organizational aspects of the percept. In essence, his system focused only on location scores, with little regard for the content or determinants or a response. Where form level determination was required, Friedman relied on Beck's or Hertz's form tables. His scores fell into either developmentally high or low categories. Friedman included six scorres for developmentally high responses: (1) W++, (2) D++, (3) W+, (4) D+, (5) Wm, and (6) Dm. The W++ and D++ scores pertained to the highest levels in which either the unitary whole blot (W++) or a unitary D area (D++) was articulated and reintegrated into a clearly differentiated percept of accurate form level. The W+ and D+ scores reflected a similar process of articulation and integration but on blot areas that were already broken down perceptually. The Wm and Dm scores referred to accurately perceived mediocre responses that were based on the general outline of an unbroken blot area. These were seen as easier responses to produce since they do not require further articulation and reintegration.

In descending order of primitivity, Friedman's ten scores for developmentally low responses began with Wv or Dv and Wa and Da categories in which the individual used either the whole blot or a D area to form a response where form is either secondary (Wv and Dv) or irrelevant (Wa and Da). W- and D- scores were given to responses in which there was a total mismatch between the content given and the form of the inkblot. DW and DdW scores referred to the confabulatory responses as originally defined by Rorschach. A FabC score referred to fabulized combination responses, à la Rapaport, in which two or more separate areas were interpreted and combined unrealistically on the basis of their spatial relationship. Finally, and more developmentally primitive, was the ConR or contamination response, in which two separate responses to the same blot area (either W or D) were merged into one bizarre response.

Friedman defined perceptual regression as the most developmentally primitive levels of functioning. He viewed W- and D- scores as indicative of syncretic functioning in which the individual's preoccupation with idiosyncratic internal issues determined the way that a person perceived and reacted to the external world. Like Hertz, Friedman considered DW and DdD responses as signs of "pars pro toto" thinking, while FabC and ConR responses reflected a primitive mode of magical thinking described by Werner (1948) as the "magic of contiguity" or by Sullivan (1953) as parataxic distortion.

Friedman's system yielded two broad summary scores, an Index of Integration and an Index of Primitive Thought. The Index of Primitive Thought or IPT was based on the sum of FabC + ConR + DW + DdD scores divided by the total number of responses, multiplied by 100.

Goldfried et al. (1971) reviewed research using Friedman's developmental scoring system and found it to be a useful measure of developmental level. Studies have supported its relevance in differentiating children at various age levels and different forms of psychopathology. Several investigators demonstrated that developmental scores could distinguish schizophrenic patients from normals (Friedman, 1952; Lebowitz, 1963) and between schizophrenic patients at different levels of severity (Siegel, 1953; Becker, 1956; Wilensky, 1959). These studies found that the developmentally low scores of schizophrenic patients were quite similar to the scores of children at different ages.

Goldfried et al. concluded that Friedman's scoring system was more appropriate for research than clinical use. They also believed that the normative data for the Friedman System was not adequate. However, aspects of Friedman's developmental approach are clearly represented in the Developmental Quotient (DQ), Z Score, and Special Scores in the Comprehensive System (Exner, 1993), which has an extensive developmental and clinical normative base.

Holt's Primary Process Scoring System

Holt (1956, 1977; Holt and Havel, 1960) pioneered a method for assessing both adaptive and maladaptive manifestations of primary process thinking. Compared to previous indices such as the Delta Index, Holt and Havel's Primary Process System had a much broader focus than that of assessing pathological thinking. Based on a psychoanalytic drive-structure model of the mind that held that schizophrenic pathology is a product of the failure of repression of primitive direct drive derivatives, Holt devised a method for assessing the nature and severity of drive intrusion into conscious thinking and experience. In essence, Holt's instrument included three component measures: (1) An appraisal of the degree of drive domination that permeates thinking; (2) A rating of the degree to which primary process ideation in the response demands; some defensive effort so as to make the response more socially acceptable and, (3) An assessment of the efficacy of defensive efforts in reducing or preventing anxiety, thus making it an adaptive response to the stress of the testing situation.

Contemporary Systems

Several mainstream and alternative systems are reviewed in the next five chapters. The mainstream contemporary approaches involve scoring systems that have enjoyed either widespread attention or acceptance and are currently used in research and clinical practice. These systems include the Rapaport System, Holt's Primary Process System, the Thought Disorder Index (TDI) (Johnson and Holzman, 1979), and the Special Scores and Schizophrenia Index (SCZI) of the Comprehensive System (Exner, 1986a, 1993). The alternative approaches are less well known and not commonly used.

Virtually all Rorschach systems for assessing disordered thinking were, and still are to a large extent, based on the work of Rorschach, Rapaport, Watkins and Stauffacher, and Holt. However, nearly all of these contemporary approaches share a common heritage that can be traced back to the contributions of David Rapaport. Figure 2.1 depicts the evolution of Rorschach thought disorder scoring systems and their linkage to Rapaport and secondarily to other investigators including Rorschach himself. The systems differ considerably in degree of complexity and thoroughness, the categories chosen and symbols used, and the extent to which they are based on a conceptual as opposed to an empirical-sign or cluster approach.

PART
2

THOUGHT DISORDER
SCORING SYSTEMS

Four different approaches to scoring thought disorder on the Rorschach will be reviewed. The systems developed by Rapaport and Holt are about 50 years old and not widely used today. Although the Rapaport method is infrequently taught in graduate or postdoctoral programs (Hilsenroth and Handler, 1995), it is still used by a segment of diagnosticians; and Rorschach studies based on Rapaport's method of administration and scoring continue to appear in the psychodiagnostic literature (Lerner and Lerner, 1988; Blatt, 1990; Lerner, 1991). Holt's system is generally too complex to use in clinical settings and is more often employed as a tool in research investigations. The Thought Disorder Index (TDI) is the only contemporary scale specifically designed to assess disordered thinking. It is a system that stands independently, focusing only on the dimension of pathological verbalization, while ignoring or deemphasizing other scoring variables. The Special Scores and Schizophrenia Index (SCZI) of the Comprehensive System are essential scoring features in the most widely used contemporary approach to the Rorschach. In developing the Special Scores and the SCZI, Exner's effort was to simplify thought disorder scoring by eliminating and consolidating many of the categories used in previous systems.

Although each of these approaches to scoring thought disorder is being viewed here as a contemporary clinical or research scoring system, I do not intend to convey that they are truly contemporaneous or even equivalent. The Rapaport System has been eclipsed by the Comprehensive System, which dominates the current Rorschach scene; and the Holt System is more than 20 years older and less frequently used than the TDI. Nonetheless, each system, whether used often or infrequently, in primarily clinical or research settings, purports to measure deviations in thinking. Thus, beginning with a detailed review and critique of thought disorder scoring in Rapaport method, I will examine the scoring criteria, empirical underpinnings, contributions to clinical diagnostic work, and limitations of these systems as they relate to the assessment of disordered thinking.

In addition to the major contemporary research and clinical thought disorder scoring systems, there are a number of less well known and relatively obscure systems for scoring thought disorder on the Rorschach. Whether developed specifically for research purposes or proposed for use in clinical practice, these "secondary" systems employ a mixture of generally accepted scoring concepts along with novel additions and modifications. Chapter 7 summarizes the contributions of these systems developed by Wynne and Singer; Harrow and Quinlan; Schuldberg and Boster; Burstein and Loucks; Athey, Colson, and Kleiger; and Wagner.

CHAPTER

3

THE RAPAPORT METHOD

Dissatisfied with contemporary psychological, psychiatric, and psychoanalytic theories that focused too heavily on thought content or dynamics, Rapaport sought instead to study the structure of thought. Rapaport believed that symbolic interpretation of Rorschach content or verbalizations was as incomplete, and possibly misguided, as dream interpretation based only on manifest or latent content. Without understanding the principles of dream work, dream interpretation can be misleading. Similarly, Rapaport felt that without understanding the formal characteristics of thought processes, symbolic interpretation of the content or verbalizations was of limited usefulness. Together with Gill and Schafer, he sought to systematize the most common kinds of deviant verbalizations that occur on the Rorschach and to explain the psychological processes that underlie them.

Assessing thought disorder through an analysis of deviant verbalizations was based on Rapaport's concept of "distance" from the inkblot. For Rapaport, thinking was always tied to the perceptual reality of the inkblot. Adaptive, reality-based thinking depended on the smooth interdigitation of perceptual and associational processes. In other words, the associations set in motion by the inkblot must not stray too far, or be too distant from, the perceptual reality of the inkblot. If associative processes are too far removed, or distant, from the inkblot, the subject was viewed as showing a disregard for the perceptual reality in front of him or her. On the other hand, rigid attunement to the perceptual features of the inkblot may lead a subject to regard it as too real, hence failing to maintain an appropriate distance or "as if" attitude towards the inkblots. Rapaport's concept of "distance" will be discussed in greater detail in chapter 8.

Rapaport (Rapaport et al., 1968) labeled all of the categories of disordered thinking on the Rorschach "deviant verbalizations." He stated that the comprehensive and systematic examination of the various types of deviant verbalization on the Rorschach was "the highway for investigating disorders of thinking" (p. 431). Although Rapaport and his colleagues borrowed several of the titles of categories of pathological verbalization from the extant Rorschach literature, they modified the scoring and extended the meaning of most of these existing categories; as well, they identified and labeled several new categories. The following list describes the scoring categories that Rapaport and his colleagues introduced under the heading of deviant verbalizations.

1. FABULIZED RESPONSES. Rapaport introduced this term to describe varying degrees of affective elaboration or embellishment that mark a progressive departure, or increase of distance, from the inkblot. Embellished responses such as "hungry animals," or an "ugly person" (as opposed to simply "animals" or a "person") suggest an increasing degree of subjectivity and subtle shifting away from the concrete reality of the inkblot. Although fabulized responses generally were said to reflect an increased distance, they were also simultaneuosly viewed as reflecting a loss of distance, especially when the subject expresses an emotion-laden conviction that the image assigned to the inkblot is not simply a symbolic representation but something vivid and real.[1] For example, the subject who looks at Card I and says "Oh no, it's a dangerous bat!" reveals both an increase in distance (the inkblot does not support the descriptor "dangerous") and a loss of distance (the subject reacts as if the image really is dangerous). Rapaport concluded that the presence of a few mild fabulized responses was not pathological. It was only when there was an abundance of such responses that one should begin to suspect autistic thinking.

2. FABULIZED COMBINATIONS. Although Hermann Rorschach identified a deviant form of combinatory response, which he called a "confabulatory combination," it was Rapaport who formalized this scoring concept and introduced the term "fabulized combination" into Rorschach language. Fabulized combination was the name given to combination responses in which separate deatails or areas of the inkblot are related

---

1. Rapaport's concept of increased and decreased distance appears in a number of later chapters. The reader is referred to this discussion to help clarify the concept.

in some arbitrary or unrealistic way.[2] The key element in these combinative responses is that the spatial relation between separate areas is taken as a fixed and real relationship. In this sense, Rapaport indicated that fabulized combinations reflect primarily an extreme loss of distance from, or concrete interpretation of, the inkblot.

The unrealistic nature of the relationship or interaction can be based on disproportionate size or an unnatural or bizarre relationship that does not occur in nature. Rapaport allowed that fabulized combinations could occur occasionally in the Rorschachs of more intact subjects; however, when present they would usually be accompanied by an appreciation of their unrealistic nature.

3. CONFABULATIONS. This represented one of Rapaport's most original contributions to scoring disordered thinking on the Rorschach.[3] Although the term itself was not new, Rapaport extended its meaning beyond its original use by Rorschach and others who followed him. Rorschach used the term "confabulatory whole response" (designated by the symbol DW) to describe those responses in which a subject begins with one detail and generalizes to a whole response. Recall his original example of the Card I, "a crab," which was based on the perceptual generalization from one small detail (e.g., "a claw") to an inaccurately perceived whole response ("a crab"). Here the confabulatory, or pathological filling in, process was based on perceptual and not ideational or associational features. Rapaport's unique contribution was based on his concept of distance from the inkblot. Confabulation responses were, in essence, fabulized responses taken too far. In other words, the confabulating subject reports seeing images that cannot be justified by realistic aspects of the inkblot. Based on either the unwarranted infusion of affect or fantasy into the response, or an inappropriate degree of specificity of the response, Rapaport believed that confabulations most always indicated severe thought pathology of at least a preschizophrenic nature.

According to Rapaport, confabulations frequently reflect combinations of pathological loss of and increase in distance from the inkblot. Aspects of the inkblot can be taken too literally and then elaborated in a manner that goes beyond any supporting features of the inkblot. Rapaport (Rapaport et al., 1968) provided such an example with the Card V response, "two people lying down, tired, resting [side figures] . . . somebody helping them [central figure], nature might be helping them . . .

---

2. The conceptual nature of fabulized combination responses is addressed in great detail in chapter 10.

3. An in-depth discussion of confabulation is contained in chapter 9.

might be God" (p. 433). The infusion of energy (or in this case, a lack of energy, i.e., "tiredness" and "resting") reflects an increase in distance that is part of a fabulizing process. Rapaport noted that the literal interpretation of the central figure as a "helper," based on its erect form and spatial relationship to the two side figures that were seen as reclining, is an example of a pathological loss of distance. Finally there is an extreme leap in fabulizing as the subject takes the concept "helper" and extends it to "nature" or "God," both of which go far beyond what is reasonably suggested by the inkblot.

Rapaport believed that confabulation responses reflected elements of both fabulized responses and fabulized combinations. He was confident that all three types of response, but especially confabulation, signaled the presence of idiosyncratic thinking in everyday common situations, in which fantasy begins to progressively encroach on one's adherence to reality. Rapaport concluded that confabulations are "the most autistic and most clearly a part of schizophrenic thinking" (p. 435).

4. DW RESPONSE. Rapaport's DW score was essentially no different from that first introduced by Rorschach as the "confabulatory whole response" and used in the same manner by subsequent Rorschach investigators. However, unlike other investigators, Rapaport did not refer to the DW response as a "confabulation," a term he reserved for the kinds of deviant elaborations and embellishments described above. DW responses, for Rapaport, were grounded in perceptual concreteness and reflected a loss of distance from the inkblot. Rapaport gave an example of a DW, the Card VI response, "a cat" based on the fact that the top detail looked like "whiskers" (p. 430). The stimulus-bounded loss of distance was reflected in the subject's reasoning that "if these are whiskers, then it must be a cat."

5. CONTAMINATIONS. According to Rapaport, the unrealistic fusion of two separate ideas or images results from a loss of distance from the card. Two separate images or concepts are merged into one based on the spatial overlap or identity of the area(s) of the inkblot (the process underlying contaminatory thinking is reviewed in chapter 11). This spatial overlap or identity is then taken to represent a real relationship between the separate images/concepts which share a common blot area. The boundary between two distinct ideas or images is lost, and the final response reflects a highly distorted and unrealistic increase of distance from the Rorschach card. Rapaport's classic example of a contamination response was his Card III response of "this bloody little splotch here . . . bloody island where they had so many revolutions" (p. 437), which fuses the images of a bloody spot and an island, both of which occupy the same blot area.

Rapaport described more subtle variations of contamination responses, but each type could be characterized by a loss of distance from the inkblot in which the spatial layout of the card is taken too literally. Like many investigators before him, Rapaport viewed contamination responses as reliable indicators of schizophrenia.

6. AUTISTIC LOGIC. Rapaport first used the term "autistic logic" to describe the types of fallacious logic that von Domarus (1944) called "paralogical" or "predicate" thinking and Arieti (1974) referred to as "paleological" reasoning (see chapter 12 for an extended discussion of this process). Rorschach used the symbol "Po," for position-determined response, to depict one common inkblot example of "paralogical thinking."

Rapaport and his colleagues elaborated on the "Po" category and defined autistic logic responses to be those in which the subject's reasoning is explicitly illogical. Typically, the subject's autistic reasoning is heralded by the word "because" as the subject makes his or her reasoning error explicit. For example, the position response to Card IX of "the north pole . . . *because* it is at the top" reflects the subject's air of certainty in reaching this illogical conclusion.[4] Although Rapaport noted the rarity of autistic logic responses, he believed that, like contamination responses, they signaled extremely disorganized thinking and impaired reality testing and, as such, were almost always pathognomic of schizophrenia.

7. PECULIAR AND QUEER VERBALIZATIONS. Whereas several of Rapaport's categories had been previously described by earlier Rorschach investigators, his effort to categorize pathological speech or language, independent of the percept involved, was pioneering. In these scoring categories, the object of study is not the process of autistic logic, but the verbal end product. Rapaport held that deviant language reflected either pathological loss of or increase in distance from the Rorschach card.[5]

"Peculiar verbalizations" are the milder of the two types of deviant communication. The criterion for peculiar responses was that the verbalization was only inappropriate or idiosyncratic in the context of the

---

4. At first blush this kind of response will probably strike most listeners as a bit odd and concrete, but it might not reach the threshold of what many would judge as "crazy" or psychotic reasoning. However, its departure from conventional logic is clear; and as we shall see in chapter 12, this type of response reflects a less differentiated form of reasoning associated with psychosis, magical thinking in primitive cultures, and developmentally immature logic.

5. Rapaport did not regard speech as independent of thought and perception. As discussed in chapter 1, the question of what determines deviant verbalizations is a complex one that lies at the crossroads of psychology, neuropsychology, and psycholinguistics.

particular Rorschach response. Outside of that context it was not remarkable. For example Rorschach verbalizations such as "a cranial skull," "an eagle view of it," "two legs raising each other," and "joined at the hands" strike the listener as odd; however, in a different context, each may have its appropriate usage. Furthermore, in each example, the oddity of expression does not disrupt the intended meaning that the subject tries to convey. Jarring though these peculiar verbalizations may be, the listener can usually follow the subject's ideas.

According to Rapaport, "queer verbalizations" are expressions that would sound strange in any context. Thus, peculiar and queer verbalizations were seen as different gradients on a continuum of severity. Response verbalizations such as "the echo of a picture," "a split color," and the Rapaport group's example of "an artistic design of a fly's boot" (p. 447) have a bizarre quality, in which the subject tries to convey meaning that is remote and strangely private. Unlike the stilted but discernible peculiar verbalization, queer responses leave the listener feeling confused. Rapaport stated that peculiar verbalizations were more common than queer ones, except in more disorganized schizophrenic patients. He felt verbal convention could mask pathological thinking and allow many psychotic patients to maintain a good front. Rapaport noted that peculiar verbalizations can occur in neurotic and normal Rorschach records but with far less frequency than in schizophrenic and preschizophrenic ones. Queer verbalizations, however, were felt to be more severe indicators of schizophrenic or, at least, preschizophrenic pathology. Rapaport went so far as to state that peculiar verbalizations, in ample frequency, were more diagnostic of preschizophrenic conditions, whereas queer verbalizations were indicative of schizophrenia proper.

8. VAGUENESS, CONFUSION, AND INCOHERENCE. The Rapaport group identified three related categories of verbalization that referred to a continuum of "response atrophy" or degradation in which the subject seems to lose hold of the response due to either a perceptual or verbal difficulty. Vagueness of verbalization reflects the subject's difficulty in articulating a response in a clear and sharp manner. In Rapaport's words, the subject has difficulty keeping a percept with a definite form alive. Subjects may reveal their vagueness of verbalization by expressing a degree of perplexity as they attempt unsuccessfully to communicate what they see. Neurotic level subjects were viewed as better able to communicate their feeling of vagueness, while psychotic individuals typically did not. Rapaport gave examples of vagueness of verbalization which included the Card I response "I can almost get a witch's face but I can't make it" and the Card IV response "a skin tacked on a wall . . . I can't quite get it but it is there some place" (p. 449). Rapaport believed that these verbalizations often betrayed a prepsychotic or psychotic condi-

tion. In these responses, the first perceptual impression of the inkblot is fleeting and seems to evaporate quickly. Rapaport suggested that the examiner, in such cases, may have the feeling as if he were "digging in quicksand."

Rapaport used the term "confusion" to refer to those responses in which subjects express confusion either in their experience of the inkblot, or in their attempt to communicate what they see, or both. According to Rappaport, the subject maintains that he perceives the inkblot a certain way but that this cannot be. In doing so, the subject reveals a distinct confusion about the apparent contradiction between what he sees and what he feels to be the truth. Confusion responses usually reveal some overt or more subtle expression of the subject's perplexity, as in Rapaport's example of a Card II response, "Clowns . . . they have three legs . . . they can't have three legs!" (p. 450). Rapaport and his colleagues viewed the confusion response as a signal of the presence of confusion in everyday life and, at worst, as an inability to maintain conceptual boundaries between contradictory experiences.

Incoherent verbalizations reflect the most severe kind of intrusion into and disruption of the response process. Rapaport reserved this scoring category for those responses that were so laden with extraneous verbiage as to make them almost incomprehensible. Rapaport's example of a Card IX response of "limbs and shoulders of men . . . always inner ambition that man could make wings and overcome gravity . . . that the card reminded me that it can be done," leaves the listener confused, a key criterion for scoring a response as incoherent (pp. 450–451). The listener might well label such a response "disorganized" because it does not follow the rules of conventional, orderly thinking, in which the initial link of a thought chain exerts a regulatory effect on the remainer of the chain of ideas and associations. In Rapaport's example, the initial percept "limbs and shoulders of men" has no logical, coherent connection with the verbiage that follows, thus leaving the listener hopelessly confused and wondering if he has misheard or missed something. Rapaport stated that incoherence is always a psychotic indication and usually diagnostic of schizophrenic or organic psychotic conditions.

9. SYMBOLIC RESPONSES. Symbolic responses reflect the subject's attempts to "interpret" abstract levels of meaning into the inkblots. Rapaport suggested that there were two types of symbolic responses, implicit and explicit, and that both types could signal the presence of a psychotic process. However, he also noted that highly imaginative normal or neurotic individuals could also produce more toned-down versions of each of these types of symbolic response. The explicit type of symbolism is clearly present when the subject indicates that something about the inkblot (or the blot as a whole) symbolizes an abstract concept.

According to the Rapaport group, psychotic-level symbolism is based on a conviction that the inkblot represents a meaningful idea or truth; however, the interpretation has an autistic and overly private quality that is usually not comprehendible to the listener. Furthermore, the symbolic ideas are not well integrated with the formal qualities of the inkblot and do not enrich the response. The Rapaport example on Card VIII of "the one who drew this must have intended to represent the similarity theory of nature" (p. 452) conveys both the subject's certainty that he has discovered the true meaning of the inkblot and the idiosyncratic nature of his symbolic thought processes, which leaves the listener feeling lost and confused. On the other hand, more intact subjects may attempt to interpret meaning based on symbolism in a way that is both more integrated and conventional. Rapaport mentioned the often seen Card II response of "Two people fighting and the red might be symbolic of the conflict" as an example of normal/neurotic-level symbolism in which the symbolic interpretation is well integrated and easily comprehended.

Rapaport described implicit symbolism as a process that occurs when a subject makes no direct reference to symbolic meaning but uses images that may symbolize libidinal or aggressive impulses. For example, he suggested that the response to the upper projection of Card IV (where, according to Rapaport, a penis is often seen) of an "erect snake ready to strike" may well represent latent phallic symbolism." Rapaport indicated that psychotic and nonpsychotic individuals use implicit symbolism when viewing the inkblots. In terms of distinguishing the higher from the lower level type, Rapaport suggested that elaborate, implicit symbolism, that does not fit with the blot area, might be a "danger signal" for the examiner to be alert to other psychotic indicators in the record.

Rapaport also cautioned examiners against making inferences about unconscious contents based on explicit or implicit forms of symbolism. Consistent with his approach to the Rorschach, it was the formal qualities of symbolic responses that were to be interpreted as indications of a particular kind of thought process (e.g., autistic/psychotic) and not as windows into the subject's unconscious conflicts.

10. ABSURD RESPONSES. For Rapaport, absurd responses exemplified the concept of pathological distance from the inkblot. Here there is no justification for what the subject associates to the inkblot. The form is, by definition, bad in that the response is clearly unrelated to the area of the inkblot chosen. Whereas the adequate response requires that the subject's perceptual and associative or ideational processes work in unison, or as Rapaport said, in a "cogwheeling" fashion, absurd responses reflect a marked dysynchrony between these two processes. The Rapaport example of the Card V response of "Could it be a hippopotamus spread out like that?" is clearly absurd (p. 458). The examiner is

left nonplussed about the origin of such a response. Rapaport viewed these kinds of patently unjustified responses as suggestive of schizophrenia.

11. RELATIONSHIP VERBALIZATIONS. Rapaport described several kinds of relationship verbalizations. He broke these up into several groups, those having to do with perceiving relationships within a card, those having to do with perceiving relationships between cards, and those in which the subject is concerned about what the inkblots might relate to. He described how the first category might reflect a pathological loss of distance from the blot, as the subject concretely perceives relationships between blot elements based on spatial contiguity. He related this to fabulized combinations. Perceiving relationships between cards may also reflect a concrete loss of distance, as the subject assumes that similarities between inkblots implies that they are somehow connected. Additionally, perceiving relationships between cards (e.g., "This one is related to the one before because of the white space in the middle") may reflect an increase in distance, especially if the subject focuses primarily on the formal characteristics of the inkblots and ignores the object images. Rapaport believed that this type of increase of distance from the inkblot reflected the subject's retreat from meaningful objects and reality in general.

The final type of relationship verbalization that Rapaport was concerned with was more subtle. These responses had to do with the subject's search for some connection between the inkblot and something else. For example, the subject who wonders what the inkblots might relate to is searching beyond the card for a connection with something else that he assumes might be obscure or hidden. Verbalizations such as "I think that this card relates to something but I'm not sure what" or "I've seen this one; this part was on the other card you showed me" reflect a paranoid quality which Rapaport was quick to point out.

12. VERBALIZATION OF REFERENCE IDEAS. When the relationship verbalization is carried to an extreme, it can become referential. According to Rapaport, referential responses are based on the perception of an arbitrary relationship between different areas of the inkblot that may even be spatially unrelated. The subject is trying to interpret the inkblot and find connections between disparate blot elements. However, he does so in an idiosyncratic manner that often defies logic. For example, Rapaport's Card III response, "Looks like a body to me . . . these are blood spots . . . I don't know why they should be there . . . might have come out of the body," is reminiscent of both fabulized combination and autistic logic responses (p. 456). Rapaport said that extreme examples of referential responses occurred almost exclusively in the records of schizophrenic patients.

13. SELF-REFERENCE VERBALIZATIONS. Rapaport meant for this score to be used when the subject indicated that some aspect of the inkblot had special reference to him. These responses were to be differentiated from more benign examples of personal associations to the inkblots. In the self-reference verbalization, the subject loses all awareness of the impersonal reality of the card or test-taking situation and responds as if the inkblot has immediate relevance to him. Rapaport gave the example of the Card II response of "menstruation" which was followed by the disgusted statement "I revolt against being a woman and not a man!" (p. 457). Although the self-reference is implicit, the subject's inability to take appropriate distance from the card is obvious.

14. DETERIORATION COLOR RESPONSES. When color is used to justify some crude or gory percept, the color deterioration score should be used. Here color stimulates socially unacceptable ideas that the subject is unable or not inclined to screen out. For example, the Card X response "Urine stains" leaves little doubt that, for this subject, color has served to evoke primitive and crude fantasies, which he felt compelled to report to the examiner. Rapaport contended that these responses were most frequently given by chronic, deteriorated schizophrenic patients.

15. EXACTNESS VERBALIZATIONS. These responses reflect an overly meticulous and critical approach to the inkblots. The subject has difficulty "rounding off" and approximating. Each card is criticized for not looking exactly like the object the subject perceives. For example, a hypercritical attitude is revealed by the Card V response, "I suppose it could be a bat, but it's all wrong; the wings are not shaped right up in this corner." Rapaport indicated that decompensating obsessionals and paranoid patients could give such responses.

16. CRITICISM VERBALIZATIONS. Rapaport believed that subjects who criticize amorphous inkblots are often displacing their hostility onto the cards. Thus, he felt that depressed subjects, for example, who have difficulty expressing anger directly, may do so by making critical comments about the inkblots. Rapaport also indicated that these subjects may lose distance from the inkblots and take them too seriously.

17. VERBAL AGGRESSION. These are comments that are not directly related to the response itself. As the name implies, these verbalizations are hostile in nature and usually directed against the examiner or some aspect of the testing situation. Rapaport stated that such comments usually are given by paranoid subjects or individuals with antisocial characters.

18. AGGRESSION RESPONSES.   In these responses, the aggression is not directed toward the examiner or test but is an integral part of the response. Aggressive action is infused into the response with descriptors such as "splattered," "smashed," "ripped apart," "fighting," and so forth. A greater degree of control is implied by integrating the aggression into the response, instead of directing it toward the examiner. Nonetheless, Rapaport concluded that aggression responses indicate that the subject is struggling with a great deal of aggressive tension.

19. SELF-DEPRECIATION VERBALIZATIONS.   Comments such as "I don't have a very good imagination" or "I'm just not very good at this" reflect a degree of self-depreciation. Subjects who are sharply critical of their capacity to respond to the inkblots may be revealing depressive and masochistic character trends.

20. AFFECTIVE VERBALIZATIONS.   Subjects who respond to the inkblots as if they were terrifying pieces of reality will lose distance from the test and utter emotionally charged responses. Dramatic side comments such as "Take it away; I can't stand to look at it" reflect the degree to which the subject has lost his proper perspective and "fallen into" the inkblots. Rapaport suggested that such verbalizations were characteristic of hysterics, anxious depressives, and overideational preschizophrenics.

21. MASTURBATION AND CASTRATION VERBALIZATIONS.   Rapaport included responses in which the subject described something as deteriorated, eroded, damaged, broken, or missing as either masturbation or castration responses. Responses such as these were taken as symbolic representations of either masturbatory guilt or castration anxiety. Rapaport stated that a preoccupation with damage or deterioration reflects a special sensitivity often in subjects who suffer from guilt about masturbation. Similarly, he pointed out that concern about missing or broken objects suggest a sensitivity to a sense of incompleteness characteristic of castration anxiety. Rapaport cautioned against applying simple formula solutions to such interpretations and offered these as only a few of the several interpretative possibilities for the examiner to consider.

Modifications of the Rapaport System

A number of Rapaport's disciples modified his scoring system and did not carry forward the elaborate list of thought disorder scores that their mentor originally described. Most of the modifications included simplifications of the thought disorder scoring system which attempted to remove some of the ambiguity that some felt plagued his original system.

Schafer's Psychoanalytic Approach

Following Rapaport, Schafer wrote extensively about the psychoanalytic interpretation of the Rorschach (1948, 1954). Of all Rapaport's disciples, Schafer remained closest to the letter and spirit of the original list of thought disorder scores that Rapaport, Gill, and he had developed. In each of his books, Schafer presented a number of case studies of thought-disordered patients and listed scores for their deviant Rorschach verbalizations under the "Qualitative" heading of the "Summary of Responses" section of the protocol.

Schafer's first book (1948) provided a shortened list of thought disorder scoring categories, which included DW; absurd form; confabulation; contaminations; autistic logic; queer content; peculiar communications; relationship, reference, and self-reference ideas; confusion; fabulized combinations; and fabulations. In addition to using many of the original Rapaport scores, Schafer (1954) introduced a few additional scores, including those he called "fluid," "irrelevant," and "perseveration" responses. Rapaport spoke of "fluidity of conceptual boundaries" when discussing confusion and incoherent responses; however, he did not list "fluid responses" as a separate scoring category. Schafer used the term "fluidity" to refer to an unstable and shifting quality of perceiving or thinking, in which the response does not "take hold" and too readily becomes something else (similar to Rapaport's vagueness and confusion responses).

Schafer also referred to responses that did not quite reach the scoring threshold as "tendency" responses. For example, a response that approached, but was not quite, a contamination was called a "contamination tendency," while a near confabulation was called a "confabulation tendency." Earlier, Rapaport had hinted that these "tendency" responses should be recognized; however, he did not use this term and never developed the concept of a continuum of severity within each type of deviant verbalization.

Allison, Blatt, and Zimet's Approach

The same year that Holt completed his revised edition of Rapaport, Gill, and Schafer's *Diagnostic Psychological Testing,* Allison, Blatt, and Zimet came out with their own text, entitled *The Interpretation of Psychological Tests* (1968). Their Rorschach thought disorder scoring approach was quite consistent with, but generally simpler than, that of the Rapaport group. Allison et al. provided brief definitions for the following scores; fab comb; fab; confab; contam; pec; autistic logic; fluid; symbolic; and self-ref. Following Schafer's lead, they defined "fluid" as "Loss of the train of thought; loose shifting from percept to percept;

inability to recall responses" (p. 181). They also seemed to be following a trend to streamline Rapaport's lengthy list of deviant verbalizations into more usable and operationally defined categories.

Mayman and Appelbaum Modifications

Mayman altered and extended several aspects of the Rapaport System. One of his students, Stephen Appelbaum, added some of his own ideas and passed these on to several generations of postdoctoral clinical psychologists at the Menninger Foundation. In the 1960s, Mayman wrote a Rorschach scoring and interpretation manual (copyrighted by Mayman in 1982); and Appelbaum subsequently revised it (Appelbaum, 1975).

Mayman developed a five point scale for identifying degrees of fabulized embellishment of Rorschach responses. The total "fab score" was intended as a measure of the frequency and degree to which the response process became infused with fantasy and departed from object reality (see chapter 9). Unlike Rapaport, Mayman used the expression "extreme loss of distance" from the inkblot to refer to those responses that were embellished with fantasy material that went far beyond what the inkblot could support. Rapaport would have referred to such responses as a product of an extreme "increase of distance" from the blot, as in the case of a confabulation response. Mayman also developed a scale for rating the blatency of oral aggressive content in Rorschach responses.

In terms of scoring thought disorder proper, the Mayman-Appelbaum manual defines only a few key scoring categories, such as fabulizations; fabulized combinations; confabulations; contaminations; peculiar and queer verbalizations.

Lerner's Modern Psychoanalytic Approach

Lerner's texts on psychoanalytic theory and the Rorschach (1991, 1998) are the latest attempts to represent Rapaport's theoretical/conceptual approach to the Rorschach. Although Lerner supplemented Rapaport's standard ego psychological interpretation of Rorschach determinant and content scores with more contemporary research regarding defenses, self and object relations, he stuck closely to Rapaport's original list of deviant verbalizations. Lerner limited his presentation to ten varieties of pathological responses, including fabulized response (Fab); fabulized combination (Fab-Comb); confabulation (Confab); contamination (Contam); autistic logic (Aut); peculiar verbalization (Pec); queer verbalization (Queer); vagueness (Vague); confusion (Conf); and incoherence (Incoh).

A CRITIQUE OF RAPAPORT'S DEVIANT VERBALIZATIONS

The methodology on which the Rapaport System was developed has been an easy, albeit appropriate, target for critics of Rorschach research (Goldfried et al., 1971; Exner, 1974, 1986a, 1993). Goldfried et al. mentioned the composition of the comparison groups and the methods of data analysis as two primary problem areas of the "Rapaport Study." They pointed out, for example, that sample groups of patients and control subjects differed along important demographic factors. In particular, the control group was significantly different from most of the patient groups in terms of education, intelligence, and social class. Regarding data analysis, Rapaport et al. performed a large number of statistical tests without consideration that conducting an enormous number of tests would affect probability levels. They also made specific comparisons and cutoff points after an examination of the data, none of which were cross validated on subsequent samples of subjects.

Exner (1974) addressed some of the problems inherent in Rapaport's efforts to categorize deviant verbalizations that justified his early decision to exclude formal thought disorder scoring from his Comprehensive System. Specifically, he noted that the overlap in categories and the lack of clear operational definitions made precise quantitative scoring extremely difficult. Even Rapaport's most loyal followers seemed to agree that his list of scores was unwieldy, both for research purposes and reliable clinical scoring, and looked for ways to simplify the scoring categories. Most followers listed roughly 10 varieties, which were the most commonly occurring types.

Reading Rapaport's original description of thought disorder categories can be confusing for a number of reasons. First, the language and concepts that they used can be difficult to grasp. As Holt (Rapaport et al., 1968) noted, the concept of "distance from the inkblot" created a great deal of uncertainty and frequently led followers to confuse pathological increases and losses of distance with one another. Their discussion of whether a particular response reflects loss or increase of distance, or both, can be difficult to follow and tends to obfuscate the more meaningful rationale for each scoring category. Additionally, the Rapaport group extended the concept of "confabulation" in ways that were both extremely helpful but also confusing because it differed from the standard way that this term was used in Rorschach testing. Confabulation was no longer regarded simply as a perceptual process, as in the DW response, but became a broad category that reflected inappropriate fantasy embellishment of the inkblot. The broader definition of confabulation allowed examiners to pick up on a type of deviant thought process that had been all but ignored in the past; however, the use of the term led to confusion among psychodiagnosticians using different Rorschach systems.

The lack of any type-scoring continua was another problem in Rapaport's original list of categories. Scores were listed as discrete qualitative variables that were considered to be either present or absent. The lack of formal recognition of nascent or subthreshold forms of a particular type of deviant verbalization eventually led Schafer (1954) to begin recording "-tendency" responses among the thought disorder scores.

To balance the ample criticisms of their methodology, it is important to recall the authors' recognition of the crudeness and limitations of their approach. In their words,

> It is not our claim that the following pages present a complete explanation or systematization of final validity of the material we have excerpted, or that the excerpt represent an exhaustive collection of all possible kinds of deviant verbalizations. We do not even maintain that the distinctions we made between different kinds of pathological verbalizations are entirely consistent or correct. . . . Our approach to the verbalizations was a gross one [pp. 425–426].

Thus, the Rapaport scoring system should be respected for what it was: a preliminary attempt to establish some order in what had been an unsystematically evaluated, and often ignored, component of Rorschach testing. Even with its methodological flaws and occasional conceptual lack of clarity, Rapaport, Gill, and Schafer's contribution to scoring and understanding thought disorder on the Rorschach is fundamental and has formed the backbone of all later efforts to measure pathological thinking with the Rorschach.

CHAPTER

4

HOLT'S PRIMARY PROCESS
SCORING SYSTEM

Like many of Rapaport's early students, Robert Holt became a prominent psychoanalytic researcher and Rorschach theoretician in his own right. During the course of his research, Holt became interested in the psychoanalytic concept of neutralization or how primary process thinking could be tamed or bound in the service of adaptation. He reasoned that thought processes, as respresented by Rorschach responses, could reflect neutralized drive energy to the extent that responses lacked evidence of libidinal or aggressive drive derivatives. Holt developed a "neutralization index" to measure the degree to which primary process material pervaded Rorschach content (Klopfer, Ainsworth, Klopfer et al., 1954). The index consisted of the sum of all content that involved oral, narcissistic, anal, voueuristic, exhibitionistic, urethral, phallic, homosexual, as well as all manifestations of aggressive or destructive contents, and divided this by R.

In examining the Rorschachs of a group of college students, Holt noticed that aspects of primary process thinking could be detected in the Rorschach responses of some students, but that these were frequently balanced by humor and cultural references in those students who were independently judged to have more flexible cognitive styles. Thus, Holt began to pay close attention to the relative effectiveness of a subject's efforts to control or defend against the emergence of primary process material in his Rorschach responses. In doing so, he found that it was possible to distinguish between unbridled breakthrough of primary process derivatives and the more modulated and socially acceptable expressions of this material.

Holt became interested in establishing a theoretically-based Rorschach scoring system that would not only assess primary process manifestations but, more importantly, measure aspects of ego control and defense. Together with his colleague, Joan Havel, he developed his comprehensive "PRIPRO Scoring System" ("PRIPRO Scoring" standing for "scoring manifestations of the primary process") as a research tool, and not a clinical instrument. With close to 100 individual scoring variables grouped together across three broad scoring categories, Holt believed that the system was too cumbersome to be used efficiently in a typical clinical setting.

Each of the three scoring categories corresponds to a different aspect of primary process thinking, as described by Holt (1956, 1970, 1977; Holt and Havel, 1960). First, since primary process thinking is characterized by its wishful quality, Holt and Havel constructed a group of *content variables* to reflect the degree of primary process wishfulness present in each response. Secondly, primary process thinking is defined by unique structural characteristics, which led Holt and Havel to modify and extend Rapaport's list of Rorschach scoring categories for formal thought disorder and develop their own group of *formal variables*. Finally, the emergence of primary process thinking prompts either effective or ineffective defensive and control efforts, which are measured by Holt and Havel's third category, *control and defense variables*.

The PRIPRO system is summarized below. Further discussion regarding the theoretical basis underlying the scoring categories will be presented in chapters 7 and 17 when the conceptual underpinnings of Holt's system and its relevance to the study of creativity is examined.

CONTENT VARIABLES

Holt was concerned with developing a scale that would measure the degree of wishfulness embedded in an idea. He assumed that Rorschach responses which contained libidinal and aggressive imagery reflect drive derivatives or wishes characteristic of primary process thinking. Holt specified two major content categories reflecting libidinal and aggressive wishes. Each of these categories was then subdivided into "Level 1" and "Level 2" responses reflecting the degree of proximity of a response to the realm of primary process experience. Level 1 responses were defined as imagery that reflected blatent, crude, and more primitive, unmodulated expressions of libidinal or aggressive impulses. On the contrary,

Level 2 responses reflected more socialized, civilized, and modulated expressions of primary process experience.

Libidinal Content

By "libidinal," Holt meant content that reflected partial sexual drive derivatives or developmental stages of psychosexual maturation. In addition, certain sexually specific contents were scored even though they did not reflect fixation at any particular psychosexual stage. Holt scored two types of material: (1) response content or imagery which itself expressed drive-related material and (2) response verbalizations, associations, and elaborations which conveyed libidinal concerns.

LEVEL 1 (LI. PRIMITIVE, CRUDE, AND BLATANT LIBIDINAL EXPRESSION)

1. *L 1 O.* Oral Receptive: Derives from early oral incorporative and passive sucking stage of development. Mouth, lips, tongue, breasts are scored when seen in isolation.
2. *L 1 O-Ag.* Oral Aggressive. Derives from the later oral-biting phase including such contents as teeth, jaws (when seen in isolation); cannibalism; castration, sadistic biting; parasites.
3. *L 1 A.* Anal. All references to excretory organs, defecation, or feces.
4. *L 1 S.* Sexual. Both phallic and genital sexual imagery are scored. Genitals are scored when seen in isolation or as a part of a person, or animal; use of the term "phallic symbol"; sexual activity.
5. *L 1 E-V.* Exhibitionistic-Voyeuristic: Any specific reference to nudity or pornography; exhibition of sexual anatomy or voyeuristic activity.
6. *L 1 H.* Homosexual; Sexual ambiguity: Overt and less blatant homosexual activity; uncertainty regarding sex of figures; hermaphroditism.
7. *L 1 M.* Miscellaneous Libidinal: This is intended as an additional category to capture libidinal response content or associative material that are not subsumed by any other category.

LEVEL 2 (L2. INDIRECT, "SOCIALIZED," AND MODULATED LIBIDINAL EXPRESSION)

1. *L 2 O.* Oral Receptive. Milder, modulated and more toned-down expressions of oral receptive issues, including percepts of breasts, lips, mouth, and tongue.
2. *L 2 O-Ag.* Oral Aggressive. Percepts having to do with poisonous foods, plants, and all animals that are feared because of their potential to bite; teeth, beak, or jaws; and verbal aggression including arguing, cursing, yelling, and spitting.
3. *L 2 A.* Anal imagery having to do with percepts of tails and buttocks when seen as part of a person or animal; intestines; toilet or sewer; disgust when attributed to a figure; mud, dirt, smearing.

4. *L 2 S.* Sexual imagery including breasts (which can also be scored as L1O or L2O); kissing (similarly scored as L1O and L2O); reference to love, marriage, romance, valentine hearts, and other socialized expressions of genital sexuality, procreation, or reproduction.

5. *L 2 E-V.* Exhibitionistic and voyeuristic impulses that are expressed in more sublimated ways including references to the concealing function of clothes; peering, looking, and peeking when emphasized; reference to actors, theater, masks.

6. *L 2 H.* Sexual Ambiguity: Percepts having to do with transvestism; sublimated homosexual activity; uncertainty about the sex of a figure.

7. *L 2 M.* Miscellaneous Libidinal. This category includes responses that have a more modulated libidinal quality (including such things as uterus, womb, pelvis, pregnancy, fetus, and bladder) and reflections when they are associated with figures looking at or admiring themselves in a mirror.

Aggressive Content

Holt and Havel divided aggressive and destructive content into three subtypes: (1) those in which the person, animal or object (central figure) is the subject who perpetrates the aggression; (2) those in which the central figure is the victim or object of the aggression; and (3) those responses which depict the aftermath or results of destructive action or aggression. When a response includes both the perpetrator and victim, Holt recommended scoring for the perpetrator.

LEVEL 1 (AG1. MORE PRIMITIVE AND OVERT EXPRESSIONS OF AGGRESSION).

1. *Ag 1 S.* Sadistic Aggression including examples of sadistic fantasies; primitive annhilation of people and animals; murder, mutilation, and torture.

2. *Ag 1 Ob.* Masochistic Aggression which is reflected in images of castration, extreme victimization and torture, sexual masochism, terrifying helplessness, and suicide.

3. *Ag 1 R.* Results of Aggression involving graphic images of death with explicit mention of hostile intent, decayed flesh or organs, and mutilation of animals or people; the aftermath of sadistic lethal action.

LEVEL 2 (AG2. SOCIALIZED AND SUBLIMATED EXPRESSIONS OF AGGRESSION).

1. *Ag 2 S.* Subject Aggression, implying aggressive acts in which the agression is expressed in toned-down and socially acceptable manner.

2. *Ag 2 Ob.* Object Aggression in which the emphasis is on the victim of Level 2 violence or aggression.

3. *Ag 2 R.* Results of Aggression in which the aggression may be only implied and not directly stated. Included are such percepts as deformed or injured persons, plants, or animals.

FORMAL VARIABLES

Holt believed that Rapaport's list of deviant verbalizations was actually a way of categorizing formal manifestations of primary process experience. The scoring manual devised by Holt (1968, 1970)[1] for assessing formal aspects of primary process thinking was thus an outgrowth of Rapaport's work. Holt and Havel initially attempted to correlate primary process manifestations in Rorschach responses with formal characteristics of dreams. They wondered how these formal characteristics of dreaming—condensation, displacement, and symbolization—might appear in Rorschach responses. However, they realized that dreaming and Rorschach thinking differ considerably and could not be considered comparable processes. Holt and Havel reasoned that without a subject's associations, it is difficult to know when condensation, displacement, or symbolization occurs in Rorschach responses. Nevertheless, they believed that crude traces of these primary process characteristics can be left behind and leave their mark on the finished Rorschach response. In these cases, the subject's failure to cover up or screen out the traces of such primary process in his or her thinking and perception can reveal deviations from the kind of logical, orderly thinking that is anchored in reality-based secondary process thinking.

In constructing their formal variables section in their scoring manual, Holt and Havel did not restrict themselves to the types of formal deviations associated with dream processes but tried to include other deviant processes that were unique to the Rorschach situation. Holt revised this manual a number of times, expanding and refining the operational definitions of the scoring categories. Beginning with the concepts of condensation, symbolization, and displacement as broad organizing categories, he derived close to 40 separate scores to measure structural deviations in the perceptual organization and verbalization of the response and the thought processes that underlie them. Like the content variables, each formal scoring category is associated with either a Level 1 or Level 2 designation, indicating the degree to which this aspect of the response represents a more primitive, unmodulated expression of primary process thinking.

Condensation

As one of the hallmarks of primary process thinking, condensation refers to the inability to keep images and ideas stable and separated in a

---

1. Holt is currently revising his PRIPRO system and may publish his latest textbook on the scoring of primary process manifestations sometime in 1999.

way that is demanded by an accurate view of external reality. Holt identified eight different types of what he termed "image-fusion," scored at either Level 1 or Level 2, or both.

1. *C-ctm*. Contamination (scored only at Level 1). Holt followed his predecessors, in identifying the contamination response as the fusion of two separate images into a single percept. Holt indicated that this category was reserved not only for rarely occurring conventional contamination response, but also for lesser versions that would be scored as "contamination-tendency."

2. *C-ctgn 1*. Contagion (scored only at Level 1). In the contagion response, there is a fusion between the nature of the percept and the experience of the subject. The subject loses a boundary between him or herself and the response so that he or she begins to feel or take on key characteristics (affects, etc.) of the response.

3. *C-int 1*. Interpenetration (partial fusion of two separate percepts) (scored only at Level 1). Instead of a total fusion or merger of two separate images or ideas, the subject is unable to decide between two percepts which are seen in the same blot area. Ideas may become intermingled in a confusing manner (e.g., "It looks like a rat but the beak area makes it look more like a bird, right here in the middle, see it looks just like a bird but the furry area makes it look more like a rat").

4. *C-co 1*. Composition (Level 1). Impossible fusions, in which parts from two or more percepts are unrealistically combined to make a hybrid creature, are the prototype of the Level 1 composite response.

5. *C-co 2*. Composition (Level 2). This category refers to composite images that exist in art, mythology, folklore, or the popular media and for fusions that may be realistic (e.g., "siamese twins").

6. *C-a-c 2*. Arbitrary Combinations of Separate Percepts (scored at Level 2). This was essentially Holt's score for "fabulized combinations." Responses in which the combination is based on physical contiguity without interpenetration of boundaries or implied meaning in the relationship (e.g., "These two ladies here are joined together down here") were referred to as "arbitrary linkage."

7. *C-arb 1*. Arbitrary Combination of Color and Form. In this particular response, the fusion occurs between two different realms, color and form. In the Level 1 response, the subject uncritically assigns inappropriate color to an object without questioning the inherent incongruity of the combination.

8. *C-arb 2*. Rationalized Inappropriate Color and Form. C-arb 2 is scored whenever a subject assigns an inappropriate color to an object, even though it may be rationalized in an acceptable manner.

Displacement

Holt indicated that displacement often had the effect of making a response more socially acceptable. As a result, some displacements come close to the secondary process end of the continuum. Holt's scoring categories for displacement included both Level 1 and Level 2 responses.

1. *D-chain 1*. Chain Associations (scored only at Level 1). Holt used this term to describe fluid associations in which the subject went from one idea to the next without the overall guidance of an organizing set or concept. He emphasized that this was the hallmark of manic thought disorder. In his manual, Holt (1970) gave the following example of a D-chain 1 response:

   A star (?) this and this . . . 6 point star. 106th division, see, I was in an ambulatory division, I wasn't a doughboy—I think it is the word KP's call them [tells story about KP]; (In what way did you mean it looked irregular?) the damn lines aren't regular on it. It's just not regular, Doc. I'm a regular guy (sings: "Here comes that guy") I'm going to have them work on my teeth today . . . ; an open womb, I think of an opening—circle—earth—reproduction—growth—birth [p. 35].

2. *D-dist 2*. Distant Association (scored only at Level 2). Here the listener may be able to follow the subject's train of thought, which may be somewhat circumstantial.
3. *D-clang 1*. Clang Association (Level 1). Instead of the typical type of associative links, the subject connects ideas on the basis of assonance from one idea to another.
4. *D-clang 2*. Puns and Malapropisms (Level 1). Usually with humorous intent, the subject substitutes one word for another of a similar sound or by a homonym. D-clang 2 is scored as long as the verbalization does not contain elements of a verbal condensation.
5. *D-fig 2*. Figures of Speech (always scored Level 2). Metaphors, hyperbole, or inappropriate similes are scored only if they have an idiosyncratic quality.
6. *D-time 2*. Displacement in Time (always scored Level 2). This category involves an anachronistic introduction of an attribute or activity from one time period into another.

Explicit Symbolism

Holt's symbolism category pertains to concrete features of the inkblot that are used to represent an abstract idea. In each case, the subject makes explicit his attempt to represent an abstract idea by using either the color, shading, spatial arrangement, or form features of the inkblot. Three specific subtyes of explicit symbolism are scored.

1. *Sym-C 1*. Idiosyncratic Color or Shading Symbolism (Level 1). When a subject uses either shading or color features to represent an idea, activity, or object in a manner that is not in line with the socially accepted meaning of the color or shading, then Level 1 Sym-C is scored.
2. *Sym-C 2*. Conventional Color or Shading Symbolism (Level 2). The use of socially or culturally sanctioned symbolic meanings or color or shading merit a Level 2 score. For example, blue is associated with depression; green with envy; yellow with cowardice; red with anger or heat; and black with evil, depression, and death.
3. *Sym S 1*. Spatial Symbolism (scored only at Level 1). Spatial relations between different parts of the inkblot can lead a subject to infer idiosyncratic symbolic meaning that is not readily apparent from the features of the blot.
4. *Sym-I 1*. Idiosyncratic Image symbolism (Level 1). This score pertains to the use of an idiosyncratic concrete image to represent an abstract idea.
5. *Sym-I 2*. Conventional Image Symbolism (Level 2). Symbolic meaning is assigned to an image in a conventional manner, that is easily recognized by the examiner.

Contradictions

Although Freud did not include "contradiction" as a formal characteristic of primary process thinking, Holt extrapolated from Freud's writing and concluded that tolerance of contradictions was a hallmark of primary process experience. Holt scored three types of contradictions: (1) Affective contradictions, (2) Logical contradictions, and (3) Contradictions of reality (formerly called Inappropriate activity).

1. *Ctr A 1*. Affective Contradiction (scored only at Level 1). The subject makes it clear that in response to a particular percept, he experiences contradictory affects at the same time. The subject's affect may fluidly shift from one extreme to another or his affect may actually appear inappropriate.
2. *Ctr L 1*. Logical Contradiction (scored only at Level 1). The subject makes one statement that is logically incompatible with another, by either assigning mutually exclusive qualities to a single percept or simultaneously asserting and denying something about the inkblot or some aspect of his response.

3. *Ctr R 1*. Contradiction of Reality (serious) (Level 1) Deliberate molding of the blot's reality. In this particular response, the subject ignores a reality feature of the inkblot and molds his response into what he wants it to be. Color, shading, or spatial realities of the blot are disregarded as the subject makes the blot into what he wants it to be.

4. *Ctr R 2*. Contradiction of Reality (less serious) (Level 2). These include less serious attributions of inappropriate activities or characterisitics to people, animals, or objects. The percept is described in ways that violate reality. The projection of color on an achromatic blot is a further example of this score.

Verbalization Scores

Holt was not sure how to classify or interpret deviant forms of speech. He believed that they were different from deviations in perception and associative elaboration and could not be readily placed under the headings of condensation, displacement, or symbolization. Nonetheless, he included five verbalization scores in his system to capture deviant forms of verbal usage. However, he felt that each should be cautiously interpreted.

1. *V I 1*. Verbal Incoherence (Level 1 only). Associations that are extremely autistic and fail to communicate the subject's ideas are considered incoherent. In responding to the Rorschach card, the subject essentially lapses into a word salad as a means of expressing his ideas.

2. *V C 1*. Verbal Condensation (Level 1 only). The subject either produces neologisms or words or phrases in which the condensed elements are apparent.

3. *V Q 1*. Queer Verbalizations (Level 1 only). The subject fails to maintain an appropriate set with regard to the subject matter, the test, or the examiner. Words are used in an extremely stilted and idiosyncratic manner that cause the listener some confusion about the subject's intended meaning.

4. *V P 2*. Peculiar Verbalizations (Level 2 only).[2] The subject uses words or phrases that strike the listener as odd, but the meaning of what is being said can be understood.

5. *V S 2*. Verbal Slips. All slips of the tongue are scored under this category, regardless of whether the subject notices and attempts to self-correct his error.

---

2. Here, Holt's use of a Peculiar, Level 2, as opposed to Queer, Level 1, follows Rapaport.

Miscellaneous Distortions of Thought and Perception

Holt grouped 11 additional scores under the rubric of this miscellaneous category. These included a number of well-known scores popularized by Rapaport and his predecessors. They did not fit neatly into any of Holt's principal categories and hence, had to be listed under this heterogeneous category of primary process responses.

1. *Au Lg 1*. Autistic Logic (Level 1 only). In addition to fallacies in syllogistic reasoning, Holt included DW and Position (Po) responses as subtypes of autistic logic.
2. *M L 1*. Memory Loosening (Level 1 only). Here a subject, who knows better, makes a factual error. Holt considered this error to signal a looseness in the conceptual organization of memory.
3. *Intr 1*. Intrusion of Irrelevancy (Level 1 only). The subject has difficulty maintaining a focus and screening out irrelevant ideas. In such a case, the subject abruptly inserts an irrelevant idea into the response (e.g., "This looks like a person; what kind of cologne are you wearing?").
4. *Impr 2*. Impressionistic Response (Level 2). The subject gives a response as a feeling or an impression, often indicating that the response is just a "feeling" or an "impression" that he has.
5. *Un Rel 1*. Unrealistic Relationship (Level 1). The subject perceives an unrealistic relationship between inkblots or between elements of one card. Here the subject actively, but erroneously, forms a relationship between things or ideas that do not belong together.
6. *Trans 1*. Fluid Transformation of Percept (Level 1). The subject actively describes a percept's changing from one thing to another.
7. *S-R 1*. Self Reference (of a magically unrealistic kind) (Level 1). The subject identifies that something in his response has personal meaning or reference for him.
8. *Au El 1*. Autistic Elaboration (Level 1). This was essentially Holt's category for confabulation. He disliked the term "confabulation" which he felt was too easily confused with the DW response.
9. *Au El 2*. Autistic Elaboration (Level 2). When a subject embellishes a response thematically but the elaboration is not bizarre or unrealistic, then the response is scored at Level 2.
10. *Do 2*. Fragmentation (Level 2). When a subject reports seeing part of a percept where most subjects see a whole percept, he is given the score Do. Rorschach referred to this as an "oligophrenic detail."
11. *F-msc 1 or 2*. Miscellaneous Formal Deviations (Levels 1 and 2). Holt listed a number of additional deviant responses including: (1) perseveration (Level 1); (2) taking the blot as reality (Level 1),

where the subject reacts to the blot as if it were the real object, person, or animal; and (3) physiognomic responses (Level 1) to some property of the inkblot other than color.[3]

CONTROL AND DEFENSE SCORES

Holt's most original contribution was his effort to operationalize control and defense variables. These categories were scored whenever a response included either content or formal variables that warranted separate scores. Holt believed that these scoring categories of defense and control represented both the subject's conscious or latent awareness that the material contained in the response is inappropriate and also his efforts to modulate the way it is expressed and communicated to the examiner. Holt assigned either a minus or plus sign to many of these scores to designate whether the efforts to tone down or control the material were successful (+) or unsuccessful (–). No sign is used if the response is not significantly improved or spoiled by the attempt at control and modulation.

Holt originally identified seven groups of control and defense categories: (1) Remoteness (R); (2) Context (Cx); (3) Reflection (Refl); (4) Postponing Strategies; (5) Miscellaneous Defenses; (6) Sequence (S); and (7) Overtness (O). He later included Reflection and Sequence under his Miscellaneous category.

Remoteness

Holt called upon Thompkins's concept of remoteness or distance on the TAT (Tompkins, 1947), in which a subject attempts to make an unacceptable impulse more socially acceptable by making the response in

---

3. At this point, readers may be wondering about the practical value of all of these finely tooled distinctions in scoring variables. Readers may ask, "Does this really make a difference in our understanding of an individual's thought organization?" or "Is it worth the effort to employ such a complex set of scores?" It is important to mention again that Holt devised the PRIPRO as a research instrument and was interested in studying subtleties of thought organization as they might pertain to a range of dependent measures. As fine as many of his distinctions may have been, they were worth making since Holt did not know beforehand how fine-grained an instrument would be needed to discriminate between different groups of patients and other subjects.

question remote in time, place, person, or level of reality.[4] Holt believed that creating distance or remoteness from primary process material reflected the adaptive process of displacement. There are 15 different subtypes of Remoteness scores. The last 9 (from R-dep on) may be scored for formally deviant responses when the remoteness has relevance to the formal quality that is scored.

(1) *R-min*. Minimal Remoteness. This score pertains to a response that involves persons (whole or part) represented in the here and now, existing in reality. (2) *R-eth*. Remoteness-Ethnic. This score is given when the ethnic or racial group of the human figures is different from that of the subject. (3) *R-an*. Remoteness-Animal (ego syntonic). When the main figures in the response are animals, the R-an score is used. (4) *R-(an)*. Remoteness-Animal (ego alien). This second R-(an) score is given when the main characters or figures in the responses are sub-mammalian (including bats and birds). (5) *R-pl*. Remoteness-Plant. Score R-pl when the main figure is any kind of a plant. (6) *R-ia*. Remoteness-Inanimate. Inanimate actions or objects (nonhuman, animal, or plant) and abstract ideas are given the score of R-ia. (7) *R-dep+*. Remoteness-Depiction. The central character or the focus of the primary process material is depicted in a painting, movie, drawing, statue, cartoon, or other. The plus sign (+) indicates that this type of response is associated with intelligence, education, and other adaptive aspects of personality. (8) *R-geo+*. Remoteness-Geographic. Geographical remoteness refers to placing people, animals, or objects at a geographical distance. Again, the plus sign (+) is associated with adaptivity.

The following categories are self explanatory and are scored either + or – depending on whether they are well articulated, integrated, consistent with reality, and used in an appropriate manner: (9) *R-time+/–*. Remoteness in Time, past or future. (10) *R-fic s+/–*. Remotesness, Fictional-Specific. (11) *R-fic n+/–*. Remoteness, Fictional-Nonspecific. (12) *R-rel+/–*. Remoteness, Religious. Religious figures or context from current world religions are subsumed under this score. (13) *R-fan+/–*. Remoteness, Fantasy. The subject attempts to gain distance by referring to dreams, daydreams, fantasy, or the imaginary. (14) *R-fig+/–*. Remoteness, Figurative. The subject employs a figure of speech in his/her response. (15) *R-cond*. Remoteness, Conditional. When the primary process material appears as a conditional part of a statement in the response, or when the whole statement is tentative, this final Remoteness score is used. Holt's two examples from his manual, "He'll

---

4. Quite obviously, Tompkin's use of the term "distance" has different, that is, more adaptive, significance than Rapaport's use of the term. For this reason, the term "remoteness" is preferred, so as to avoid any confusion.

get well again—*unless* he dies of starvation" and "It might look like a vagina, if I stretched my imagination," reflect distancing that occurs through a conditional or tentative toning down of primary process material (Holt, 1970, p. 68).

Context

The context in which the response is presented may either effectively or ineffectively justify or "tone down" the primary process aspect of the response. Holt identified four kinds of contextual scoring categories which could either be scored plus (+) when a given context successfuly justifies the deviant elements, or minus (–) when the context is so inappropriate as to make the response worse than it would have been without an attempt at providing a context.

Finally, the context scores that follow may be given without either a + or a – if the context is viewed as somewhat forced and unconvincing but not inappropriate. (1) *Cx C.* Cultural Context. Primary process aspects of a response can be made more acceptable by couching them in the context of culture, ritual, mythology, folklore, an occupational or social role. (2) *Cx E.* Aesthetic Context. Reference to artistic context enables a subject to achieve distance from primitive aspects of a response. (3) *Cx I.* Intellectual Context. A scientific and technical backdrop may reflect the subject's efforts to intellectualize more highly charged issues. (4) *Cx H.* Humorous Context. Appropriate humor and fanciful elaboration may aid in the control or "taming" of primary process response material.

Postponing Strategies

Holt identified two types of postponing strategies, both of which had the effect of buffering the emergence of primary process material: (1) *Del.* Delay. Holt assumed that when primary process material emerged after some period of delay, there was an inhibitory process that was containing or modulating its expression. Del was scored when the first emergence of primary process material occurred in the inquiry (or as an additional response), with no mention of this in the original response. (2) *Blkg.* Blocking. When a subject struggles for at least two minutes protesting an inability to see anything and then gives a response containing scorable primary process material, a more primitive defensive effort has come into play.

Miscellaneous (Mostly Pathological) Defenses

Holt included a number of heterogeneous scores that reflected familiar defense mechanisms. A number of these were considered maladaptive and as such were assigned minus signs. Others were viewed as more adaptive. Holt drew upon Schafer's work (1954) to help identify relevant defensive processes that could be inferred from Rorschach responses. In addition to defenses such as negation, denial, rationalization, repudiation, minimization, and undoing, Holt included a number of other variants of defensive activity. (1) *Eu.* Euphemism. (2) *Vulg.* Vulgarity of Verbalization. Subjects use shocking and crude terms in an apparent effort to shock the listener for defensive purposes. (3) *Mod+.* Adaptive Modification of Response (toward secondary process). Reflective of the process of undoing, the subject begins by giving a response with scorable primary process material and then edits or modulates it so that it changes from Level 1 to level 2 or to a response that is not scorable for any level of primary process manifestation. (4) *Ratn.* Rationalization. Rationalization is scored when a subject delivers a response with either primary process content or formal qualities and then spontaneously adds more detail that he seems to hope will make the response more acceptable or plausible. (5) *Neg.* Negation. Holt described this as the conscious appearance of an idea with an immediate denial of its existence. Negation may also be scored when a subject attributes benign qualities to something threatening in an attempt to tame or detoxify it. (6) *Minz.* Minimization. Here threatening material (usually content) is allowed into consciousness but made more acceptable by either seeing it in tiny areas of the blot or by making it "small" and less threatening. (7) *Cphb-.* Counterphobic Defense. In the context of threatening content or images, the subject attempts to manage anxiety by belittling the response content or disparaging the threat as silly or amusing. Holt gave this score a minus sign (–) but allowed that responses demonstrating more adaptive counterphobic attempts to master anxiety may be scored without the minus sign. (8) *Self-D-.* Self-Deprecation. These subjects do not hesitate to give a response containing primitive material; however, they appear to take distance by criticizing themselves in inappropriate ways for giving such responses. (9) *Rep-.* Repudiation or Disavowal of a Response. The subject tries to rescind part or all of a response, either asking that it not be written down or by simply stating that he did not really mean to say whatever was considered to be objectionable. (10) *Va-.* Vagueness of Percept or Communication. After giving an objectionable response, the subject indicates that he did not really see it in the first place or can only barely make it out. (11) *Proj-.* Projection. Subjects may demonstrate projection either by externalizing responsibility for the response or by rejecting or devaluing the response, test, or examiner. (12) *Obs-.* Obsessional Defense. Obsessional defenses against primary process material may themselves become maladaptive when they reflect excessive doubting, hypercritical perfectionism, or ruminative vacillation. (13) *Iso-.* Isolation.

Decompensated manifestations of isolation occur when a subject expresses significant emotional detachment from the highly-charged response material or when he separates ideas or percepts that are normally connected or related. (14) *Eva-*. Evasiveness and Avoidance. These responses reflect the subject's attempts to avoid being pinned down or to commit to a response. (15) *Imp-*. Impotence. This score pertains to a subject's inability to explain a response when the examiner attempts to get clarification, usually during the inquiry. (16) *S*. Sequence. Subjects may defend by interspersing primary process responses with more neutral secondary process material. The individual may alternate between either a Level 1 or Level 2 response and an unscorable response or go from a Level 1 to a Level 2 response.

Overtness

Holt based this category on the distinction between potential and active expressons of primary process material. Primary process content can be expressed along a continuum of overtness from wishes and thoughts, to words, and to actions. The more a primary process impulse is expressed in the form of action, as opposed to thought, the more it is presumed to be overt, and less well defended. (1) *O-beh*. Overtness-Behavioral. When primary process material gets expressed through behavioral action of the characters in a response, overtness occurs on a behavioral level. (2) *O-vbl*. Overtness-Verbal. Verbal statements of desire, intention, or emotion that are attributed to characters in a response merit this score. For example, instead of saying "This guy is attacking this guy over here" (which would be scored *O-beh*), a subject might say "This guy says to the other guy "I'm going to attack you" (scored *O-vbl*). (3) *O-exp*. Overtness-Experiental. When primary process material is expressed as a wish, feeling, sensation, or fantasy, the level of overtness is further attenuated (for example, "hungry wolf" or "angry face"). (4) *O-pot*. Overtness-Potential. In this final level of overtness, the primary process material is expressed only as a potentiality. Movement might be expressed as static, potential, or about to happen (for example, "A giant getting ready to get me" or "Snipers about to shoot").

RATINGS OF THE TOTAL RESPONSE

In the 1970 draft of his scoring manual (Holt, 1970), Holt presented three rating scales that could be applied to each response. These included rating the form level of the response, the quality of combinations and integrations, and the level of creativity. Holt (1977) later indicated that scoring creativity and combinations/integrations was optional and not necessary to calculate the overall effectiveness of defensive capacity in containing primary process material. Holt used Mayman's multi-tiered scale (Mayman, 1964) for assessing form level and added quantitative ratings as follows:

FL. Form Level Scoring

Rating   Form Level

7	F+	Sharp and convincing form that can be seen easily.
6	Fo	Popular and near-popular.
5	Fw+	Reasonably plausible with some stretching.
4	Fw–	Bearing only slight resemblance to the blot.
2	Fs	On the way to an F+ or Fo but the subject spoils the response by introducing something that downgrades the acceptability of the form level.
1	F–	Arbitrary form with little or no resemblance.
5	Fv+	Vague forms that fit the blot well and nondefinite form that is combined with appropriate use of color or shading.
4	Fv	Vague form with no other determinant.
3	Fa	Amorphous responses in which form does not play any role (e.g., pure C, C', or Ch responses).

DD: Demand for Defense

Rating for Demand for Defense (DD) represents an elaboration of the Level 1 vs Level 2 distinction. The degree to which a response (the content or formal qualities) demands that some defensive or controlling provisions be made in order to make the response more socially acceptable is quantified under the heading of DD. At one extreme, blatant Level 1 content and frankly illogical thinking that is captured by some of the formal scores, place significant demands on the subject to explain away the primary process primitivity embedded in the response. At the other extreme are those responses that do not even merit a Level 2 content score and contain no deviations in formal reasoning or logic. Thus, each response is rated quantitatively on the degree of defense demand.

Holt recommended using the following 6-point DD rating scale for each response as a whole. (1) *No apparent need for defense*, including responses that indirectly contain aspects of primary process material that almost go unnoticed. (2) *Slight need for defense*, in which formal or content variables strike the listener as slightly unusual, or any response that contains both Level 2 content and formal scores is rated at this level. (3) *Moderate need for defense*, includes formal or content variables that might cause some tension or embarrassment in a social situation are rated at this level and any response that includes Level 1 content and Level 2 formal or Level 2 content and Level 1 formal variables would be scored at this DD level. (4) *Considerable need for defense*, for reference to sexual organs or any response combining Level 1 content and Level 1 formal aspects is always rated at this DD level. (5) *Great need for defense*, for ideas that are always inappropriate in social conversation (usually suggestive of psychosis because they imply impaired social judgement). (6) *Greatest need for defense*, for responses that depict the most extreme combinations of primitive content and psychotically impaired reasoning (e.g., contains both content and formal deviations rated at the previous highest rating).

DE: Defense Effectiveness

Holt also rated the effectiveness of defensive or controlling measures in each response that contained either primary process content or formal qualities. According to Holt (1977), Defense Effectiveness (DE) is rated along a multipoint scale, ranging from +2 to –3, by half-point increments. The positive values indicate adaptive regression and effective control, while the negative ratings indicate ineffective defenses and pathologically regressive shifts in functioning. Holt attempted to distinguish successfully defended responses from response creativity, which was rated on a separate scale.

In addition to numerical ratings, some responses are assigned the letter "a" to distinguish undefended responses, in which the subject makes no attempt to control or defend against the primary process material. If the response is, in most respects, successful, the lack of scorable defensive or control measures is not necessarily considered a liability. Mature individuals who are not threatened by primary process thoughts and images may not feel a need to defend against it.

ARS: Adaptive Regression Score

The Adaptive Regression Score (ARS) is the product of DD and DE, response by response, summed and divided by the number of primary process responses. The mean DD and DE can also be obtained by dividing the sum of DD and DE by the total number of primary process responses. Other useful indices include the percentage of responses that contain primary process material (percent total primary process); the percentage of responses containing primary process content (percent content) or the percentage containing formal indications of primary process (percent formal); percentage of responses at Level 1 or 2 (percent Level 1 or Level 2); and mean form level rating.

EMPIRICAL FOUNDATION OF HOLT'S PRIMARY PROCESS SYSTEM

Lerner and Lewandowski (1975) reviewed the characteristics and empirical underpinnings of Holt's scoring system. They evaluated the scoring system by reviewing various reliability and validity studies. Lerner and Lewandowski attempted to score protocols provided in Holt's manual to see the degree of concordance they could achieve with Holt. Scoring agreement was high for content but less so for formal scores. The reviewers concluded that scoring formal variables was possibly too complex, requiring too many variables to be kept in mind. As their familiarity with the system increased, however, the reviewers were able to improve the accuracy of their scoring in this area. Lerner and Lewandowski also found that the control and defense ratings were less difficult to score provided that the formal and content variables were initially scored accurately. Finally, the reviewers commented on the difficulties they encountered with Mayman's form level scoring. Specifically, they tended to overuse the Fs (spoil) category and to have problems distinguishing Fw+ from Fw- responses. Once again, however, they found that with increased practice and more comprehensive inquiries, they could make finer discriminations in form level ratings.

Lerner and Lewandoski reported Holt's own findings (Holt, 1966) that R (the total number of responses in the record) correlated positively with Level 2 libidinal and aggressive content categories for both a composite sample of 121 normal males and 81 schizophrenic patients. Holt presented correlations for his summary scores and R in his manual and found them to range between .25 and .78. Gray (1969) used Holt's scoring system with the Holtzman Ink Blot Test instead of the Rorschach in order to try to control for the effect of R. However, even with the number of responses controlled, verbal productivity was not, resulting in a correlation of .77 between verbal productivity and a primary process summary score.

In addition to Lerner and Lewandowski's review, Holt (1966, 1977) reviewed a number of studies that measured interrater reliabilities of different components of his primary process scoring system. Reliability studies have unearthed a common problem in evaluating complex rating scales such as Holt's primary process system. Although typically judges can reach an acceptably high level of concordance on summary scores, they do much more poorly when it comes to individual scoring categories or response by response measures of interrater reliability. Six studies (McMahon, 1964; Rabkin, 1967; Bachrach, 1968; Benfari and Calogeras, 1968; Russ, 1980) showed that the content variables, formal variables, and the mean DD (Defense Demand) were all higher than .80.

Mean DE (Defense Effectiveness) scores from these studies were more variable, ranging between .56 and .90. However, this spread is a bit misleading, because if one excludes the McMahon (1964) study, which yielded the reliability coefficient of .56, the average mean DE in the other five studies is .88.

Holt (1966) reported personality correlates of his content scores and found substantial construct validity for his libidinal and aggressive content scores. However, one surprising finding was the degree to which Level 1 Oral content was associated with personality resources, in particular feelings of adequacy and enthusiasm and an openness to taking in information. Level 2 Oral content was also associated with positive attributes such as cognitive competency and ego autonomy. Only the sum of Level 1 Aggressive content was associated with negative characteristics, which Holt referred to as pathological regression in thinking and behavior.

A large number of studies have contributed to the construct validity of the PRIPRO. Holt's system has been used in over 10 specific areas of investigation, establishing a relationship between adaptive regression and the thought processes of people who have undergone religious experiences (Maupin, 1965; Allison, 1962); the capacity for cognitive flexibility and coping with cognitive complexity (Von Holt et al., 1960; Blatt, Allison, and Feirstein, 1969; Murray and Russ, 1981); creativity and divergent thinking (Cohen, 1960; Pine and Holt, 1960; Russ, 1988; Russ and Grossman-McKee, 1990); the capacity to tolerate unrealistic experiences (Feirstein, 1967); emotional sensitivity and nonverbal communication (Weiss, 1971); empathic behavior in therapists (Bachrach, 1968); the ability to tolerate sensory deprivation (Goldberger, 1961; Wright and Abbey, 1965; Myers and Kushner, 1970) and teachers' ratings of coping abilities and achievement scores in second and third graders (Russ, 1980, 1981, 1982).

Interestingly, the majority of these diverse studies have demonstrated that the capacity to integrate primary process material in a controlled and adaptive manner is associated with an array of positive findings for males but not females. Male subjects who have controlled access to primary process thinking, as reflected by their Rorschach responses, seem able to deal more effectively with cognitive complexity, to shift problem-solving strategies flexibly, and to demonstrate divergent thinking, which in turn is positively associated with coping and anxiety management ratings.

It is not clear why these findings do not seem to apply to female subjects. Holt indicated that several researchers (Pine and Holt, 1960; Holt, 1970) have attempted to explain this finding that has been replicated in a number of controlled studies.

Silverman conducted a series of studies that employed the PRIPRO as a dependent variable in research examining the effects of experimental conditions on thinking (Silverman, 1965, 1966; Silverman and Goldweber, 1966; Silverman and Spiro, 1967; Silverman and Candell, 1970). These studies suggested that there is a significant increase in pathological and primitive thinking following the presentation of drive-related stimuli, especially when the subjects are psychotically organized and when the stimuli are of an aggressive as opposed to libidinal nature.

Silverman, Lapkin, and Rosenbaum (1962) studied adolescents with schizophrenia and indicated that the percentage of formal primary process manifestations (as opposed to content scores) was a primary indicator of psychosis and an effective measure of thought disorder. Zimet and Fine (1959) looked at the differences in quantity and quality of thought disorder between reactive and process schizophrenic individuals. As expected, they found that the process group exhibited more Level 1 and 2 scores than the reactive group. Finally one early study used the Holt System to demonstrate the positive effects of drug therapy on the treatment of schizophrenic patients (Saretsky, 1966).

Critique of the Holt System

In general, empirical support for the Holt system has been broad based and impressive. Studies over a 30-year period have demonstrated that various aspects of the system are reliable and valid measures, not just for disordered thinking per se, but for the degree to which primary process thinking is controlled and available for adaptive use, which itself has been shown to relate to a variety of cognitive and affective capacities. Thus, one can see that as a simple measure of thought disorder, the PRIPRO offers much more than a clinical index of pathological thinking.

As can be seen from this chapter, the Holt system offers one of the most comprehensive methods for assessing the quality of thought organization. Holt devoted much of his career to refining the system and completed at least 10 revisions of his scoring system. This fact alone may present some difficulties for researchers attempting to use his system. Although many of the changes he made in his scoring criteria were subtle, research teams using different vintage scoring manuals may encounter difficulties with reliable scoring.

Regarding the formal aspects of thought organization, Holt's effort to group his scores into three broad categories, consistent with Freud's theory of primary process thinking, was a creative and scholarly effort to advance and to empirically evaluate one aspect of psychoanalytic theory. However, with close to 40 separate scores, Holt's formal variables are nearly double the number of scores that Rapaport proposed. Although Holt must be credited with broadening the conceptual realm of thought disorder, his system is an enormously difficult one to learn and score. Furthermore, the introduction of new terminology for describing many of the formal aspects of primary process thinking, though consistent with Freudian concepts, may be intimidating to students of the Rorschach who are tasked with trying to keep straight an array of different terms for similar processes.

Holt's system is surely not an efficient method for the clinical assessment of disorganized thinking. However, Holt never intended for his system to be used as a clinical instrument but as an investigative tool to study the manifestations of adaptive and maladaptive regressive thinking and to contribute further to an understanding of the Freudian concepts of primary and secondary process thinking.

CHAPTER

5

THE THOUGHT DISORDER INDEX (TDI)

Recognizing the complexity and continuum nature of thought disorder phenomena, Johnston and Holzman (Johnston, 1975; Johnston and Holzman, 1979) developed the Thought Disorder Index (TDI) as a summary measure of pathological thinking. First introduced in 1975 as part of an unpublished doctoral dissertation, (Johnston, 1975), the TDI later formed the basis of a book entitled *Assessing Schizophrenic Thinking* (Johnston and Holzman, 1979), which presented empirical support for the reliability and validity of the TDI.

Taking Rapaport's deviant verbalization categories on the Rorschach as a starting point, Johnston and Holzman looked for a way to quantify the assessment of schizophrenic thought disorder. They found a suitable precedent for quantifying Rapaport's thought disorder categories in the Delta Index that was developed almost 25 years earlier by Watkins and Stauffacher (1952). Johnston and Holzman applauded the innovative work of their predecessors, who quantified Rapaport's scoring categories, but felt that the Delta Index was overly narrow in its scope and stated purpose (to differentiate schizophrenic from nonschizophrenic subjects).

The Delta Index consisted of 15 scoring categories, three of which were dropped by Johnston and Holzman because they were considered either too rare or too difficult to identify reliably or because the scoring category was not actually an indication of thought disorder (fabulized responses, deterioration color responses, and mangled or distorted concepts). To the 12 remaining scores of the Delta Index, Johnston and Holzman added eight other categories to capture a wider range of thought disorder phenomena encountered in verbal interactions with psychotic patients (inappropriate distance, word finding difficulty, clang, perseveration, incongruous combination, looseness, fluidity, and neologism). Unlike Watkins and Stauffacher, Johnston and Holzman used four, instead of three, weighted levels of severity (.25, .50, .75, and 1.0 as compared with .25, .50, and 1.0 used in the Delta Index). In 1986, Holzman and a group of colleagues at McLean Hospital (Solovay et al., 1986) further refined the scoring categories of the TDI, renaming some categories and adding three additional ones (flippant responses, playful confabulation, and fragmentation), bringing the total number of scoring categories to 23.

Initially, Johnston and Holzman used the TDI to assess thought disorder on verbal subtests of the WAIS in addition to the Rorschach, believing that the less structured subtests of the WAIS and the Rorschach would be equally likely to provide a context for eliciting disordered thinking. Eventually, Holzman and his colleagues (Solovay et al., 1986) concluded that the WAIS was not as rich a context for eliciting thought disorder as the Rorschach. Although most contemporary studies with the TDI use the Rorschach only, some researchers have scored deviant thinking using the WAIS-R and WISC-R (Armstrong, Silberg, and Parente, 1986; Harris, 1993; Skelton, Boik, and Madero, 1995).

TDI Scoring

Johnston and Holzman (1979) established reliability and validity for the TDI based on the Rapaport method of Rorschach administration, which requires the Inquiry to be conducted after each card. They limited the number of responses to five or six per card (after Card I, on which the subject was allowed to give as many responses as desired) and inquired about each Rorschach response and deviant verbalization. The Rorschach administration was tape recorded in order to provide a complete verbatim record of the subjects' verbalizations. The transcript was scored using the TDI by trained raters who were blind to group membership.

Johnston and Holzman (1979) recommended that multiple scores could be assigned to a single response. This recommendation was further clarified in the 1986 revision of the scoring manual, which specified that scorers should "tag" the category that best captures the pathological process most characteristic of the response. More than one category of thought disorder should be scored only when there are distinct and qualitatively discrete kinds of thought slippage within the same response.

For example, a response may contain an incongruous or fabulized combination, but if it is part of a confabulation, only the confabulation would be scored. If the subject also produced other types of thought disorder that are not part of the combinatory process, such as a peculiar verbalization, then the other processes are scored as well.

Because many of the scoring categories seemed to exist along a continuum of severity, Johnston and Holzman used Schafer's (1948; 1954) "tendency" designation for responses that did not quite reach scoring threshold. These "tendency" scores are weighted at a level just below the one containing the standard score. For example, a full confabulation is weighted at the .75 severity level, whereas a confabulation tendency would be given a .50 weighting. TDI categories in the mildest severity level (.25) are not scored at the tendency level.

Like the Delta Index, the mildest instances of thought disorder are given the lowest weight (.25); moderate instances receive intermediate weights (.50 or .75); and the most severe instances are given the highest weight (1.00). The total TDI score is derived by summing the product of each severity level and the number of thought disordered responses at that level, dividing by the number of Rorschach responses and multiplying by 100.

$$\frac{(Sum\ weighted\ scores)}{R} \times 100 = \text{Total TDI Score}$$

Many of the 23 scoring categories include subcategories that further refine the principal category. The authors emphasized the heuristic value of these subcategories, which were not meant to be scored separately. In fact Johnston and Holzman indicated that a number of these subcategories could not be reliably distinguished from one another. The 23 scoring categories, and subcategories, of the TDI are summarized.

.25 Level

The mildest severity level is reserved for minor instances of thought slippage that may go unnoticed in conversation. There is little interpretative significance attached to scores at this level, unless such instances are unusually frequent or malignant. Categories included in the .25 level are the most frequently scored examples of thought deviance in all subjects, including acutely psychotic individuals, and, as such, the most reliably scored categories.

1. *INAPPROPRIATE DISTANCE.* Based on Rapaport's concept of "distance" (Rapaport et al. 1968), this category includes five subscores that refer to the perceptual and ideational "distance" that separates a subject and the inkblots.

(a) "Loss or Increase of Distance." A subject may *lose distance* from Card I and say, "Oh God! That looks like a werewolf; I don't want to look at it because it scares the hell out of me!" Here, the inkblot loses its symbolic property and is taken as a literal depiction of something so threatening as to evoke an emotional response. Conversely, another subject may demonstrate an *increase of distance* on the same card and respond, "That looks like a werewolf. Wow! werewolves make me think of that creepy movie with all those people changing into creatures and going after people; it just gave me the creeps!" In this case, the subject's emotional reaction is triggered by increasingly distant and personalized associations to the original response. (b) "Excessive Qualification," based on Rapaport's "exactness verbalization" score, refers to those occasions in which the subject's rigid perfectionism intrudes into the response. The subject may appear troubled that the inkblot does not resemble perfectly the image he or she had in mind. (c) "Concreteness." Here again the inkblot is taken as a literal depiction of reality, as the subject fails to take the distance necessary to represent symbolically the inkblot. (d) "Overspecificity." Although there is a similarity to excessive qualification responses, the overspecificity response involves an arbitrary and irrelevant specification of details that ruins the response. According to the Holzman's research group (Coleman, personal communication, June 1992), these responses are rare and may approach the level of absurdity because the subject's attempt to be overly precise gives the response a bizarre quality. (e) "Syncretistic Response." Whereas overspecificity involves the inclusion of inappropriate detail, syncretistic responses tend to be inappropriately abstract and overinclusive.

2. *flippant responses.* Flippant responses were added to the scoring system in the 1986 revision to capture those instances in which the subject interjects inappropriately humorous, sexually tinged, or sarcastic remarks that reflect a lack of seriousness about the task.

3. *VAGUENESS.* According to the Holzman's group (Coleman and Levy, personal communication, June 1992), vague responses tend to be relatively rare. They are characterized by a poverty of expressed meaning in the response. Subjects who deliver vague responses have trouble elaborating any clear percept or may give a response without stating clearly what they are seeing.

4. *PECULIAR VERBALIZATIONS AND RESPONSES.* The revised TDI scoring manual describes three subtypes of peculiar responses/verbalizations, including:

(a) "Peculiar Expressions," characterized by odd combinations of words within a phrase resulting in redundant, contradictory, incongruous, or inappropriate verbal expression. Most listeners will hear the odd quality of these expressions, but will be able to comprehend what the subject is trying to convey. (b) "Stilted and Inappropriate Expression," including awkward, overly intellectualized, or pseudo-scientific terms or expressions that have a stilted and wooden quality. Again, the meaning may not be lost, but the phrasing is distracting. (c) "Inappropriate Word Usage" includes odd word substitutions or inappropriate metonymy.

5. *WORD-FINDING DIFFICULTY.* Subjects may merit this score, providing they give two wrong words first before finally producing the correct word or clearly stating that they know the word but are not able to think of it. To give this score, the examiner must be clear that the difficulty is not just due to simple lack of knowledge.

6. *CLANGS.* This comparatively rare scoring category, described previously in Holt's system, applies to responses in which the subject's verbalization is based on the sound rather than the meaning of the word.

7. *PERSEVERATION.* Overvalent ideas that linger across cards and compulsively intrude into consecutive responses reflect a perseverative process. To be scored, the same poor form quality response is given on at least three cards.

8. *INCONGRUOUS COMBINATIONS.* Johnston and Holzman incorporated four subtypes of Incongruous Combinations into the TDI. (a) "Composite Response," in which parts from two or more percepts are unrealistically combined to make a hybrid creature or object. (b) "Arbitrary Form-Color Response," scored when the subject does not seem to be aware of, or concerned by, the inappropriate combination of form and color. (c) "Inappropriate Activity Response," in which the condensation occurs between an object and an activity that is incongruously ascribed to it. (d) "External-Internal Responses," which were given a severity rating of .50 because they reflect a more extreme manifestation of strained reasoning.

.50 Level of Severity

Whereas responses scored at the .25 level may occur in the records of normal individuals (especially under conditions of stress, anxiety, or fatigue), responses at the .50 level convey increasingly odd thinking not typically found in nonpsychotic individuals. Eight scores are represented at this level of severity.

9. *RELATIONSHIP VERBALIZATION.* Relationship verbalizations occur rarely on the Rorschach (Coleman, personal communication, June 1992). In order to be scored the subject must make it clear that the new response is connected with a response given earlier.

10. *IDIOSYNCRATIC SYMBOLISM.* In the revised scoring manual, the criterion for scoring this category requires only that the subject delivers the idiosyncratic symbolization response with conviction and without awareness of its inappropriateness. Two subtypes are specified:

(a) "Color Symbolism" is scored only when color is interpreted symbolically in an odd or bizarre manner. (b) "Image Symbolism" is scored when concrete images or spatial details are treated as symbolic representations of abstract ideas in a strained and bizarre-sounding manner.

11. *QUEER RESPONSES.* Whereas peculiar verbalizations may be overlooked or go unnoticed in everyday speech, queer responses strike the listener as odd and difficult to comprehend. A useful rule of thumb for distinguishing between the two forms of deviant verbalization is that peculiar responses include real words that are used inappropriately or awkwardly, but convey meaning that the listener can grasp, whereas queer responses include real words whose meaning is unclear or made-up words whose meaning is clear. There are three subtypes of queer responses in the TDI:

(a) "Queer Expressions" are those in which the subject uses an extremely odd expression with a sense of certainty and conviction, but the listener does not know what the subject means. (b) "Queer Imagery" is scored when the image, as opposed to the verbal expression, is bizarre and hard to understand. Examples might include images such as "glorified rain," "the intestines of the tunnel," or "colorful numbers." The words are unremarkable by themselves; however, the image depicted makes little sense. (c) "Queer Word Misusage" involves more extreme versions of idiosyncratic word usage that leave the listener uncertain what the respondent means.

12. *CONFUSION.* Unlike other pathological forms of verbalization, the listener/scorer's confusion is not relevant for scoring Confusion responses. Instead, it is the subject who conveys confusion in his or her experience of the inkblot and/or what is seen.

13. *LOOSENESS.* Holt's formal category of Displacement included scores that pertained to degrees of associative looseness. Johnston and Holzman refined Holt's ideas and introduced the looseness category to describe a loss of cognitive focus, in which the subject's associations depart from the task at hand and become tangential or irrelevant.

14. *FABULIZED COMBINATION.* This well-known score represents unrealistic relationships that are attributed to two or more separate objects on the basis of spatial contiguity.

15. *PLAYFUL CONFABULATION.* A less severe variant of confabulation responses, playful confabulations have a whimsical or fanciful quality. The percepts show good form quality, but they are embellished in a playful and humorous way that reflects greater control over the ideational process than occurs in a confabulation.

16. *FRAGMENTATION.* Organizational and integrative failures occur rarely but may be found in the records of patients with right cortical damage (Kestenbaum-Daniels et al., 1988). Fragmentation may occur when a subject is unable to verbalize spontaneously an integration of several details into a coherent perceptual whole. For example, a subject might say to Card III, "I see legs here, and these could be arms, I guess; maybe feet or shoes at the bottom" without being able to integrate these disparate parts into a whole object, in this case a human figure.

.75 Level of Severity

Scores at this level reflect clear disturbances in thinking that usually reflect a psychotic experience. Wild combinatory thinking, unstable and absurd ideas, and severely strained logic are characteristic of the four response categories at the .75 level.

17. *FLUIDITY.* Fluid responses are rare scores that may be viewed as the perceptual counterpart of associative looseness. Fluidity is scored when the subject indicates that one percept is changing into something else. Additionally, an inability to remember or locate a previously described percept may be scored fluid because it appears that the percept has disappeared and cannot be found again.

18. *ABSURD RESPONSES.* By definition, absurd responses are necessarily scored at a minus form level and reflect psychotic experience. The absurd response may not sound bizarre in content or syntax, but essentially it has no discernible objective support in the inkblot, even though it is quite specific.

19. *CONFABULATION.* Johnston and Holzman retained Rapaport's term, "confabulation," to depict responses that demonstrated excessive distance from the task primarily through extravagant embellishment. Both the DW response and the overembellished response are included in the TDI. Johnston and Holzman distinguish between a full confabulation (.75) from a confabulation-tendency (.50) response on the basis of how

extreme is the associative elaboration, and the extent to which the response had any grounding in the inkblot.

20. *AUTISTIC LOGIC.* The score, Autistic Logic, requires an explicit statement of illogical reasoning, often signaled by expressions such as "because" or "it must be."

1.0 Level of Severity

Rarest of all responses, some researchers have found 1.0 level responses to occur in less than three percent of Rorschach records (Koistinen, 1995). Although there are only three scores at this level, each can be taken to be almost pathognomic of severe psychosis.

21. *CONTAMINATION.* Found in all scoring systems since Rorschach (1921), contamination is scored when at least two distinct percepts are merged into a single, bizarre-sounding response.[1]

22. *INCOHERENCE.* Taken from Rapaport's original list, the incoherent response is impossible for the listener to comprehend and may even be considered to be unrelated to the task. These responses have a "word salad" quality.

23. *NEOLOGISMS* refer to newly coined words that may be the result of verbal condensation. To be scored, it must be clear that the subject lacks the critical capacity to observe the inappropriateness of the invented word. These scorable neologisms constrast with the kind of creative word-play that one finds in the "night language" of James Joyce, where purposefulness, control, and clever, subtle meaning distinguish such efforts from those reflecting a psychotic process. (The subject of creativity versus psychosis is explored further in chapter 17.)

RELIABILITY STUDIES

Johnston and Holzman (1979) based their interrater reliability data on the ratings of two independent scorers, who achieved agreement on Total TDI scores based on the Rorschach Pearson r's of .82 (controls),

---

1. The contamination response will be discussed in greater detail in chapter 11. Here, however, it is interesting to note that not all "contaminated" responses are necessarily bizarre and pathognomic of psychosis. Some have clear meaning and are examples of well-known commercial figures or products (e.g., "spider-man" or "war-bird"), while others may reflect the creative process of "Janusian thinking" (see chapter 17).

.87 (relatives of patients), .90 (schizophrenic patients), and .93 (nonpsychotic patients). Interrater reliability was slightly lower for TDI scores based on data from the WAIS. Spearman-Brown correlation of internal reliability or consistency of TDI scoring on the Rorschach was .78 (p < .001). Correlations between TDI scores based on the Rorschach and WAIS were considerably lower (ranging from .13 for controls to .51 for schizophrenic patients [p < .001]), leading researchers to conclude that the tests are not equally sensitive to eliciting thought disorder. The greater sensitivity of the Rorschach to the broad range of disordered thinking also makes it a more efficient context for evaluating cognitive slippage.

Using only TDI scores based on the Rorschach, Solovay et al. (1987) conducted a comparative study of thought disorder using the TDI and reported two-scorer interrater reliabilities of .89 for Total TDI score (with a Spearman-Brown correction); .81 for individual scoring categories; .79 for levels of severity; and coefficients ranging from.84 to .89 for factor structure scores (for four factor groupings).

Four teams of raters from the McLean Psychology Research Laboratory and Hillside Hospital (Coleman et al., 1993) conducted a comprehensive interrater reliability study on a variety of features of TDI scoring including total TDI score, severity levels, and qualitative factors. The intraclass correlation among the four teams for Total TDI scores was .74, and the Spearman rank correlations between the different rating teams ranged from .80 to .90 (p < .01). In comparing ratings across different severity levels, intraclass correlations ranged from .72 for the .25 level to .77 for both the .50 and .75 levels (scores at the 1.0 level of severity were too rare to be assessed). Reliability between different rating teams yielded Spearman coefficients ranging from .86 to .93 for .25 level scores (p < .01); .50 to .75 for .50 level scores (p < .02 or p < .01); and .50 to 1.0 for .75 level scores (p < .02 or p < .01).

Using factor groupings of TDI categories (Shenton et al., 1987), Coleman et al. (1993) reported that rating teams achieved average intraclass correlations of .86 on the "Irrelevant Intrusions" factor; .76 on the "Combinatory Thinking" factor; and .58 on the "Idiosyncratic Verbalizations" factor. All comparisons of the rating teams yielded correlations at the .02 or .01 level of significance.

In comparing the mean total TDI derived by each team, Coleman et al. found there to be different thresholds between teams in "tagging" thought disorder. Teams generally agreed about whether a record was thought disordered and about the ranking of the amount of thought disorder in a record relative to other records, but absolute scores for the total amount of thought disorder in any one record may differ across raters.

Other reliability findings are worth noting. Arboleda and Holzman (1985) demonstrated adequate interrater reliabilities between two teams' scores for the Total TDI score for severity levels in a sample of children and adolescents. Carpenter et al. (1993) studied interrater reliabilities between four- and 10-card Rorschach protocols and found highly significant correlations, suggesting that the four-card forms yield highly adequate composite indexes of total TDI, severity levels, and serve to identify more frequently occurring qualitative scores. Finally, in a large Finnish study (N = 583), Koistinen (1995) found statistically significant interrater reliabilities between two teams of raters, each scoring 59 Rorschachs, quite similar to those found in previous studies by the McLean research group.

Validation Studies

Social Class and Culture

Johnston and Holzman found that Total TDI scores were not related to the sex, ethnicity, or socioeconomic status of the subjects. It is not surprising, however, that they found that TDI scores based on responses to verbal subtests of the WAIS were negatively correlated with IQ. In a separate study, Haimo and Holzman (1979) found that the TDI was a valid measure for assessing disordered thinking, distinguishing it from subcultural language patterns, in nonwhites from lower socioeconomic groups. Total TDI scores accurately differentiated schizophrenic patients and parents of schizophrenic patients from normal controls in both Black and Caucasian subjects.

Thought Disorder in Nonpsychotic Relatives of Psychotic Patients

Johnston and Holzman (1979) demonstrated that the parents of schizophrenic patients have higher Total TDI scores than normal controls, suggesting that familial and genetic factors may play a role in the transmission of disordered thinking. Holzman and colleagues used the TDI specifically (Shenton et al., 1989) and examined TDI scores in first-degree relatives of a broad range of psychotic patients. They found that schizophrenic, manic, and schizoaffective patients with high TDI scores tended to have first-degree relatives with high scores as well, and that the quality of the thought disorder was similar in both patients and their relatives. Studying thought disorder in children, Arboleda and Holzman (1979) found equally high TDI scores among nonpsychotic, nonhospitalized children with psychotic mothers (deemed high-risk children) and hospitalized psychotic children.

Normative Data and the TDI

A number of researchers have attempted to establish cutoff scores on the TDI that would correctly identify psychotic individuals. Edell (1987) found that a cutoff of 9.0 discriminated between normal controls and psychiatric patients, but that this cutoff incorrectly identified 25% of the normals as psychiatric patients. Koistinen (1995) set out to establish a cutoff point that would discriminate healthy subjects from psychiatric patients; however, he also was unable to achieve such a cutoff point. Thus far, efforts to establish cutoff points have not been terribly useful because the sensitivity and specificity of these cutoffs have yielded unacceptably high false negatives and false positives.[2]

Johnston and Holzman (1979) reported that their normal control group had a mean Total TDI score of 4.46. A later sample of normal controls had a mean TDI total of 5.9 (Holzman et al., 1986). Among Edell's (1987) normal controls, the average TDI score was 6.1. In a large sample of Finnish subjects, Koistinen (1995) found a higher mean TDI of 11.7 in healthy subjects but concluded that his group of normal controls was more heterogeneous and did not screen out subjects with minor cognitive deficits or psychopathology.

Arboleda and Holzman (1979) established norms for a sample of 79 normal children and found that the mean TDI scores decreased with age. They found that children aged 5 to 6 (n = 16) had a Total TDI mean of 9.30; children 8 to 10 (n = 23) a mean of 9.42; 11– to 13-year-olds (n = 22) a mean of 7.78; and that 14– to 16-year-olds (n = 18) had mean TDI scores of 5.34.

Several of the Holzman research group have established a rough hierarchy of severity for different TDI totals (Coleman and Levy, personal communication, June 1992). Scores of 0 to 10 suggest low thought disorder; 11 to 16, mild thought disorder; 17 to 22, moderate; and 22+, severe levels of thought disorder.

Factor Structure of the TDI

In order to study the qualitative features of various forms of thought disorder, Holzman and colleagues looked at four sets of TDI factors that were derived by different statistical methods (Holzman et al., 1986;

---

2. I am grateful to Dr. Deborah Levy for reminding me that all cutoffs must take into account the scoring thresholds of a particular group of scorers. The cutoff that maximizes sensitivity and specificity has to be empirically determined by each group and is transferable to the extent that other groups share a similar scoring threshold.

Shenton et al., 1987; Solovay et al., 1987). The group began with an a priori grouping based on combining conceptually meaningful TDI categories into four dimensions or factors. This a priori classification, based on Johnston and Holzman (1979), is presented in Table 5-1. The four conceptually-based a priori factors included (1) Associative Thinking, (2) Combinatory Thinking, (3) Disorganization, and (4) Deviant Verbalizations.

Using a principal-components analysis with a variance maximization rotation, the research group derived a second set of factors using 97 psychotic patients. Six conceptually meaningful factors emerged from this analysis, each with eigenvalues greater than 1.0. These factors were named Combinatory Thinking, Idiosyncratic Verbalization, Autistic Thinking, Fluid Thinking, Absurdity, and Confusion. Holzman and his colleagues referred to this classification as the "empiric factors," which are presented in Table 5-2.

A third classification, referred to as post hoc factors, was derived from the TDI categories that best differentiated manic from schizophrenic patients. The post hoc factors, presented in Table 5-3, were called Irrelevant Intrusions, Combinatory Thinking, Fluid Thinking, Confusion, and Idiosyncratic Verbalizations.

The fourth set of factors was derived from the four severity levels of the TDI, with eight scores at the .25 level; seven at the .50 level; five at the .75 level; and three at the 1.0 level.

Differential Diagnosis of Thought Disorder

Johnston and Holzman found that both schizophrenic and manic psychotic patients obtained the highest Total TDI scores. Essentially, manic and schizophrenic patients did not differ in the absolute amount of thought disorder, but chronic deteriorated schizophrenic patients tended to have higher Total TDI scores than any of the other nonschizophrenic psychotic patients. Although Johnston and Holzman suspected that there were qualitative differences between different diagnostic groups, their original research did not present empirical data to buttress this speculation.

Such data came about half a decade later in the studies by Holzman and colleagues (Shenton et al., 1987; Solovay et al., 1987). Using a large and carefully diagnosed sample of 107 subjects (43 schizophrenic patients, 20 manic patients, 22 schizoaffective patients, and 22 normal subjects), the research team studied TDI features of the different diagnostic groups using the factor analytic methods described above. Table 5-4 shows the mean Total TDI scores for the patient groups and normal controls.

Table 5-1 A Priori Classification of TDI Categories

Factor	Severity Level			
	.25	.50	.75	1.0
ASSOCIATIVE	Inappropriate Distance Flippant Clang Perseveration	Relationship Verbalization Looseness	Fluidity	
COMBINATORY	Incongruous Combination	Fabulized Combination Playful Confabulations Idiosyncratic Symbolism	Confabulation Autistic Logic	Contamination
DISORGANIZATION	Vagueness Word-Finding Difficulty	Confusion Fragmentation		Incoherence
IDIOSYNCRATIC VERBALIZATIONS	Peculiar	Queer	Absurd	Neologism

From Holzman, Shenton, and Solovay, 1986.

Table 5-2 Principal Component ("Empiric") Classification of TDI Categories

Factor	Categories (Loading)	Eigenvalue
COMBINATORY THINKING	Playful Confabulation (.83)	2.11
	Incongruous Combination (.60)	
	Flippant (.58)	
	Fabulized Combination (.53)	
IDIOSYNCRATIC VERBALIZATION	Peculiar Responses (.83)	4.06
	Queer (.69)	
AUTISTIC VERBALIZATION	Autistic Logic (.79)	2.04
	Incoherence (.72)	
FLUID THINKING	Fluidity (.71)	1.53
	Contamination (.69)	
ABSURDITY	Neologism (.86)	1.24
	Absurd (.49)	
CONFUSION	Vagueness (.76)	1.18
	Confusion (.76)	

From Holzman, Shenton, and Solovay, 1986.

The four "factor structures" were statistically evaluated to determine which factors distinguished various groups. Discriminant function analyses were used to assess how well each set of factors was able to classify subjects as schizophrenic, manic, or schizoaffective. All factor sets successfully classified patients above chance expectation (33.3%). The post hoc factors best discriminated the three groups, correctly classifying 57.7% of the patients. When only schizophrenic and manic patients were compared, the post hoc discriminant function analysis correctly classified 82.2% of the schizophrenics and 70.7% of the manics, or a total of 76.5% of all patients. Thus, Holzman and his group concluded that the TDI is a sensitive instrument that can identify qualitative differences in thought disorder among three of the most common diagnostic groups of psychotic patients.

Various researchers have used the TDI to investigate disordered thinking among borderline and schizotypal individuals (Edell, 1987; Harris, 1993; Coleman et al., 1996) and have found elevated Total TDI scores among these groups (see chapter 15). In perhaps the most ambi-

Table 5-3 Post Hoc Classification of TDI Categories

Factor	Categories
COMBINATORY THINKING	Playful Confabulation Incongruous Combination Fabulized Combination
IRRELEVANT INTRUSIONS	Flippant Looseness
FLUID THINKING VERBALIZATION	Relationship Verbalization Fluidity Contamination
CONFUSION	Word-Finding Difficulty Confusion Absurd Responses Incoherence Neologism
IDIOSYNCRATIC VERBALIZATION	Peculiar Verbalization

From Holzman, Shenton, and Solovay, 1986.

tious study, Koistinen (1995) examined thought disorder features among a large group of subjects from a Finnish family adoption study. Koistinen compared TDI results among patients with schizophrenia, schizophrenic spectrum disorders, affective disorders, nonspectrum personality disorders, neurotic disorders, and no psychiatric disorders and concluded that the quantity and quality of Rorschach TDI scores predicted levels of psychopathology along a continuum.

TDI and Medication Effects

Two studies have addressed the impact of neuroleptic medication on TDI scores in psychotic patients (Hurt, Holzman, and Davis, 1983; Spohn et al., 1986). Hurt et al. demonstrated that within as few as 3 days after the initiation of treatment with haloperidol, Total TDI scores and the Brief Psychiatric Rating Scale (BPRS) decrease significantly for schizophrenic patients. Spohn's group used the TDI to assess thought disorder in medicated schizophrenic, schizoaffective, and bipolar patients and normal controls. One group of subjects was withdrawn from neuroleptics and placed on a placebo for a 10-week period, while

Table 5-4 Mean TDI Scores for Diagnostic Groups and Normal Controls

Group	N	Mean	(SD)
Schizophrenic	43	34.6	(38.8)
State Hospital	16	37.8	(33.0)
Private Hospital	27	32.6	(42.3)
Manic	20	35.0	(16.2)
Schizoaffective	22	22.8	(21.4)
Manic	12	31.0	(25.6)
Depressed	10	13.0	(8.6)
Normals	22	5.9	(4.5)

From Holzman, Shenton, and Solovay, 1986.

the other group continued taking its prescribed neuroleptic over the same time period. The major finding of their study was that antipsychotic medication reduced the frequency of the severe categories of thought disorder (those scored at the .75 and 1.0 levels of severity), while milder levels of thought pathology (e.g., scores at the .25 level) persisted independent of clinical remission. This finding supported the conclusion that antipsychotic medications treat floridly psychotic, or state-related, manifestations of schizophrenia but do little to affect thought disorder that is trait-related, that which is associated with the syndrome but not its exacerbation. Finally, working with a sample of adolescent-onset schizophrenic patients, Makowski and colleagues found that recent exposure to neuroleptic drugs did not mask the sensitivity of the TDI in discriminating among different diagnostic groups and between psychotic patients and controls (Makowski et al., 1997). More important, the same kinds of thought disorder found in adult-onset schizophrenic patients were found to occur in early adolescent-onset patients with schizophrenia.

CRITIQUE OF THE TDI

Developed roughly 20 years ago, the TDI has become recognized as a robust clinical and research tool for assessing and quantifying varieties of disordered thinking. Despite its empirical sturdiness and increasing utility as a clinical diagnostic instrument, a number of potential difficulties have been identified. One difficulty concerns the manner in which scores are assigned to different levels of severity. The basis of assignment was not empirically founded and is not always conceptually clear. Wahlberg (1994) agreed with Holzman's (1978) earlier comment that the TDI may construct an artificial continuum of thought disorder by assuming a linear relationship between certain scores at different levels of severity. Athey, Colson, and Kleiger (1993) suggested that the distinctions between the levels of severity themselves are not always consistent with the nature of the different scores contained within each level. Each level assumes a measure of homogeneity of severity for all scores within that level, which may not always be the case. For example, a severe, incongruous combination, such as "a bat with landing gears" would be weighted the same as a mild peculiar verbalization, such as "that looks like a hornlike construction on its head." Because the TDI does not recognize varying levels of severity within a particular scoring category (with the exception of noting when there is a tendency to a certain score), both responses would receive a score of .25. However, most people would agree that the first sounds qualitatively more bizarre.

Other researchers have questioned whether each of the individual categories of thought disorder scores exists as a unitary entity or should include a severity continuum. As indicated above, by placing all examples of a particular scoring category within the same severity level, an assumption is made as to the unitary nature of these responses. In other words, the TDI assumes that all incongruous combinations are of equal severity; that all fabulized combinations are of .50 and all contaminations are of 1.0 level of severity. It is reasonable to consider the possibility that some types of incongruous combinations are more common in normal records (i.e., playful popular incongruous combinations), while others have a more malignant quality and are found primarily in the records of psychotic patients.

Other researchers have argued for a different weighting of several items on the scale (Wahlberg, 1994; Koistinen, 1995). Wahlberg suggested that a more suitable weighting for incongruous combinations would be .50 because of its basic similarity for the fabulized combination response. Blatt, Tuber, and Auerbach (1990) extended this point when they argued that an incongruous combination is a more severe manifestation of disordered thinking than a fabulized combination and should be considered more like a contamination tendency. However, it seems that this is more of an empirical question which may be answered, in part, by examining the frequency with which these responses occur in nonpsychotic and normal records. We know from Johnston and Holzman's original study that incongruous combinations occur more frequently in the records of normal and nonpsychotic subjects than do either fabulized combinations and contaminations.

Likewise, Exner (1991) found that incongruous combinations (INCOMs) occurred more frequently in the records of 700 nonpatient adults than did fabulized combinations (FABCOM's). These findings suggest that most incongruous combinations are a less serious manifestation of disordered thinking than fabulized combinations and that the lower severity level assigned to them may, indeed, be appropriate.

Koistinen (1995) also raised questions about the weighting of individual items on the TDI. He presented empirical data to support his contention that perseveration responses should receive a higher weighting by showing that subjects with schizophrenia-spectrum disorders had the highest scores on the perseveration item. In concluding that perseveration is a typical score of subjects with schizophrenia (and of high-risk adoptees with schizophrenic mothers), Koistinen suggested that perseveration scores should be given a weighting of .75.[3]

The TDI (and nearly all Rorschach thought disorder scoring systems, for that matter) lacks anything like Holt's detailed effort to operationalize control and defense variables. Thus, the TDI offers no method of systematically evaluating either the subject's conscious or latent awareness that the material contained in the response is inappropriate, or his or her efforts to modulate the way it is expressed and communicated to the examiner. By not doing so, the scope of the TDI is limited to measuring a single component of ego impairment, the absolute presence, quantity, and type of thought disorder, while giving little systematic consideration to concomitant ego resources and controls, which may modulate the negative impact of the absolute elevation of a given TDI score. In fairness to the developers, however, their task was, by design, more limited in scope than that of Holt. Their intention was not to devise a comprehensive system for studying the conceptual nature of primary and secondary process thinking, but to develop a reliable and valid measure of thought disorder. Nonetheless, it is possible that applying something like Holt's Defense Effectiveness (DE) rating scale to TDI protocols would help to identify important differences in adaptive and pathological regression in subjects with similarly high TDI scores.

---

3. Debbie Levy (personal communication, December 1997) questioned Koistinen's recommendation on two counts. First, because perseveration is a relatively rare score, there is some question of whether these responses were scored correctly. Secondly, even if they were scored correctly and were found to occur frequently among schizophrenic subjects, this is not a valid reason to increase the weighting. Peculiar responses are the most frequent TDI score in schizophrenic Rorschachs, but that is not sufficient grounds for increasing the weighting of this score which is found in a wide range of non-schizophrenic records as well.

Aside from the considerations described above, what can be said about the empirical basis and utility of the TDI? Clearly, the TDI rests on a solid empirical foundation. It has repeatedly been demonstrated to be a psychometrically sound instrument that has contributed mightily to the understanding of thought disorder and to the nature of psychotic syndromes, schizophrenia in particular. Like the Holt system, the TDI was constructed as a research instrument and applied in clinical settings only later. Although less intricate and easier to learn than the Holt system, potential users must invest significant time in mastering the scoring, which can be difficult and time-consuming. Holzman's group recommends learning the system directly from members of its research team and calibrating one's scoring threshold to this group. Although interrater reliability has been shown to be high, raters may be discouraged to find that their reliability for rating individual responses tends to be much lower than their rating for levels of severity or the total TDI score. Some researchers, finding the scoring system cumbersome and time consuming, have opted for interview techniques or global clinical rating scales like the BPRS to assess thought disorder (Andreasen, 1979a,b; Harrow and Quinlan, 1985; Marengo et al., 1986).

As a clinical instrument, the TDI shows promise as a focal diagnostic tool to help clinicians discriminate among different types of psychotic disorders. At Mclean Hospital, clinicians often request a "TDI" on their patients in order to make a differential diagnosis before instituting pharmacological treatment. In some cases, four-card Rorschach sets are used to answer differential diagnostic questions. The validity of this modification rests on empirical findings that demonstrated high correlations between TDI features of 10- and four-card sets of Rorschach cards (Carpenter et al., 1993).

In summary, the TDI is an empirically sound instrument that recognizes the complexity of thought disorder. It has been used in a wide variety of studies that have contributed to the construct validity of thought disorder and has also advanced the knowledge base of schizophrenia. One might hope to see further revisions of the scoring manual, as researchers continue to evaluate the weights assigned to different categories and to drop other categories that occur infrequently and are less reliably scored. Whatever the case may be, the TDI has become the "gold standard" for Rorschach-based thought disorder scoring systems.

CHAPTER

6

EXNER'S SPECIAL SCORES AND SCHIZOPHRENIA INDEX (SCZI)

By synthesizing the most reliable and valid variables from existing Rorschach systems, Exner (1974, 1978, 1986a, 1990, 1993; Exner and Weiner, 1982, 1995) successfully addressed previous criticism that had questioned whether the Rorschach was a psychometrically sound and clinically valid instrument (Buros, 1965). No higher praise for Exner's contributions to the survivability of the Rorschach could have been given than that which was offered by Margarite Hertz, the grand dame of Rorschach testing herself, who stated that Exner and his colleagues had "brought discipline into our ranks and a sense of optimism to our field" (Hertz, 1986, p. 405).

It may seem surprising that Exner's initial effort to construct a comprehensive Rorschach system (1974) omitted any formal scoring for thought disordered responses. Although he referenced the scoring systems of Rapaport and Holt, Exner questioned whether many of these scores could be reliably coded and supported by the empirical literature. Reliability of scoring was, after all, one of Exner's most significant concerns about the Rorschach. Thus, at the time he published his first text on the Comprehensive System (1974), Exner concluded that thought disorder scores generally lacked clarity in definition and were too unreliable to score in a system that prized itself with psychometric precision. At the same time, however, he maintained that unusual verbalizations could be interpretively significant. Despite his decision to exclude formal thought disorder categories from his original Comprehensive

System, he included several "Fabcomb" and "Incomb" scores in one of the sample protocols in his case examples (Exner, 1974).

It was not long before Exner began a serious study of thought disorder scoring, seeking ways to incorporate reliable and valid "special scores" into his Comprehensive System. Shortly after the publication of his introductory text (1974), Exner, Weiner, and Schuyler (1976) began to develop scoring criteria for thought disorder scores that would allow for acceptable levels of interrater reliability and empirical validity. Exner was heavily influenced by Weiner who had 10 years earlier written extensively about the Rorschach characteristics of disordered thinking (Weiner, 1966). Exner and his colleagues eventually developed two broad categories of special scoring in the Comprehensive System: Perseverations and Unusual Verbalizations. Later Exner (1986) labeled these two broad realms of Special Scores (1) Unusual Verbalizations and (2) Perseveration and Integration Failure.

Unusual Verbalizations

Exner et al. (1976) initially described three categories of Unusual Verbalizations: Deviant Verbalizations, Inappropriate Combinations, and Inappropriate Logic. They felt that these scores were not specific to any particular diagnosis and that, while often found in the records of schizophrenic patients, they could occur in the records of nonschizophrenic and normal subjects as well. Exner and his colleagues also noted that these scores might be more common in younger children and that they shouldn't necessarily be taken as indications of psychopathology across the developmental spectrum. Eventually, Exner elaborated these three categories of Unusual Verbalizations into six critical Special Scores. Each is described below.

Deviant Verbalizations

DEVIANT VERBALIZATIONS (DVs). DVs were said to be characterized by "distorted language usage or idiosyncratic modes of expression that impede the subject's ability to communicate clearly" (Exner et al., 1976, p. 47). The group included two fairly broad and nonspecific subtypes of DV responses that subsumed Rapaport's categories of peculiar and queer verbalizations and the neologisms of the TDI. Exner et al. initially used the terms "queer" and "peculiar" in describing these two subtypes of DV responses; however, they defined these terms somewhat differently than did Rapaport and seemed to obscure the distinction.

In defining their first subtype of DV, which they loosely referred to as the "queer response," both Exner et al. (1976) and Weiner (1966) before him relied on Holt's statement that queer verbalizations result from a failure to maintain an appropriate set in talking about the subject matter at hand. Their example of such a response, "A crab *but I was hoping for an octopus*," depicts this odd type of loss of focus, in which the patient interjects an irrelevant phrase which clearly detracts from the original subject.

Their second form of DV was characterized by odd use of language that is not explained on the basis of subcultural idioms. Exner et al. referred to these as "peculiar" responses, which are distinguished by their stilted or redundant quality. Although some of these words or expressions may be appropriate in the context of the Rorschach test, they almost always strike the listener as odd. Exner and colleagues went on to list neologisms as a common manifestation of the peculiar DV.

In his 1978 text, Exner attempted to refine and elaborate upon his distinctions between the subtypes of DVs. He dropped the somewhat confusing use of the terms "peculiar" and "queer" in distinguishing the different forms of DV responses and presented four overlapping subtypes of DV as follows:

(1) An "inappropriate commentary" DV, in which the subject interjects a highly personalized association as an afterthought. An example of this would be the response, "A crab, *but I was hoping to see an octopus.*"

(2) The "loss of appropriate set" DV, in which the subject loses focus in describing the object that he/she perceives. Exner's example of this form of DV was "A monster *that no one has ever seen*" (Exner, 1978, p. 22).

(3) The "odd use of language" DV, in which the subject responds in a stilted or redundant manner, as in the response, "A slide of *microscopic aspects of some organism*" (stilted response) or "A *male penis*" (redundant response).

(4) The "neologistic" DV, in which the subject uses an incorrect word in place of a correct word.

Exner (1986a) eventually streamlined the DV category to eliminate the overlap and unclarity of his earlier attempts to delineate subtypes. He did away with the "inappropriate commentary" and "loss of appropriate set" DVs (which he placed in a new category, the Deviant Response, or DR) and ended up with two clear-cut, albeit comparatively narrow, subtypes of DV: neologisms and redundancy responses.

DEVIANT RESPONSES (DRs). Exner introduced the Deviant Response in 1986 (Exner, 1986a) to describe answers that have "a strange and peculiar quality" manifested in one of two ways:

1. "Inappropriate phrases" were originally subsumed under the DV category as "queer" responses and later as "inappropriate commentary" DVs. They include irrelevant or personalized interjections such as the familiar, "A crab, but *I was hoping for an octopus*" and a host of other examples as well. This subtype of DR also includes what Exner had previously referred to as "loss of appropriate set" DVs, typified by his above mentioned example, "A monster *that no one has ever seen.*"

2. "Circumstantial responses." Exner added this new subtype of deviant verbalization to capture those responses that were fluid, rambling, vague, or inappropriately elaborative. Exner gave numerous examples of circumstantial DRs that were all characterized by a tendency for the subject to wander off target into some overly personalized, excessively detailed, or inappropriately elaborative verbalization that had little to do with the inkblot or initial response. The subject may deviate from his or her original focus without ever returning to the point. The language that the subject uses may not be bizarre by itself. It is, instead, the process of wandering off track that distinguishes this subtype of DR.

Exner and Weiner (1995) subsequently elaborated on the definition of the Deviant Response. Exner and Weiner invoked Rapaport's concept of "increased distance" by emphasizing the rambling and disjointed nature of DRs in which the subject loosely associates to her or his initial response and ends up taking excessive distance from the inkblot. They also referred to inappropriate phrase DRs as "queer responses," again attempting to link this category to Rapaport's concept of queer verbalizations.

Exner and Weiner added a third subtype of DR to include those responses characterized by the subject's vagueness in responding to the examiner's questions. They noted that this type of deviant verbalization results in a discontinuity or communication breakdown between the examiner's questions and the subject's answers. The following exchange is an example of this confusing communication process:

Subject: I see a lady here.
Examiner: (Inquiry) You said, "I see a lady here."
Subject: Yes, right here.
Examiner: I'm not sure where you're seeing it.
Subject: She's up a tree actually, actually it's a woman.
Examiner: A woman?
Subject: Actually she looks like a witch, here's her broomstick.
Examiner: Could you show me the parts you're describing?
Subject: What is it you'd like to know about it? [pp. 137–138].

Exner indicated that some DR answers would simultaneously contain a DV; but he cautioned that when this occurs, only the DR is scored.

Exner did not say any more about these cases or explain what he had in mind by offering examples of such responses.

Inappropriate Combinations

Exner et al. (1976) introduced the term "Inappropriate Combinations" to depict a category of cognitive slippage that Weiner (1966) referred to as "combinative thinking." Following Weiner's lead, Exner and his colleagues listed three types of Inappropriate Combinations: (1) Incongruous Combinations (INCOMs), (2) Fabulized Combinations (FABCOMs), and (3) Contaminations (CONTAMs).

INCONGRUOUS COMBINATIONS (INCOMs). The INCOM Response in the Comprehensive System includes some scores from Holt's Condensation category and overlaps considerably with the Incongruous Combination score in the TDI. Exner remained consistent with these other systems by defining INCOMs as the inappropriate condensation of blot details or images into a single incongruous and unrealistic object.

However, Exner's definition of INCOM is somewhat narrower in scope than the Incongruous Combination category in the TDI. This more precise definition of INCOM may have been an effort to increase the reliability of the scoring. For example, the TDI includes two incongruous combination subtypes (the external-internal and inappropriate activity responses) that are not clearly specified as examples of INCOMs in the Comprehensive System. Unlike the TDI, Exner includes external-internal Responses under the FABCOM category, which he considers to be a more serious sign of disturbed thinking. Furthermore, Exner has not been consistently explicit about whether the combination of objects and inappropriate actions (e.g., "A laughing insect") should be scored as an INCOM. In his original description of the larger category of inappropriate combinations (Exner et al., 1976), Exner indicated that these responses occurred when subjects inferred unrealistic relationships "between images, blot qualities, objects, or *activities attributed to objects*" (emphasis added, p. 48). In his subsequent texts (Exner, 1978, 1986a, 1993), however, Exner has not specifically referred to inappropriate activity responses while discussing INCOMs. Although he has consistently mentioned the inappropriate combination of color and form as a special example of the INCOM, he has not clearly included the incongruity between an object and its action as a subtype of the INCOM response.

FABULIZED COMBINATIONS (FABCOMs). Like Johnston and Holzman, Exner and Weiner followed Holt's lead in delineating three different kinds of impossible relationships that subjects may infer between different blot elements—those based on (1) size discrepancy; (2) putting together things that do not occur together in nature or reality; and (3) mixing natural and supernatural frames of reference. One noteworthy difference, however, is that Exner's FABCOM category includes implausible transparencies, which are scored as severe variants (.50 vs .25 level) of the Incongruous Combination category in the TDI (i.e., the External-Internal Response). Because such responses unrealistically condense different blot elements into a single incongruous object, Weiner (1966), too, originally designated such transparency responses as Incongruous Combinations.

Given that Exner's definition of INCOM also indicates that blot elements are merged into a single object, it would appear more consistent to score the transparency response as an INCOM instead of a FABCOM. It is reasonable to assume that Exner allowed for this apparent inconsistency and designated these responses as FABCOMs in order to capture what he and others (Johnston and Holzman, 1979) believed was a more severe manifestation of disturbed thinking.

CONTAMINATIONS (CONTAMs). In describing the fusion or merging of two or more impressions or blot elements into a single bizarre response, Exner presented the metaphor of a photographic double exposure, in which one response has been psychologically superimposed or overlaid on another. In his earlier work (Exner et al., 1976), Exner maintained that all CONTAM responses were assigned a minus form quality; however, he subsequently (Exner, 1986a) changed this rule by distinguishing perceptual processes (depicted by form quality) from ideational activity (depicted by the merging of two ideas or percepts into one). This distinction is consistent with Rapaport's ego psychologically based dialectic between perceptual and associational processes, and implicitly recognizes a range of severity in the types of contaminated responses.

Inappropriate Logic

AUTISTIC LOGIC (ALOG). Exner's ALOG is essentially the same score as the Autistic Logic scores in the Rapaport System, the TDI, Weiner's Rorschach indices of disturbed reasoning, and Holt's PRIPRO. However, whereas Weiner's earlier description of Autistic Logic and the TDI definition of this category both suggested that milder forms of Autistic Logic responses may be scored, Exner is closer to Holt in maintaining that there are no milder forms of ALOG. In both the Holt and Exner systems, there is no Level 1 versus Level 2 severity distinction given for ALOG responses.

Perseveration and Integration Failures

Exner described two lesser categories of Special Scores indicative of cognitive dysfunction, perseverations (PSVs) and confabulations (CONFABs).

Perseveration (PSV)

Initially, Exner et al. (1976) described only two types of perseveration, "within card" and "content" perseveration. Exner later added a third type, which he called "mechanical perseveration." No distinction between these three varieties is made in the scoring system as each incidence of perseveration receives a score of PSV.

(1) "Within Card Perseveration" is scored when a subject uses the same location, determinant(s), content, Developmental Quality (DQ), Form Quality (FQ), and Z score as had been used in the preceding response. Even though the content may vary slightly, the general content category is the same. For example, seeing Card V first as a "bat" and then as a "butterfly" warrants the score of PSV when all the features mentioned above are the same.

(2) "Content Perseveration" is scored when a subject indicates that a response is the same as one seen earlier. The two responses are often not consecutive or even given within the same card and do not have to share any scores in common. This kind of perseverative activity would be scored as a relationship verbalization in the Rapaport System and TDI, which is given a higher severity weighting (.50) than a perseveration score (.25).

(3) "Mechanical Perseveration." Exner noted that this third kind of perseveration may reflect either neurological or intellectual impairment or a defensive avoidance of the task. In both cases, subjects may give the same simple response on several cards without consideration of the goodness of fit.

Confabulation (CONFAB)

Exner introduced the CONFAB into his Comprehensive System in 1986 to describe the kind of perceptual overgeneralization originally referred to as the Confabulated DW response by Rorschach (1921). Unlike Rapaport and the developers of the TDI, Exner's CONFAB does not refer to ideationally embellished responses but only to the traditional DW process in which the subject generalizes inappropriately from one blot detail to a larger area or the entire inkblot. The form level of these responses is almost always poor because of the arbitrary nature of the generalization.

SPECIAL CONTENT SCORES

Exner added six special content scores to the Comprehensive System to identify response features that may reflect specific psychological characteristics. Of the six, his Abstractions (AB) score may be most indicative of pathological thought processes.

Abstractions (ABs)

Initially referred to as "Abstract Content," the special score AB is used for responses that either describe human emotion, sensory experience (coded under content as Hx), or clearly specify symbolic representation. The latter class of responses may reflect the kind of idiosyncratic symbolizing that Rapaport, Holt, and Johnston and Holzman tried to capture in their thought disorder scoring systems. Exner and Weiner (1982, 1995) indicated that intellectually oriented normal subjects often attribute symbolic meaning to Rorschach cards. Roughly 14% of nonpatient adults give symbolic responses. When they occur in the records of nonpatients, Exner and Weiner pointed out that they occur as second or third responses or are given as whimsical elaborations of completed responses. According to Exner and Weiner, when AB scores become more prevalent and occur as first or primary responses, which are delivered with an air of certainty, the subject has demonstrated a pathological preoccupation with inappropriate levels of abstraction.

Although there are no specifically designated subtypes of AB or pathological symbolism in the Comprehensive System, Exner and Weiner described two classes of deviant symbolism which they referred to as "idiosyncratic symbolism" and "overly abstract elaborations." Idiosyncratic symbolism is based on referents that are peculiar to the subject and quite distant from consensually validated experience. This class of responses would include both the unconventional color and image symbolism responses scored at the .50 level of severity in the TDI.

Overly abstract elaborations include highly elaborated responses in which abstract ideas take on a life and reality of their own. The authors give several examples of this type of response, including the Card IX response, "It gives me a feeling of nature up here and of Hell down here, one against the other, beauty against evil, with a sense of really high ideals coming out of the whole thing" (Exner and Weiner, 1995, p. 140). Clearly Rapaport and the TDI would score such a response as a severe confabulation. Exner and Weiner also agree that in addition to giving the Special Score AB, such a response would merit a DR score as well.

INADEQUATE M RESPONSES

Exner pointed out that Human Movement responses are sensitive indicators of the quality of an individual's thinking. He recognized two types of inadequate M responses as possible signifiers of deviant thought processes. The first of these is the M– response. Normatively, M– responses are rare in adult nonpatients (roughly 3%) and quite common in the records of different patient groups, such as character disorders (32%), depressives (40%), and schizophrenics (80%). Following Rorschach tradition, Exner maintained that even one M– may be suggestive of peculiarities in thinking, and more than one M– response raises the likelihood of "disoriented, very strange thinking" (Exner, 1993, p. 482). Paying attention to whether the M– is of a passive or active sort may also be important in evaluating the quality of the disordered thought process. According to Exner, passive M– responses may reflect the potential for "delusional operations." Exner recommended studying the content of M– responses to find possible clues about the nature of the delusional material. He added that patients suffering from reactive psychoses often give homogeneous content in such passive M– responses, reflecting "well-fixed delusional systems."

The second type of inadequate M, indicative of disordered thought, is what Exner termed the formless M response. These are usually highly symbolic responses that focus on some aspect of emotion or sensation. For example, responding to an inkblot as if "It looks like depression" or "It reminds me of the joyful feeling of togetherness" all but ignores the critical features of the blot. Formless M responses will also receive the Special Scores of AB and possibly DR (given the confabulatory embellishment that cannot be supported by stimulus aspects of the inkblot). Exner mentioned that formless M's may "have features that are quite similar to a hallucinatory-like operation" (Exner, 1993, p. 482).

SCHIZOPHRENIA INDEX (SCZI)

Exner's first attempt to develop a composite index to detect schizophrenia occurred shortly after he introduced Special Scores into the Comprehensive System in 1976. Exner based his experimental index on Weiner's conceptually based criteria for characterizing schizophrenia. Following Weiner's lead, Exner identified the four Rorschach indicators of schizophrenia: (1) disturbed thinking (poor human movement responses [M–] and/or examples of the five Special Scores—DV, INCOM, FABCOM, ALOG, or CONTAM); (2) impaired reality testing (poor form level or low X+ and F+%); (3) poor emotional controls

(CF+C > FC); and (4) interpersonal ineptness, absence of pure H responses or (H) > H. Exner found that 91 of 125 cases of schizophrenic patients were positive on all four features of this experimental index.

Over the next six years, Exner used the Research Diagnostic Criteria (RDC) (Spitzer, Endicott, and Robbins, 1977, 1978) to refine his sample of schizophrenic subjects and converted his experimental index into a formula that consisted of five variables. As available cases increased, Exner revised the experimental index in 1981 and then again in 1984 (Exner, 1981, 1984). When he added the sixth Special Score (DR), he found that the discriminating power of the formula improved. In 1984, Exner introduced the original Schizophrenia Index, called the "SCZI," which was made up of five variables.

The six critical Special Scores had each been weighted according to relative severity as follows: DV = 1; INCOM = 2; DR = 3; FABCOM = 4; ALOG = 5; and CONTAM = 7. Along with a low X+% and the presence of at least one M–, the weighted sum of these six scores (WSUM 6) was one of the key components of the SCZI. In 1986a, the SCZI was made up of the following five variables related to disturbed perception and thinking:

(1) X+% < 70 (the sum of good form level responses is less than 70%);

(2) Sum X– > sum Xu or X – % > 20% (the sum of poor form level responses is greater than the sum of unusual form level responses or poor form level responses are greater than 20%);

(3) M– > 0 or WSUM 6 > 11 (poor human movement responses are greater than zero or the weighted sum of critical special scores is greater than eleven);

(4) DV+DR+INCOM+FABCOM+ALOG+CONTAM>4 (the unweighted sum of critical special scores is greater than four);

(5) Sum DR+FABCOM+ALOG+CONTAM > Sum DV+INCOM or M–>1 (the sum of Deviant Responses, Fabulized Combinations, Autistic Logic Responses, and Contaminations is greater than the sum of Deviant Verbalizations and Incongruous Combinations or poor human movement responses total more than one).

The original SCZI showed diagnostic accuracy rates between 72% and 89%; however, false positive rates were shown to be unacceptably high for some patient groups. A score of 5 on the SCZI was considered quite diagnostic of schizophrenia, whereas a score of 4 produced many false positives. Investigations designed to make the SCZI a more sensitive and specific index of schizophrenia continued over the next six years.

The SCZI was revised again in 1990 (Exner, 1990) in order to improve the false positive and negative rates. The improvement was greatly advanced by the addition of Level 1 and 2 scores (described below) and S – % (minus form white space responses) variables to the index. Based on correlational and discriminant function analyses, Exner settled on six items consisting of a total of 10 variables for his revised SCZI.

(1) X+% < 61 and S–% < 41 *or* X+% < 50

(2) X–% > 29

(3) Sum X– > Sum Xu *or* Sum X– > Sum(Xo+X+)

(4) Sum Level 2 Special Scores > 1 and FABCOM2 > 0

(5) Sum 6 Special Scores > 6 *or* WSum 6 Special Scores > 17 (cutoff adjusted for children > 1SD above the mean)

(6) M– > 1 *or* X–% > 40

The critical interpretative value of SCZI is a score of 4, which indicates a significant probability of schizophrenia but also a fair possibility of having a false positive. For this reason, scores of 4 are interpreted with caution. According to Exner's research, scores of 5 or 6 indicate a much stronger likelihood of schizophrenia, while minimizing the probability of receiving a false positive.

LEVEL 1 AND LEVEL 2 SCORES

After the SCZI was developed, Exner concluded that the weights assigned to the six critical Special Scores did not reflect the appropriate degree of severity of each score. For example, some INCOMs were quite severe in nature whereas others were more benign and developmentally not unusual, often found in the records of children. Exner recognized that these two expressions of the same Special Score needed to be differentially weighted. The simplest, best way to address the variability within each scoring category was to assign a value of 1 or 2 to the following four Special Scoring categories, DV, DR, INCOM, and FABCOM. Level 1 ratings reflect mild or modest instances of illogical, peculiar, or fluid slippage in thinking. Most of these responses would merit similar TDI scores from the .25 level of severity.

Level 2 ratings refer to moderate to severe fluidity in thinking, lapses in logic, or more bizarre examples of reasoning or judgment. These responses would receive comparable TDI scores from the .50, .75, and potentially, 1.0 levels of severity. Because ALOGs and CONTAMs fall at the more severe end of the Rorschach thought disorder scoring continuum, Exner considered them, by definition, to be Level 2 Special Scores.

Since nearly 81% of nonpatient adults gave at least one Level 1 special score, and nonpatient children gave an even greater number, Exner viewed the presence of Level 2 scores as cause for greater concern. However, he found that at least one Level 2 score was also often found in the records of normal children (for example, in almost 25% of the records of 13-year-olds) and even more frequently in the records of non-schizophrenic patient groups (71% of inpatient depressives and 38% of a mixed sample of outpatients). Based on these normative findings, Exner concluded that Level 2 scores may have no specific diagnostic significance, other than as general indicators of more severe cognitive slippage, and that the presence of a single Level 2 score should not be viewed as a pathognomic sign of thought disorder.

INTERSCORER RELIABILITY

As early as 1978, Exner began to gather interrater reliability data on Special Scores (Exner, 1978). He reported two early studies, one with 20 schizophrenic and 20 nonpatients and another based on 75 responses selected from 250 protocols. In both studies, the reliabilities ranged from .81 to .91 for each of five Special Scores (DR had not yet been introduced into the Comprehensive System). In 1986 (Exner, 1986a), Exner provided additional data on scorer agreement for Special Scores. The results of two separate reliability studies were presented. The percentage of agreement between scorers in both studies was extremely high, ranging from 93% to 99%.

NORMATIVELY BASED CONTINUUM OF SEVERITY

Using frequencies and means from patient and nonpatient adult and developmental age groups, Exner was able to construct a rough hierarchy of severity for the Special Scores according to their relative frequency in his large nonpatient and patient samples. In essence, his normative data provided some basis for an empirically derived continuum of severity for the critical Special Scores. For example, over half of his 700 nonpatient adults (53%) had at least one DV1; 46% had an INCOM1; 15% a DR1; 16% a FABCOM1; 1% a DV2; .5% an INCOM2; 4% an ALOG; 2% a DR2 or FABCOM2 and none of the normal subjects had a CONTAM in their records. Of the 320 schizophrenic subjects, 227 had at least one Level 2 score; 63% gave at least one FABCOM2; and 5% gave at least one CONTAM (a rare score under any circumstance). In this schizophrenic sample, the mean number of Special Scores per record was 9.

Extensive normative data for patient and different age groups can be found in volume 1 of Exner's text (1986a, 1993). Additional norms for samples of borderline and schizotypal subjects that Exner collected prior to the differentiation between Level 1 and 2 Special Scores (Exner, 1986b) are available.

Since almost 81% of the nonpatient adults (and the majority of normal children) in his sample had at least one Special Score in their records, Exner cautioned that low frequencies of Special Scores in patients' records should not necessarily be interpreted as evidence of disturbances in thinking, unless the scores in question are DR2s, FABCOM2s, or CONTAMs. Based on his normative findings, Exner offered the following rough continuum of severity of Special Scores:

DV1 INCOM1 DR1	DV2 FABCOM1 INCOM2 ALOG	DR2 FABCOM2 CONTAM
MILD	SERIOUS	SEVERE

Exner felt that as many as three DV1s may mean little in a record but that the presence of a single DV2 might be cause for concern. He also indicated that a few INCOM1s in a record are not highly interpretable unless the subject begins to give more bizarre condensations (INCOM2). As for FABCOMs, Exner pointed out that they are common in the records of children, schizophrenic, and character disordered patients and should only be regarded as a negative sign in adults and adolescents if the FABCOM1s number two or more or if there is a single FABCOM2. The presence of DR2s, ALOGs and CONTAMs, of course, suggest more serious disturbances in thinking. In summary, Exner concluded that the presence of greater than five Special Scores in the records of adults and greater than one standard deviation above the age mean for younger children suggest that a thought disorder may exist. He offered a rough cut off for WSUM 6 of 9 to demarcate the normal range of cognitive slippage from clinically meaningful pathology of thinking. However, he also cautioned against a strictly quantitative approach and recommended that clinicians examine each incidence of Special Scoring separately.

COMPARING SPECIAL SCORES WITH OTHER THOUGHT DISORDER SCORING SYSTEMS

The Comprehensive System was developed by incorporating empirically valid aspects of other Rorschach systems and systematizing them into a standardized format. As has been previously mentioned, Exner relied heavily on Weiner's (1966) earlier contributions to the Rorschach thought disorder literature; and Weiner, of course, drew from both Holt's and Rapaport's seminal work in this area. However, there has been little effort to examine possible relationships between Exner's Special Scores and other Rorschach systems for assessing disordered thinking. One notable exception is the work of Meloy and Singer (1991) who attempted to link selected Special Scores to the Rapaport System and psychoanalytic theories of development and psychopathology.

Meloy and Singer looked at the convergence and divergence between seven Special Scores in the Comprehensive System and the deviant verbalizations first described by Rapaport. Table 6-1 summarizes their rationally based comparison between thought disorder scoring in the two systems.

In addition to comparing Exner's Special Scores with those of the Rapaport group, Meloy and Singer reviewed research pertaining to each scoring category in an attempt to build conceptual and empirical bridges between the Special Scores in the Comprehensive System and psychoanalytic theories of thought disorder.

It is interesting to compare and contrast the Exner's Special Scores with the thought disorder categories of the TDI. Table 6-2 presents such a comparison between the Special Scores and some of the factors that Holzman and his group derived from the factor analytic studies of the TDI (Holzman et al., 1986).

In this comparison, one can see that the DR score is overrepresented. Of the 14 different TDI scores that contribute to this five-factor structure, DR appears to be the Special Score equivalent for half of these and is present in four of the five factors.

CRITIQUE OF THE COMPREHENSIVE SYSTEM SPECIAL SCORES

Exner quickly grasped the significance of his oversight in excluding thought disorder scoring from his original Comprehensive System (1974). As early as 1976, he began working to address this critical gap in his original hybridized system. Exner can be credited for his effort to develop a normatively based set of thought disorder scores that attempt to capture Rapaport's major categories of deviant verbalization in a simplified, parsimonious, and reliably scored format. Like many of the Rapaport loyalists who felt that his 23 categories of deviant verbalizations were too unwieldy to score, Exner tried to scale down Rapaport's list to roughly 10 categories or fewer. By limiting his list of Special Scores to those that could be reliably differentiated from one another, Exner tried to address his earlier criticism that the overlap in Rapaport's categories and the lack of clear operational definitions made precise quantitative scoring extremely difficult (1974).

Table 6-1 Comparison of Special Scores and Rapaport, Gill, and Schafer's Categories of Deviant Verbalization

Description of Response	Special Scores	Deviant Verbalizations
Two percepts combined in an impossible way	FABCOM	Fabulized Combination
One percept with impossible details	INCOM	Fabulized Combination
Extensive arbitrary elaboration of a response	DR	Confabulation
Fusion of two percepts into one	CONTAM	Contamination
Illogical cause-effect relation	ALOG	Autistic Logic
Peculiar, non sequiturs	DV	Peculiar, Queer
Inappropriate perceptual generalization	CONFAB	DW

From Meloy and Singer, 1991.

Unlike Holt's system or the TDI, Exner's Special Scores can be learned and reliably scored with relative ease. As with all features of the Comprehensive System, the Special Scores are bolstered by extensive normative data that allow for comparisons with large samples of developmental age groups: ages 5–16 (N = 1390), nonpatient adults (N = 700), character disorders (N = 180), outpatients (N = 440), inpatient schizophrenics (N = 320), inpatient depressives (N = 315), schizotypals (N = 76), and borderlines (N = 84).

Exner's normative data laid the foundation for a continuum of severity of Special Scores based in part on the relative frequency with which different scores occurred in nonpatient and clinical samples. Furthermore, Exner recognized a limited continuum of severity within several of the categories of Special Scores. His efforts to capture a range of severity within scoring categories led to the introduction of Level 1 and 2 ratings for four of the six critical Special Scores. Meloy and Singer (1991) suggested that the high retest reliabilities and interjudge agreement with regard to Level 1 and 2 differentiations can increase both the sensitivity and specificity of the DV, DR, INCOM, and FABCOM scores.

Table 6-2 Comparison of Special Scores with TDI Post Hoc Factors

Factor	TDI Categories	Special Scores
IRRELEVANT INTRUSIONS	Flippant	DR1
	Looseness	DR2
COMBINATORY THINKING	Incongruous Combination	INCOM1&2
	Fabulized Combination	FABCOM1&2
	Playful Confabulation	FABCOM1&2 or DR1&2
FLUID THINKING	Relationship Verbalization	PSV
	Fluidity	DR2
	Contamination	CONTAM
CONFUSION	Word-Finding Difficulty	
	Confusion	DR2
	Absurd Responses	DR2
	Incoherence	DR2
	Neologisms	DV2
IDIOSYNCRATIC VERBALIZATION	Peculiar	DV1

From Molzman and Singer, 1986.

Extensive research has gone into refining the SCZI in order to maximize accurate identification of schizophrenic patients and minimize false positive and negative rates. The SCZI has been shown to identify the presence of schizophrenia with accuracy rates between 75 and 90%. False positive rates among several of Exner's large samples (1990) ranged from 0 to 11%, depending on which group was being studied. False negative rates were found to range from 12 to 22%, with most of the false negatives occurring among constricted records (with fewer than 17 responses). Exner's key variables approach to interpretation (1990) sets up a strategy for viewing the significance of SCZIs with a value of 4, 5, and 6. This format may provide quantitative support for diagnostic inferences of varying degrees of certainty. In other words, Exner's studies suggest that a SCZI of 4 should be interpreted with great caution, while a SCZI of 6 indicates a much greater likelihood that schizophrenia is present.

Despite the many strengths and the appeal of the Special Scores in the Comprehensive System, Exner's efforts to simplify thought disorder scoring and to develop a set of reliably scored categories may have

limited the scope of scorable deviant responses. In his effort to be parsimonious, Exner either condensed or simply overlooked discrete types
of pathological verbalizations that may have particular diagnostic significance. Several examples of this possible tendency to condense or
oversimplify categories exist among the Special Scores. For example, the
DV category appears to be rather narrowly defined. By limiting DV
scores to either redundancies or neologisms, a broader array of idiosyncratic verbalizations may be overlooked. Technically, many of the examples of odd and stilted expressions and idiosyncratic word usage and
images, scored as peculiar and queer verbalizations in the TDI, may not
be scorable as DVs in the Comprehensive System because they are neither redundancies nor neologisms. For example, responses such as "two
legs raising each other," "potential ears," "a perverted jack-o'-lantern,"
"a foxed comic dog," or "an echo of a picture" include neither redundancies nor neologisms per se, and as such, may not merit a Special
Score of DV.

The DR scoring category is even more problematic in terms of its
lack of specificity and crispness of conceptual boundaries. Meloy and
Singer (1991) equated the DR score with the concept of confabulation
in Rapaport's original scoring schema but acknowledged that DR was a
slightly more expansive category. Although intended to capture
responses in which the subject "wanders off target," I believe that
Exner's DR is more than "slightly expansive" and has become so broad
in scope that it risks becoming a "wastebasket" category for a variety of
different responses. The crude comparison between Special Scores and
scoring categories in the TDI, depicted in Table 6-2, reflects the breadth
of the DR category, which may subsume a number of separate scoring
categories in the TDI. For example, TDI categories roughly equivalent
to DR1 and 2 may include such disparate scores as inappropriate distance, flippant responses, vagueness and confusion, looseness, playful
confabulations and confabulations, fluid, and incoherent responses. The
separate factors of Irrelevant Intrusions, Combinative Thinking,
Confusion, and Fluid Thinking all contain scores that would likely be
scored DR1 or 2 in the Comprehensive System.

Besides the overly broad quality of the DR category, there is a para-
doxically narrow aspect to Exner's definition of DR. By defining DR as
a "wandering off target," in which the subject either produces an "inappropriate phrase" (e.g., "It's a bat but I was hoping for a butterfly") or
a "circumstantial response," Exner has restricted the meaning of DR,
focusing primarily on those responses in which the subject essentially
departs from the task and becomes inappropriately discursive or loose.
However, some subjects do not "wander away" from the blot but
become inappropriately immersed in it. These subjects are not circumstantial in Exner's sense but become lost in an elaborate description of

the blot itself. For example, consider the response "Looks like a beetle that's been injured. It looks frightened, angry, and aggressive. An uh . . . very intent on . . . attacking in um . . . in retaliation for something that's bothering it." This response is clearly not an inappropriate phrase DR and it is also not circumstantial; the subject does not wander away from the response but becomes immersed in the fantasy of the response. Most would agree that such a response should receive a DR score; however, this type of "fantasy immersion" response is not clearly described under the realm of DR in the Comprehensive System. Exner could have benefited from sticking to Rapaport's distinction between "increased distance" and "loss of distance." Highly elaborated and embellished DRs can reflect either one or the other kind of problem in maintaining appropriate distance from the blot or both together. Exner's category of DR seems to address only the "wandering away" phenomenon (i.e., increased distance or, in his terms, "circumstantiality") but does not fully develop the concept of "fantasy immersion." Kleiger and Peebles-Kleiger (1993) addressed this conceptual difficulty with the DR response, noting Exner's failure to describe adequately this latter type of deviant response process (more on this in chapter 9).

Exner further confuses an already confusing issue by retaining the score CONFAB but applying this only to the DW score that appears in most Rorschach systems. In their effort to link Special Scores with psychoanalytic theory, Meloy and Singer (1991) recommended that the CONFAB category be scrapped, due to its rarity and lack of sensitivity and specificity to psychopathology, and that the DR category be renamed CONFAB because they felt that DR is essentially synonymous with Rapaport's confabulation concept. Kleiger and Peebles-Kleiger disagreed with Meloy and Singer's equating DR with confabulation and felt that Meloy and Singer did not sufficiently recognize the heterogeneity in Exner's DR category. In their detailed critique of the DR score, Kleiger and Peebles-Kleiger proposed a modification of DR scoring in order to make this a more precise score and to capture the different nuances of the process of confabulation (that appears to be broadly subsumed under the DR category). Table 6-3 presents their proposed scoring changes, which included moving the inappropriate phrase DRs back to the DV category (where they were originally contained); introducing an "overly embellished" (OR) category that would be the domain of highly embellished responses; and placing circumstantial self-reference responses under the category of Personalized Responses (PERs).

There are also aspects of Exner's continuum of severity that do not make clinical sense. For example, DR2 scores are considered in the midrange of severity, along with FABCOM1, INCOM2, and ALOG scores. However, neologisms in the TDI, surely scored DV2 in the Comprehensive System, receive the highest severity weighting (1.0) in

Table 6-3 Kleiger and Peebles-Kleiger's Proposed Modifications for the DR category

DVs	a.	Neologisms, typically scored as Level 2.
	b.	Redundancies, scored as Level 1 or 2.
	c.	Inappropriate/tangential phrases, previously scored as Level 1 or 2 DR.
ORs	a.	Embellishment tendency, previously scored Level 1 DR.
	b.	Severe embellishment, previously scored as level 2 DR.
PERs	a.	Self-reference, scored PER.
	b.	Circumstantial self-reference, previously scored Level 1 or 2 DR.

From Kleiger and Peebles-Kleiger, 1993.

the TDI. The research of the Holzman group (Shenton et al., 1987) on qualitative distinctions in thought disorder among different psychotic groups demonstrated that schizophrenic patients' thought disorders were characterized primarily by confusion and severely idiosyncratic verbalizations, most likely scored as DV2 in the Comprehensive System. Furthermore, according to Exner's norms for nonpatient adults, DV2s occur in only 1% of the protocols, making this an extremely rare score in normal records. Thus, it is difficult to understand why DV2s are not viewed among the most severe examples of deviant thinking in the Comprehensive System.

Scoring of PSVs is less precise than it could be. Three kinds of perseveration responses (PSV) are distinguished but only one PSV score is given for each subtype. However, there are differences between some of these subtypes in degree of severity and frequency of occurrence. For example, within card perseveration appears to reflect a different and less malignant kind of process than the other two types. Within card PSVs are not unusual in records of nonpsychotic patients and may reflect a defensive process of tying to "play it safe" by giving essentially the same response consecutively on a given card. On the other hand, content and mechanical PSVs may reflect more serious disturbances in cognitive functioning. Content PSVs would be scored as relationship verbalizations in the TDI (receiving a severity weighting of .50). Exner indicated that mechanical PSVs are often given by intellectually or neurologically compromised subjects. Thus, one could make the case that the latter two subtypes of PSV reflect more serious disturbances in thinking. A reasonable solution would be to assign Level 1 and 2 ratings to PSV scores, depending upon whether the PSV is the more benign, within card subtype (Level 1) or the more malignant content or mechanical subtype (Level 2).

Although there is abundant normative data pertaining to the Special Scores, there are no data bases of patient groups most relevant for making differential diagnosis of thought disorder. Exner presents extensive norms of schizophrenic patients, inpatient depressives, character disorders, and outpatients; however, the most frequent diagnostic questions do not concern discriminating between these groups or simply determining whether the patient has a thought disorder. Many times referral questions ask whether the thought disorder is more consistent with schizophrenia, a bipolar psychosis, schizoaffective disorder, or other psychotic condition. Future studies concerning the Special Scores and SCZI could profitably focus on the qualitative differences between thought disorder patterns between these psychotic groups (similar to Exner's earlier study in 1986 constrasting borderline, schizophrenic, and schizotypal subjects).

Finally, some of Exner's inferences about M– and the formless M response are not yet supported by data. According to Exner, passive M– responses may reflect the potential for "delusional operations," patients suffering from reactive psychoses often give homogeneous content in such passive M– responses, reflecting "well-fixed delusional systems," and formless M's may "have features that are quite similar to a hallucinatory-like operation" (Exner 1993, p. 482). These are intriguing hypotheses about the nature of an individual's disordered thinking, and they deserve to be studied empirically.

Criticisms nothwithstanding, Exner should be credited with developing an easily scored and reliably coded set of Special Scores that capture most of the major categories of deviant thought on the Rorschach. The ease with which Special Scores can be learned and scored makes them an attractive alternative to more intricate and cumbersome methods like the TDI and Holt's PRIPRO. When faced with more difficult questions of differential diagnosis in patients already suspected of being psychotic, however, clinicians may have more confidence using a more complex scoring system like the TDI. Furthermore, if it is important diagnostically to describe the specific nature of the psychotic process in a given patient, the TDI may offer clinicians a wider variety of categories from which to choose in attempting to score different nuances of disordered thinking.

CHAPTER

7

ALTERNATIVE THOUGHT

DISORDER SCORING SYSTEMS

In addition to the major contemporary research and clinical thought disorder scoring systems, there are a number of atypical and relatively obscure systems for scoring thought disorder on the Rorschach. Whether developed specifically for research purposes or proposed for use in clinical practice, these "secondary" systems employ a mixture of generally accepted scoring concepts along with novel additions and modifications. I include among these secondary systems Wynne et al.'s (1978) scoring of "communication deviance" on the Rorschach; the research-based scoring system of Harrow and Quinlan (Quinlan et al., 1972; Harrow and Quinlan, 1977, 1985); the clinical approaches of Aronow, Reznikoff, and Moreland (1994) and Schuldberg and Boster (1985); the psychoanalytically rooted system of Burstein and Loucks (1989); Wagner's TRAUT System (1998); and the recently devised Menninger Thought Disturbance Scales.

COMMUNICATION DEVIANCE

In the 1950s, schizophrenia researchers became interested in the familial transmission of pathological thinking in schizophrenia. In their seminal investigation, Lidz and his coworkers (Lidz et al., 1958) demonstrated the surprisingly bizarre nature of the reasoning of a sample of nonpsychiatric parents of schizophrenic patients. Singer and Wynne

(1966) pioneered a Rorschach method for scoring disordered styles of communication and developed Rorschach and TAT scoring manuals for the concept they termed "communication deviance" in families. Communication deviance was said to differ from the concept of "thought disorder" and pertained, instead, to those aspects of naming and explaining that distract and confuse a listener who is attempting to understand what the speech is communicating. In other words, instead of being able to understand a line of thought and visualize what a speaker is describing, the listener gets confused by what he or she is hearing.

In order to study communication deviance, Singer and Wynne employed the Rorschach almost as a structured interview. They took only the first response to each card and conducted the inquiry after all ten cards were administered. The inquiry procedure was an open-ended one, designed to explore the subject's point of view and the reasoning behind the percepts seen.

In their original manual (Singer and Wynne, 1966), Singer and Wynne presented 41 categories of scorable communication deviance, which clustered into three groups: (1) closure problems, characterized by incomplete communication; (2) disruptive behavior, in which the speaker distracts attention away from the task at hand; and (3) peculiar language and logic, in which idiosyncratic language and reasoning interfere with the listener's ability to comprehend the thoughts or perceptions that the speaker had in mind.

Closure Problems

The nine categories of closure problems may cause the listener to be uncertain about whether the speaker has completed his or her idea or response. The speaker has difficulty sharing a focus with the listener, leaving the listener unsure about the meaning that the speaker was trying to convey. Singer and Wynne reasoned that the subtle and covert ways in which a shared focus of attention is hindered has a more detrimental impact on the listener than do the more blatantly bizarre disruptions. They hypothesized that children subjected to closure problems in communication with their parents grow up with difficulties trusting and interpreting their own perceptions and those they hear from others.

Disruptive Behavior

Clear interruptions and distractions, in which the speaker breaks set and shifts abruptly from the task at hand (interpreting the inkblots), are scored under this grouping. In normal social discourse, frequent interruptions and distracting comments create confusion for the listener who is led astray and put off course by these shifts in attentional foci.

Peculiar Language and Logic

Grouped under this heading are all those instances in which words, syntax, and logic are used in strange and idiosyncratic ways that interfere with sharing meaning with another person. Formal aspects of the response, not the content, are scored under this category. Singer and Wynne cautioned raters to be familiar with cultural idioms and the effects of lower education on the language so as to not over-rate responses in this category.

The communication deviance (CD) score was obtained by dividing the total number of scored categories by the number of transactions, which was defined as the number of first responses plus responses to inquiries into these responses. The original scoring manual was revised twice (Singer, 1973; Wynne, Singer, and Toohey, 1978) and the scoring categories were subsequently grouped into the following five clusters: commitment problems, referent problems, language anomalies, disruptions, and contradictory, arbitrary sequences (Singer, 1977).

Validity Studies

All but nine of the original 41 scoring categories differentiated (p < .01) the parents of schizophrenic patients from other parents (Wynne et al., 1978). Nine categories were eventually eliminated because they did not statistically discriminate between the parents of schizophrenic offspring and other parents. In some of their earlier studies (Wynne, 1967; Wynne et al., 1976), they found that the frequency of parental CD on the Rorschach correlated with the severity of illness in their offspring. Even if the parents of schizophrenics themselves did not suffer from a diagnosed psychiatric illness, their CDs were significantly higher than the CDs of parents of normal, neurotic, and borderline subjects. Parents of normal and neurotic subjects had low CDs; parents of remitting and non-remitting schizophrenic subjects had high CDs; and parents of borderline subjects scored both high and low (one parent high, one parent low).

Communication Deviance or Thought Disorder?

Because of the interpersonal or systemic context of their examination, Singer and Wynne advocated the use of the term "communication disorder" rather than thought disorder. A communication disorder connotes an interpersonal transaction in which thinking and language are both embedded. However, Singer and Wynne argued that what was most important here was not the psychopathology of the speaker, per se, but the psychological impact of the speaker on the listener, in this case the offspring, whose schizophrenia was thought to have been etiologically influenced by impaired communication patterns within the family.

Although Johnston and Holzman (1979) acknowledged that Singer and Wynne approached the whole question of thought disorder and schizophrenia from interactional and family systems, as opposed to intrapsychic and individualistic tradition, they wondered whether communication deviance was simply the transactional transmission of thought disorder. Although tempting to view thought disorder and communication deviance as different names for the same phenomenon, Johnston and Holzman acknowledged that Singer and Wynne's research supports the distinction between these two concepts. For example, while parents' CD scores correlated highly with illness severity ratings in their psychotic offspring, they did not correlate with ratings of severity of illness in the parents themselves. Furthermore Wynne and his colleagues (1976) discovered that CD scores of the parents predicted illness severity ratings of psychotic offspring better than the CD scores of the offspring themselves! Parents frequently scored in categories not usually associated with formal thought disorder. In contrast, schizophrenic offspring most often scored in categories associated with psychotic symptoms.

Johnston and Holzman believed that the greatest overlap between thought disorder and communication deviance occurred in Singer and Wynne's third class of communication deviance, namely Peculiar Language and Logic. The particular scoring categories subsumed under this heading share considerable space with typical forms of thought and language disorders identified by the Rorschach. Johnston and Holzman also described how the two other classes of communication deviance (Disruptive Behavior and Closure Problems) could, in some cases, be associated with formal thought disorder. Closure Problems reflect difficulties in thought organization that might become manifest in thought disorder when disorganization leads to confusion, looseness, unintelligible remarks, and fluid or unstable perceptions of the external world. On the other hand, Disruptive Behavior can lead to loss of distance or concreteness and inappropriate remarks.

Quinlan and his colleagues (Quinlan et al., 1978) examined the relationship between communication deviance on the Object Sorting Test and a variety of other measures of thought disorder. They found a significant correlation between CD scores and conceptual overinclusion and bizarre-idiosyncratic thinking. They concluded that communication deviance was a broad concept that overlapped, but was not isomorphic, with thought disorder. In other words, some individual communication deviance scores do not seem to reflect thought disorder; however, the scoring system as a whole is highly correlated with disordered thought.

HARROW AND QUINLAN'S RORSCHACH THOUGHT DISORDER CATEGORIES

Although probably not as well known as their more clinically oriented colleagues in the field of personality assessment, Harrow and Quinlan have been leading scholars in the scientific study of schizophrenia and thought disorder in particular. Their research has explored the underlying mechanisms of thought disorder, the longitudinal progression of schizophrenic thinking; and it has challenged the earlier notions of the diagnostic specificity of thought disorder.

In their earliest studies (Quinlan et al., 1972), Quinlan and Harrow identified three theoretically relevant dimensions of thought disorder including: (1) impairment of logical and coherent verbalization; (2) appearance of irrelevant or overspecific associations; and (3) appearance of affect-laden material, including affect attributed to the card or the patient's own affective response to the inkblot. Using scoring categories from the Rapaport and Holt systems, the researchers developed these dimensions into three Rorschach scales: Thought Quality, Overspecificity, and Affective Elaboration. For each scale, they included different levels of severity, with different weights assigned to each level (Quinlan, Harrow, Tucker, and Carlson, 1973).

Thought Quality (TQ)

Deviant Thought Quality (TQ) was thought to be similar to concepts of positive thought disorder and "bizarre-idiosyncratic language and thinking," a term that Harrow and Quinlan (1985) introduced at a later date to describe a variety of diverse types of speech and behavior that are most frequently associated with acute thought disorder. Harrow and Quinlan reasoned that coherent verbalization is a feature of ego functioning that is affected in a number of syndromes, especially during acute phases of psychoses. The researchers sought to identify molar variables that unified different aspects of disordered thinking with the hope of discovering the underlying cognitive mechanism common to the varied aspects of thought pathology.

Harrow and Quinlan scored deviant thought quality according to the coherence of the response and whether the verbalization had a strange, peculiar, or illogical component, without reference to the accuracy of the percept. Language that is referred to as peculiar and loose was subsumed under this broad category of bizarre-idiosyncratic speech and thinking, as was disordered and autistic logic, neologisms, and overinclusive behavior. The TQ scale included a wide array of formal thought disorder scores from the Rapaport and Holt systems and was scored on a 5-point scale (0-absent; 4-most severe). TQ1 was scored for minor variations in coherent speech. TQ1 and TQ2 were given for peculiar and queer responses respectively. TQ1 and TQ2 scores were also assigned to some confabulations and fabulized combinations, whereas TQ3 and TQ4 scores were reserved for responses which included more bizarre verbalizations, including autistic logic and contaminations.

Overspecificity (OS)

Harrow and Quinlan based this category on Rapaport's concept of "loss of distance," in which the subject associates to the inkblot as if it had some concrete reality. Scored along a 4-point scale of severity (0-absent; 1-mild; 2-moderate; 3-severe), OS subsumes varying degrees of fabulation and confabulation. It is scored whenever the subject describes details that are either more *specific* or *embellished* than can be justified by the stimulus properties of the inkblot. "Specificity" implies inappropriate precision or detail, whereas embellishment connotes the degree of extraneous (and unjustifiable) elaboration of details. Quinlan and Harrow believed that overspecificity may be related to the concept of overinclusive thinking, in which the subject is unable to separate relevant from irrelevant details.

Like Rapaport's concept of fabulation, level 1 OS responses (or OS1) reflect a mild degree of ideational (as opposed to affective) specificity that goes beyond the stimulus features of the blot. According to Harrow and Quinlan, these are not necessarily pathological responses but may reflect the subject's special interests. For example, a response to the middle detail of Card VII such as "This looks like some kind of dog; I'd say a Yorkshire Terrier" may be more specific than indicated, but it is not necessarily inappropriate and certainly not at all bizarre.

Level 2 (moderate) responses are essentially confabulation tendencies that exceed mild embellishment and begin to reflect the extent to which the subject's idiosyncratic preoccupations overshadow the reality of the stimulus. The form level of the response may still be preserved, but the subject provides specific details that go far beyond what can be justified by the inkblot. An example of an OS2 response (F+/o) to Card V would be "A hungry vampire bat that is flying in the dark of night to suck the blood of mammals in order to feed its young."

Finally, the OS3 response (severe) is dominated both by unseen elements and by idiosyncratic perception (F−). These responses would be scored as full confabulations in the TDI.

Affect Elaboration (AE)

Affective Elaboration responses reflect another aspect of Rapaport's concepts fabulation-confabulation. Harrow and Quinlan scored three levels of AE (1-mild, 2-moderate, 3-severe) to capture both the varying degrees of affective elaboration of and affective reaction to the inkblot. Mild, moderate, and severe AE of the first type parallel different degrees of overspecificity as the subject goes from producing an affect-laden fabulized response (e.g. "A sad clown"—level 1 AE) to a severe affectively driven embellishment that reflects both perceptual distortion and the intrusion of emotional elements that are not present in the card (level 3 AE). Inappropriate affective reactions reflect the subject's emotional loss of distance from the card or their response to the card. These, too, range from mild (level 1) affectively-tinged comments (e.g. "A bat; it looks kinda scary") to near catastrophic reactions (level 3) in which the subject reacts with strong affect as if the inkblot were a real stimulus (e.g., "Oh God, that's so bloody, it's just like my bloody wrists when I cut myself" [subject throws the card onto the table]).

The total thought disorder score would be the weighted sum of TQ, OS, and AE for all responses. Later, in their 1985 book, Quinlan and Harrow reported another method for computing an index score for each type of disordered thinking, similar to the way in which Johnston and Holzman (1979) computed the total TDI.

Reliability and Interscale Correlations

Quinlan and Harrow subjected their scales to empirical study in the early 1970s on a diagnostically heterogeneous sample of 70 psychiatric inpatients (Quinlan et al., 1972). The researchers found that TQ was significantly correlated with OS and moderately with AE. OS and AE were also significantly related but at a lower level than the other interscale correlations. Despite these correlations, the group of researchers concluded that the three scales represented independent constructs and should, as such, be examined separately.

In addition to examining the relationships between their three scales, the Quinlan group studied the relationship between their scales and a number of other relevant Rorschach variables including form level, drive content, fabulized combinations, and contaminations. They found that all three scales correlated significantly with F–, suggesting that impairment of thought processes tended to be accompanied by a decline in reality testing. Both TQ 2–4 and OS correlated highly with fabulized combinations and contaminations, suggesting a relationship between pathological thinking and difficulties maintaining conceptual boundaries. TQ 2–4 and OS also correlated with primary process content, pointing to a relationship between pathological thought and failure of repression. AE correlated at a lower level with some, but not all, of these other Rorschach variables.

Validity Studies

In comparing the mean scores of the three scales for their neurotic depressive versus their schizophrenic group, Quinlan et al. (1972) found that all three scales significantly discriminated between these two patient groups. The researchers also examined the relationship between their scales and an independent rating of bizarre behavior. As expected, they found a highly significant correlation between bizarre behavioral ratings and TQ, followed by lower and nonsignificant correlations with OS and AE respectively.

Harrow and Quinlan subsequently made a significant contribution to the thought disorder literature by demonstrating that milder levels of thought disorder were frequent in many types of acute psychiatric disturbances (Harrow and Quinlan, 1977). Based on their findings, Harrow and Quinlan were among the first researchers to conclude that disordered thinking falls along a continuum of severity and is by no means diagnostically specific to schizophrenia.

In an effort to study the nature of thought disorder, Harrow and Quinlan (1985) factor analyzed scores for five groups of patients on their three scales along with a number of other Rorschach scores, including form level, color responses, human movement, combinations, fabulized combinations, contaminations, drive manifestations from Holt's PRIPRO scoring system, and barrier and penetration scores (Fisher and Cleveland, 1958). They were primarily interested in examining whether there was a unitary dimension underlying thought disorder and if mild levels of disordered thinking were on the same dimensions as scores reflecting more severe degrees of thought disorder. Using a principal axis solution they derived three factors with eigenvalues greater than 1.0 that accounted for 46% of the variance.

Factor I had high loadings of variables that are traditionally associated with severe disorders in thinking, including TQ, OS, AE, contaminations, fabulized combinations, and primitive Level 1 drive material. Harrow and Quinlan labeled this factor "ideational disturbance," which, in addition to accounting for the greatest variance of any of the factors, also differentiated schizophrenic patients from others. Harrow and Quinlan believed that these severely deviant responses could be influenced by an "impaired perspective" and suggested that the lack of structure on the Rorschach makes it difficult for more disturbed patients to take a proper social perspective when looking at the inkblots and attempting to communicate their responses to others. They proposed that the major factor in the bizarre verbalizations of schizophrenic patients involved an "impaired perspective" about the social appropriateness of their own speech and behavior.

Factor II loaded for barrier and penetration scores, combinations, mild TQ, OS, and F+ form level, and Level 2 drive content. Termed "productive richness," Quinlan and Harrow related this factor to the degree to which the subject responded to the card with nonextreme elaboration.

Finally, Factor III, labeled "affective/perceptual diffuseness" yielded high loadings on pure color, mild AE, amorphous and F– form level. They felt that Factor III provided less information about thought disorder, but that this kind of diffuse productivity itself may provide useful diagnostic information. In particular, they noted that depressed patients tended to see fewer percepts and to say less about their responses than other subjects. Quinlan and Harrow also believed that Factor III represented affective lability.

Regarding the question of whether mild forms of each type of positive thought disorder are tied to more severe types, Quinlan and Harrow's data supported the separation of different levels of severity. Only Factor I distinguished schizophrenic patients from other groups. By contrast, the researchers found that mild signs of thought disorder tended to occur in the records of a variety of acute psychiatric patients without indicating the presence of a positive thought disorder or schizophrenia. As a result of these findings, Harrow and Quinlan (1977) stated that milder levels of disordered thinking on the Rorschach are not diagnostic features of schizophrenia. Like their TDI contemporaries, Harrow and Quinlan believed that the more severe types of thought disorder should be more heavily weighted than the milder forms, since only the former were diagnostically significant for schizophrenia.

Eventually, Harrow and Quinlan abandoned the Rorschach in their investigations of deviant thinking. They concluded that the Rorschach was too time consuming to administer, score, and transcribe to be efficacious in their research. Furthermore, problems in the reliable scoring of thought disorder with the Rorschach led them to adopt a simpler method of recording and scoring disordered thinking. In 1986, they teamed up with another group of researchers (Marengo et al., 1986) to develop a reliable and valid system for scoring bizarre-idiosyncratic verbalizations from two short verbal tests, the Gorham Proverbs Test (Gorham, 1956) and the Comprehension subtest of the WAIS (Wechsler, 1955).

Schuldberg and Boster's Two Dimensional Model of Thought Disorder

Schuldberg and Boster (1985) reanalyzed original thought disorder data from 106 of the 108 of Rapaport et al.'s subjects with schizophrenia and "preschizophrenia." By examining the structure and interrelationships of the original categories of disordered thinking, Schuldberg and Boster sought to specify the psychological processes underlying pathological Rorschach responses.

Schuldberg and Boster criticized Rapaport for his lack of clarity and conceptual confusion in describing thought disordered responses on the Rorschach. According to these researchers, nowhere was this confusion more prominent than in Rapaport's introduction of his concept of "distance" in the response process. Since the concept of distance formed a pivotal basis for Rapaport's conceptualizion of the psychological process underlying pathological responses on the Rorschach, Schuldberg and Boster set out to conduct an empirical analysis of the data on which Rapaport's theoretical construct was originally based.

Considering changes in diagnostic practices over the four decades since the Rapaport group conducted their seminal study, Schuldberg and Boster concluded that the original subjects were likely comprised of individuals suffering from schizophrenia, affective psychoses, and schizotypal and borderline personality disorders. The researchers used a smallest-space analysis technique (Guttman, 1968) which enabled them to form a spatial representation of the co-occurrence of 19 of Rapaport's categories across subjects. This technique tends to maximize the polarities between contrasting categories. The researchers then checked their results with a multi-dimensional scaling technique. Based on their statistical analysis, they found that the thought disordered responses of Rapaport's subjects did not form a unidimensional measure of pathological thinking and verbalization. Instead, they determined that two dimensions provided a reasonably economical representation of the structure of Rapaport's thought disorder scoring categories and his concept of distance.

The first dimension contained scoring categories having to do with objective versus personalized meaning. The low end of this dimension (Dimension 1) was typified by confusion responses, in which the subject struggles to find the real meaning inherent in the inkblots. Subjects who give confusion responses have difficulty interpreting the inkblots and instead attempt unsuccessfully to recognize the "pictures" that they believe the inkblots reflect. The high end of Dimension 1 is represented by self-reference and incoherence responses, two categories that reflect the intrusion of unrelated personal associations into the task. Thus,

Dimension 1 contrasts responses that reflect an overly literal approach to the blot (taking the inkblot as something "real" to be recognized) with responses that reflect the infusion of overly personalized (and idiosyncratic) meaning into the response process. Other examples of scores low on this dimension include position responses, reference ideas, and perseveration. Other scores at the high end of Dimension 1 are neologisms, and autistic logic.

Dimension 2 is related to verbal productivity and refers to rigid versus fluid sets in approaching the task. Responses at the low end of this dimension reflect excessive rigidity in being able to break a mental set to create new ideas. Perseveration and relationship verbalizations both reflect rigidity, stimulus-boundedness, and set shifting difficulties. At the high, or fluid, end of Dimension 2 are scoring categories that reflect a departure from the stimulus field and a focus on emotionally charged or overly specific associations. Confabulations and absurd responses have little grounding in the reality of the inkblot. Thus, categories low on this dimension reflect an excessive narrowing or rigidity in associational and attentional processes, whereas categories on the high end reflect a disorderly, unstable, and overly elaborated response process.

Schuldberg and Boster combined the Rapaport categories into a composite thought disorder score which correlated 0.29 with the Dimension 1 composite score (P = .002, one-tailed test) but not significantly with the Dimension 2 composite score (r = −0.09, P > .10). The authors concluded that the global amount of thought disorder manifested on the Rorschach is more closely associated with Dimension 1 than with Dimension 2. This correlation implies that disordered thinking, as measured by the Rorschach, may reflect primarily either those efforts to interpret the blots either in an inappropriately concrete manner or an overly personalized and idiosyncratic manner.

Schuldberg and Boster concluded that Dimension 2 was less clearly associated with thought disorder but more closely related to verbosity and the presence of affective illness. They also suggested that the test behaviors on this dimension are conceptually closer to Singer and Wynne's (1966) concept of communication deviance.

The researchers also noted that Goldstein's classic theory of schizophrenic concreteness (Goldstein and Scheerer, 1941) reflects verbalizations that would be low on both dimensions (i.e., rigidity and objective meaning responses), which are essentially two forms of pathological loss of distance from the inkblot. In other words, concreteness on the Rorschach could be characterized both by an inability to shift sets away from one focus of attention (low Dimension 2) and also by a stimulus-boundedness or tendency to ascribe literal meaning to the inkblots (low Dimension 1).

Responses that occur at the high end of both dimensions reflect marked departures from the stimulus as well as idiosyncratic associations to the inkblots. Scores high on Dimension 2 reflect fluid sets, characterized by overly elaborated responses that are independent of the stimulus qualities of the inkblot. Schuldberg and Boster indicated that this flamboyant, overassociational style has been shown to be diagnostic of borderline psychopathology (Singer, 1977; Singer and Larson, 1981) and mania (Solovay et al., 1987).

In their analyses, peculiar and queer responses did not emerge as part of a distinct dimension. Instead, these two scores were located near the center of both dimensions, supporting Rapaport's assertion that they reflect both increase and loss of distance.

Aronow, Reznikoff, and Moreland (1994) employed Schuldberg and Boster's dimensions as the chief organizing framework for their taxonomy of Rorschach thought disorder scores. They believed that the two-dimensional model organizes many types of scores in a parsimonious manner that can be linked to theory.

The two dimensions discussed here may seem to some readers quite similar and difficult to tease apart. On the one hand, "rigid responses" overlap with "objective meaning responses," both of which result from a stimulus-bounded relationship to the inkblot. On the other hand, "fluid" and "personal meaning responses" both reflect a lack of appreciation for the stimulus properties of the inkblot. Perhaps another way of characterizing the differences between the two dimensions is to think of Dimension 1 as a contrast between overinclusive thinking (fluid and shifting sets with permeable boundaries), on the one hand, and inflexible thinking (rigidly narrow sets with impenetrable boundaries), on the other. Dimension 2 could be thought of as a contrast between "autistic certainty" (i.e., expressed certainty in one's autistic associations), on the one hand, and "confused concreteness" (perplexity resulting in one's inability to interpret the inkblot playfully or imaginatively), on the other.

Some readers may also have difficulty understanding why certain scores were assigned to the specific categories. For example, some may ask why confusion and vague response were assigned to the "objective meaning" response category, if this category is supposed to reflect a tendency to respond to the blots in an overly concrete and literal manner. In other words, the link between the the subject's vagueness or confusion in responding to the inkblot and an overly concrete or objective response process may be a bit hard to grasp. The linkage is based on the fact that the subject attempts to interpret the blot in an overly objective, literal manner but fails in this effort and consequently becomes confused because he or she cannot "play" with the blots as representations, versus literal depictions, of some object in the real world.

In addition to the absence of any means of weighting or quantifying the severity of thought disorder, what is apparently missing in this two-dimensional classification is any category for peculiar or queer verbalizations. Schuldberg and Boster found that these scores did not load heavily on either of the dimensions, and as such, could reflect either a loss of or a pathological increase in distance. Aronow et al. make almost no mention of these scores either, making it difficult to know where to classify them in their system.

Psychoanalytic System of Burstein and Loucks

Burstein and Loucks developed this relatively obscure psychoanalytic approach in the 1970s. Much of the apparent motivation for their development of a new Rorschach system was their dissatisfaction with extant approaches to the Rorschach that were "theory free" and relied too heavily on a correlational sign approach to interpretation. Burstein and Loucks (1989) were explicit in their emphasis on the critical importance of blending a coherent theory of personality with the Rorschach test itself. In addition to the absence of a theoretical matrix for the Rorschach, they objected to "irrationalities and omissions" that they believed characterized contemporary approaches to scoring the Rorschach. Their answer to these identified difficulties was to develop a system strongly rooted in Kernberg's psychoanalytic ego psychological and object relational theories (1966, 1980).

The authors criticized all of the past and present Rorschach systems because of what they believed were conceptual omissions in the scoring categories and a lack of attention to subtle nuances of cognitive functioning on the Rorschach. For example, their system distinguishes between determinants that justify a percept on the basis of features of the inkblot that are physically present (e.g., form, color, shading) and those that interpret some imaginal aspect of the blot that is not physically present (such as movement and texture).

Each response is scored according to its location, cognitive complexity, determinants, form quality, content, interpersonal variables, psychosocial drive and defense effectiveness, and perceptual cognitive characteristics. It is this last category that is most relevant to the topic of thought disorder. Burstein and Loucks reserved the term "perceptual-cognitive characteristics" to describe a taxonomy of noteworthy perceptual and cognitive features of the response. What other systems classify as cognitive slippage, deviant verbalizations, or Special Scores, Burstein and Loucks called perceptual cognitive characteristics.

In evaluating a subject's thought organization, the authors stressed that it is critical to understand all aspects of cognitive-perceptual functioning. More than just assessing the subject's reality testing, the Rorschach clinician needs to evaluate the individual's style of information processing and success in responding appropriately to the inkblots. In order to capture both the adaptive and pathological aspects of perceiving, thinking, and reasoning, Burstein and Loucks created their own list of 23 idiosyncratically named categories of perceptual cognitive features. Their list included scoring categories such as (1) Affective Toning (AT); (2) Bizarre Content (BC); (3) Card Description (CD); (4) Concrete Perseveration (CP); (5) Contradiction of Reality; (6) Cluster Thinking (CT), for responses that contain ideas, themes, and concepts that are so severely interpenetrated or inappropriately combined; (7) Deterioration Color (DC); (8) Cut-off Detail (DX); (9) Egocentric Justification (EJ); (10) Fixed Concept Perseveration (FCP); (11) Loss of Distance (LD); (12) Lost Response (LR); (13) Popular (P); (14) Pantomime (PM), in which the subject substitutes actions and gestures for words (typically adjectives); (15) Perceptual Stabilization Defect (PSD), where the subject merged or confused figure and ground; (16) Predicate Thinking (PT); (17) Card Rejection (Rej); (18) Figure-Ground Reversal (S); (19) Incorporated on White Space ((S)); (20) Self-Reference (SR); (21) Transposition Response (TR), where the subject manages to avoid seeing a percept in its usual location by displacing it to another location; (22) Extreme Verbal Peculiarity (VP); and (23) Mild Verbal Peculiarity ((VP)).

Similar to the Holt system, each response is also scored on the basis of both the drive content and the level of defense effectiveness. Drive content is rated on two levels of severity, or degree of primitivity (levels 1 and 2). Defense effectiveness is determined on the basis of cultural and literary context, social appropriateness, and a shift from a covert level of drive manifestation or none at all.

In their text (1989), Burstein and Loucks included tables of Rorschach data for nine normative groups, which included both normal and clinical samples of adults and children. They indicated that each record was independently scored by two individuals who received a minimum of 12 hours of didactic instruction and practice with their scoring system. Their normative groups, based on sample sizes ranging from 20 to 241, included healthy adults; children ages 6 and 7; children ages 8, 9, and 10; children ages 11 and 12; foster adolescents, talented college students, referred children, hospitalized adults, and transsexuals.

The authors reported no reliability data, except to say that their raters were subjected to a "stringent and demanding" system for collecting normative data. Burstein and Loucks also did not report any data on the validity of their perceptual-cognitive scores or their scoring system in general.

By introducing a whole new set of symbols and an idiosyncratic scoring language, the authors have come close to throwing out the baby with the bath water. Instead of building on the psychoanalytically rooted systems of Rapaport, Schafer, or Holt, Burstein and Loucks created their own approach, which borrowed heavily from these earlier systems while renaming much of what was familiar and standard fare in Rorschach scoring systems. The majority of the perceptual-cognitive scoring categories are present in other systems in some form or another, but they appear here with new labels. The end result is an interesting approach but one that may ultimately contribute to further confusion in Rorschach scoring.

THE MENNINGER THOUGHT DISTURBANCE SCALES

Based primarily on the contributions of Rapaport, Holt, and Johnston and Holzman, Athey, Colson, and Kleiger (1992, 1993) developed a scoring system that not only reflected the full continuum of severity *among* different types of thought disorder scores but also expanded the concept of a range of severity *within* each type of thought disturbance category. In addition to describing six primary and four miscellaneous scoring categories, the Menninger group developed a set of supplementary measures. The "Supplementary Attitude Scales" involved measurement of two specific attitudes that were felt either to accompany, or, in some cases, to influence manifestations of thought disorder.

The Menninger team believed that existing systems did not adequately take into account the range of severity within each scoring category. To address this limitation, the group defined three levels of severity (mild, moderate, and severe) within each category. By defining levels of severity within each type of scoring category, the Menninger group hoped to study a broader range of thought pathology beyond what is traditionally described by the term "thought disorder." The group adopted the term "thought disturbance" to reflect the use of scales in studying the processes underlying each category and in describing the lower levels of severity that could conceivably aid in the early detection of different forms of psychopathology.

The major categories of deviant thinking in the proposed Menninger system include (1) Fabulized Combinations (FBC), (2) Confabulations (CFB), (3) Composite Figure (CPF), (4) Contamination (CTM), (5) Peculiar Verbalization (PEC), and (6) Disturbed Communication (DC). Two additional scales were devised to assess attitudinal factors that may influence the nature and degree of scorable thought disturbance. The first of these was called "Spoiling-Decompensation" to denote those instances in which the subject seems to passively "fall into" spoiled versions of what are potentially adequate responses. Spoiled responses occur when a subject is close to delivering an adequate response but suddenly veers off track and produces a spoiled version, typically in form level.

The second supplemental scale was called "Arbitrariness-Egocentricity" to describe instances in which a subject takes liberties with the task or the patient-examiner relationship in a self-indulgent, flippant, sarcastic, or oppositional manner. Even though the patient may be able to produce a more precise and appropriate response or demonstrate a more cooperative and self critical approach to the test, he or she fails to utilize these capacities. The subject may be motivated to say outrageous things for shock value or simply feel that he or she is exempt from the usual dictates of conventional logic, reality adherence, or social expectations. The subject may engage in excessive elaborations that fail to improve the response but feel that the examiner should be impressed with this verbosity. Such individuals are often described as arbitrary, egocentric, self-centered, and self-absorbed.

Viewing each thought disorder category along a continuum of severity is a novel and intriguing notion that distinguishes this approach. Although others have alluded to levels of severity within *certain* thought disorder categories, the Menninger Scales incorporated this concept into *each* scoring category. Thus, each manifestation of thought disorder exists along a continuum from mild to severe. Manifestations at the milder end of the continuum may be thought of as "disturbances in thinking," as opposed to the more forbidding term "thought disorder." Broadening the concept of "thought disorder" to capture more subtle manifestations of "thought disturbance" may provide an opportunity for studying vulnerabilities in thinking that may, under certain conditions, predispose an individual to more severe expressions of thought disorder.

Another interesting aspect of the Menninger scales is the intention to correlate traditional Rorschach thought disorder scores with test taking attitudes and psychological experiences that may be associated with different scoring categories. In particular, systematically scoring test taking attitude, separate from formal or content variables, is an interesting approach to studying an important aspect of the response process. Quantifying what has been, up to now, an elusive variable reflecting the subject's mind set in taking the test and responding to the examiner may help bring into focus important background issues that influence our interpretation of the response itself. Schafer (1954) addressed these factors in his discussion of the interpersonal dynamics in the testing situation:

It therefore seems important to note whether and to what extent the patient is kind or cruel to his responses, proud or disparaging, orderly or sloppy, generous or stingy, trivial or ambitious, flashy or drab, driven or inert, optimistic or pessimistic, and the like. How he presents, evaluates and treats his responses reflects how he presents, evaluates and treats himself inwardly and in his relationships [p. 46].

Stated somewhat differently, how serious is the subject in taking the Rorschach? Does the person "play" with the blots or, while taking them seriously, suddenly lose distance and abruptly depart from a realistic set? Is the subject trying to shock or control the examiner by willfully flouting reality and social convention? It seems quite possible that the Attitude Scales have the potential to answer some of these questions that have a bearing on how the response is eventually interpreted.

Unfortunately, the Menninger scales are lacking in empirical support. The diagnostic utility of a comprehensive intrascore continuum of disturbed thinking or the value of systematically evaluating the subject's attitude while giving a response, though intuitively appealing, are essentially unknown. Psychometrically, the scales remain untested.

In addition to the dearth of empirical support, there are other difficulties with the Menninger scales. By choosing to rename some of the traditional and more widely accepted scoring categories, our Menninger group may have contributed to the potential confusion that has plagued the Rorschach over the years. Namely, by creating new labels for scoring categories, researchers risk diluting the knowledge base of the Rorschach and making it difficult for comparisons across scoring systems.

In the end the validity of the Menninger scales will have to be determined by empirical investigations aimed at discovering whether this proposed new approach offers anything beyond that which is offered by the existing Rorschach thought disorder scales. Until such time, the Menninger Thought Disturbance Scales must be viewed as experimental and used cautiously in clinical settings.

TRIPARTITE CLASSIFICATION OF AUTISMS (TRAUT)

Wagner (Wagner and Rinn, 1994; Wagner, 1998) developed his TRAUT System as an empirical and theory-free method to detect "autisms" on the Rorschach. By "autisms" he meant the kinds of perceptual aberrations and absurd responses indicative of thought disorder. Wagner was critical of current trends in thought disorder scoring. He found Rapaport's "distance" rationale unwieldy and criticized the Comprehensive System for the absence of any logical rationale for viewing a response as thought-disordered. Furthermore, he believed that the WSUM6 in the Comprehensive System lacked sufficient temporal stability and sensitivity to identify subtle and transient manifestations of disordered thought. To remedy these perceived conceptual and psychometric difficulties, he developed the TRAUT as an empirical method that viewed "autisms" in the context of Rorschach task demands. Responses were considered autisms when the subject deviates from the explicit or implicit requirements. Viewing the Rorschach strictly as a test of perception, Wagner concluded that any violations of the standard instruction "Look at this and tell me what it might be" would signal autistic thinking. Thus, he limited his study to perceptual anomalies, while excluding linguistic oddities.

Wagner proposed three major categories of TRAUT which included what he termed "HYPOs," "HYPERs," and "RELERs." Each category subsumed four to six subdivisions, making for a total of 16 subscores in the TRAUT. HYPOs ("hypo-attentional errors") are scored when the subject ignores to varying degrees the shapes and contours of the blot and instead uses the stimuli as a springboard to private fantasies, images, or sensations. HYPERs ("hyper-attentional") reflect the subject's tendency to ignore differentially recognizable shapes and search for tiny, hidden, or impossible to find percepts to confirm private interpretations without regard for consensual validation. Whereas HYPOs ignore the reality of the blot, HYPERs overinterpret tiny or insignificant aspects of the inkblot. RELERs ("relationship errors") involve questionable relationships between and among inkblot areas based on spatial proximity instead of logically based events and objects. RELERs include inappropriate combinations (INCOM, FABCOM, CONTAM), ALOG, AND CONFAB responses.

Wagner summarized interrater reliability data from three studies in which reliability coefficients ranged from 80% to the high 90s for the three categories of scores. He also presented normative data from 19 samples, totaling 890 participants from various clinical groups, students, police academy cadets, pain clinic patients, and patients with brain damage. N's in each reference group ranged from 25 to 100 subjects.

None of Wagner's 175 nonpsychiatric subjects produced a single HYPO, whereas 50% of the inpatient schizophrenic patients gave at least one. RELERs were found in all clinical groups but most often in borderline patients (51% produced more than one).

Wagner has constructed a simple and practical method for screening disordered thinking on the Rorschach. His TRAUT System appears to offer a reliable alternative to traditional mainstream approaches. As with the other systems presented in this chapter, however, one should consider whether the advantages of adopting a new system outweigh the disadvantages of abandoning traditional and more broadly studied approaches. Although this decision is best left up to the reader, there appear to be several issues that might raise questions about the widespread utility of the TRAUT.

First, like each of the alternative systems in this chapter, the development of a new classification system with different names for old categories runs the risk of confusing clinicians who may already be sufficiently confused by thought disorder concepts and scoring categories. To adopt a new language, a system must offer a conceptual structure or some other unique feature that cannot be found in existing systems. Thus, the reader should ask whether Wagner's categories and rationale are sufficiently unique and not addressed adequately in other scoring systems. My belief is that much of what Wagner described can be accounted for with concepts and scoring categories that already exist. For example, many of the HYPOs he described could be conceptualized as variants of confabulatory thinking (see chapter 9). Furthermore, Wagner asserted that the TRAUT can account for unusual responses that other systems cannot. He gave the example of a patient who saw Card III as "These are two people beating on drums [usual side and middle Ds], and these are the drums that they threw in the air [top side red Ds]" (p. 740). When asked, the subject indicated that he saw the drums both as stationary and simultaneously as being in the air. Wagner described this response as a "heretofore unknown subspecies of RELERs" (p. 740). However, such a response can already be understood as a contamination (see chapter 11) in which two distinct conceptual and spatial frames of reference (here and there) are merged.

Finally, the exclusion of all deviant verbalizations seems to be a significant omission. Wagner indicated that verbalizations may be "interesting in their own right"; but perception, and not secondary verbalization, is what constitutes thought disordered responses. Wagner's strict adherence to a perceptual model of the Rorschach limits the TRAUT's ability to account for distinctly thought disordered responses such as peculiar and queer verbalizations, or DVs, incoherent responses, and neologisms. These linguistic anomalies have not only been widely associated with the presence of disordered thinking, but, as we shall see in chapter 13, they may have differential diagnostic implications as well.

PART

3

CONCEPTUAL AND

THEORETICAL

UNDERPINNINGS

Much has been written about the role that conceptualization and theory can play in making inferences and integrating data from psychodiagnostic testing (Schafer, 1954; Holt, 1968; Jaffee, 1990; Lerner, 1990, 1991; Sugarman, 1991; Kleiger, 1992a,b). Weiner (1986) indicated that conceptual approaches to the Rorschach not only offer clinicians the pleasure of understanding what lies behind test scores, but they also broaden the horizons of our knowledge of Rorschach psychology by encouraging clinicians to explore linkages between test variables and nontest behavior. In enumerating the benefits of conceptualization, Weiner concluded that coherent, integrated theories of personality functioning can contribute greatly to empirically validated inferences about the meaning of Rorschach data.

The following chapters examine ways in which researchers have attempted to link Rorschach thought disorder systems to underlying theories of mental functioning. Beyond developing reliable and valid measures of identifying disordered thinking, these conceptual approaches have focused on the meaning of disordered styles of thinking. Not content with restricting the meaning of thought disorder scores to their traditional definitions, the researchers in this section have attempted to

gauge the psychological processes that underlie different scoring categories and to link these to broader theories of personality and psychological functioning.

Chapter 8 highlights those approaches most noted for their conceptual and theoretical underpinnings. A pluralistic psychoanalytic framework, based on Pine's (1990) approach, will aid in organizing the
various approaches into different conceptual groupings. Chapters 9
through 12 review the psychological processes that are believed to be
represented by several of the major thought disorder scoring categories.

CHAPTER

8

PSYCHOANALYTIC UNDERSTANDING OF THOUGHT DISORDER SCORES

Five Psychologies Related to
Rorschach Thought Disorder Scores

By choosing to write about the four psychologies of psychoanalysis (drive theory, ego psychology, object relations, and psychology of the self) in an integrated way, Pine (1990) was attempting to evolve a unifying perspective that represented the diverse phenomena that clinicians encounter in their work. Almost all clinical phenomena can be understood from multiple perspectives; and at different times, one perspective may have greater narrative truth than others.

Pine's integrative approach to understanding clinical phenomena can be applied to Rorschach data as well (Kleiger, 1997). In what follows, thought disorder scores and systems will be examined through the four lenses of drive theory, ego psychology, object relations, and psychoanalytic self psychology. A "fifth" and overlapping lens, developmental psychology, will be added to complete the review. The analysis is not exhaustive and is intended only to be a sampling of the most prominent theory-based approaches to understanding the psychological processes associated with Rorschach thought disorder concepts.

PRIMARY PROCESS: ENERGY FORCES AND DISORDERED THINKING

Although Freud (1895) introduced the terms "primary" and "secondary" processes in his "Project for a Scientific Psychology," he laid out his principal understanding of these processes in "The Interpretation of Dreams" (1900). Freud maintained that primary process thinking involves energies that are uninhibited, free (vs. bound), and not neutralized, while secondary process energy is inhibited, bound, and neutralized. Freud equated primary process with both drive-dominated and wishful thought content. In his "Interpretation of Dreams," he described condensation, displacement, and symbolization as the formal mechanisms of dream work and primary process mental activity.

Various researchers attempted to conceptualize thought disorder as the intrusion of uninhibited drive energies, or primary process material, into secondary process thinking. The use of the Rorschach to study free versus bound psychic energy is represented primarily in the work of Holt (see chapter 4), and subsequently in the writings of Meloy (1984, 1986).

Holt: The Content and Mechanisms of Primary Process Thinking

Guided by dual-instinct theory, Holt originally considered only libidinal and aggressive drive material in response content as manifestations of primary process thinking. Blatant manifestations of primary process were given Level 1 scores, and more socialized expressions were scored Level 2. Holt was primarily interested in distinguishing between adaptive (e.g., creative) and maladaptive (e.g., thought disordered) regression in thinking.

Holt organized his formal scoring variables around Freud's three mechanisms of primary process—condensation, displacement, and symbolization. Holt noted that Freud said little about the primary process manifestations represented by peculiarities in verbalization. Because these were historically associated with thought disorder, Holt decided to include them under a separate formal scoring category made up of verbalization scores.

Holt believed that condensation was represented by Rorschach scores that reflected arbitrary and inappropriate combinations (fabulized and incongruous combinations, or "composition" responses) and contaminations. He indicated that displacement was represented by scores reflecting fluid or inappropriate associative thinking, such as chain, distant, and clang associations or inappropriate figures of speech, puns, or malapropisms. Finally, Holt presented several types of scores that he believed to be reflections of the mechanism of symbolization. He viewed symbolization as a special subtype of displacement in which socially shared objects and images became the structuralized representatives or substitutes for certain ideas.

Meloy: Linking Primary Process to Thought Disorder

Meloy (1986) examined the relationship between the concepts of primary process and formal thought disorder. He conceptualized two dimensions which he believed linked these terms together, one defined by the mechanism of condensation and the other by that of displacement.

Meloy pointed out how von Domarus's (1944) concept of "predicate thinking" and Arieti's "paleologic thinking" (1974) were related to the primary process mechanism of condensation. In Aristotelian logic, predicates denote only a similarity between objects or concepts, whereas in primitive paleologic, they denote identification or equivalence. According to Meloy, condensation is "a horizontal condensing of abstract, functional, and concrete representations that violates conceptual boundaries of Aristotelian logic and compels identification and equivalence of only similar representations" (p. 54). In this process, only the common element, represented by the predicate, becomes the dominant focus of attention, while other relevant characteristics of the objects are ignored.

Meloy understood disturbances in the association of ideas as thought disorder expressions of displacement. He inferred displacement from the rapid and fluid shifting of associations based on verbalizations or the symbols that are used. Reviewing the three levels of language, connotation (thoughts), denotation (things), and verbalization (symbols), Meloy suggested that the thought disordered individual experiences impairment in the ability to connote. Ideas are grouped together or associated on the basis of verbalization, not conceptual meaning. Thus, Meloy suggested that the second dimension linking primary process with formal thought disorder is the mechanism of displacement that represents "a vertical shift from abstractions (connotations) to objects and functions (denotations) to phonemes (verbalizations)" (p. 54).

Efforts to employ Freud's energic theory of primary and secondary processes to the study of thought disorder ran into conceptual difficulties. Holt's understanding of the role that drive processes played in the psychoanalytic theory of thinking changed significantly. Viewing the scores from his PRIPRO system as manifestations of unbound drive energies gave way to a revised understanding of primary process more consistent with ego psychology. Over time, Holt (1967) became a leading critic of Freud's economic, energy-based, model of primary process. He indicated that the concepts of neither primary nor secondary process could be understood without including structural aspects of psychic functioning. Energy concepts, by themselves, are meaningless without attending to the structures that generate, transmit, conduct, use, or transform the energy. Holt claimed that the formal manifestations of primary process thinking could be viewed as structural components without invoking the concept of free versus bound cathexis. Eventually, Holt (1989) concluded that the phenomenon of drive-dominated thinking reflects the operation of the pleasure principle without the need to invoke the concept of drive neutralization.

Holt (1989) struggled with certain discontinuities between psychoanalytic theory of primary process and some of the empirical findings that his PRIPRO system yielded. For example, he eventually questioned the theoretical basis for entertaining two degrees or levels of primary process scores. Holt suggested that Level 1 scores might more accurately reflect primary process thinking, while Level 2 responses might be more appropriately thought of as manifestations of secondary process thinking. Holt wondered whether socialized and attenuated Level 2 expressions of wishful content could really be considered primary process manifestations at all.

Holt also questioned the theoretical basis for understanding cases in which thought products contain wish-related content but are neither illogical nor inconsistent with reality. Likewise, he wondered about the theoretical underpinnings of the reverse case, in which a thought product evidences no sign of drive-dominated content but reveals lapses in secondary process logic and realism. Although Holt had essentially resolved this question by separating the formal from the content variables, either of which was a sufficient criterion for primary process activity, he wondered about the logic of doing so. He suggested that primary and secondary processes may be best understood as three continua: one reflecting wishfulness or drive-dominated content and the others reflecting consistency with reality and logical clarity (Holt, 1989).

If there are different components of primary process ideation, one might ask whether primary process form and content are equally consistent with the presence of thought disorder. In terms of disordered thinking, Harrow and Quinlan (1985) demonstrated that the presence of drive-dominated content was not a key factor in thought disorder, whereas bizarre-idiosyncratic thinking (reflecting disruptions in formal aspects of thinking) was much more characteristic of psychotic patients.

Thought Disorder as a Disturbance in Ego Functioning

Ego psychology is probably the most widely used model for understanding the conceptual underpinnings of thought disorder. Links between ego pathology and psychotic disturbances in thinking and reality testing were hinted at by Freud (1911), before he developed his tripartite model of the mind; the links were subsequently elaborated by Tausk, who viewed schizophrenia as a loss of ego boundaries and deficiency in ego strength (1919). After the advent of his structural model (Freud, 1923), Freud stressed that disturbances in the ego play a determining role in symptom formation in schizophrenia. Hartmann (1953) extended the role of ego impairments in the process of schizophrenia but indicated that it was important to specify which ego functions were impaired. Federn (1952) developed a distinct school of ego psychology by attempting to apply psychoanalytic principles to understanding psychotic patients. Although his concept of "ego" differed significantly from the "ego" of Freud and Hartmann, Federn used the term "ego boundaries," or loss of ego boundaries, to explain schizophrenic symptomatology.

Early ego psychologists enumerated lists of various ego functions (Freud, 1937; Hartmann, Kris, and Loewenstein, 1946; Bellak, 1949). Beres (1956) included seven functions in his list, which included a separate category for "thought processes"; Arlow and Brenner (1964) also listed "thought" as a central function of the ego. With thought and reality testing being key domains of the ego, it naturally followed for "disturbances in thinking" to be considered a constituent of ego functioning as well.

Rapaport and Holt

Rapaport viewed psychoanalytic ego psychology as the only theoretical guide with sufficient depth and breadth to illuminate the nature of thought processes. He was an early critic of a theory of psychic energy that did not include structural mechanisms as well. Motivational considerations alone could not adequately explain normal or pathological thought organization. Not only was the concept of "ego" necessary to understand the vicissitudes of thinking, but Rapaport insisted that disturbances in thought processes involve all aspects of thinking, including the component ego functions of perception, attention, concentration, concept formation, and reasoning.

In discussing the cognitive processes that underlie the formation of Rorschach responses, Rapaport focused on two related aspects of ego functioning, perception and association. He used the term "association" to mean an ideational process whereby the subject draws on internal images, ideas, and memories in response to the stimulus inkblot. According to Rapaport, the response process involves a delicate "cogwheeling" of the processes of perception and association. When these critical ego processes are not in synch, the subject's associations may wander excessively from the inkblot or become overly constrained by the perceptual reality of the blot. As was seen in chapter 3, Rapaport believed that all thought disorder scores could be understood in terms of either a pathological increase or loss of perceptual distance, or some combination of the two, from the inkblot. Disturbances in thinking were always related to the perceptual reality of the inkblot. Subjects who showed little consideration for basic features of the inkblot, such as contour, size, color, and so on, or embellished their responses with details that went beyond these basic features were said to have responded with an increase of distance from the inkblot.

In contrast, subjects who failed to view the inkblot as a symbol or representation of reality and, instead, took the inkblot as a concrete reality that could not be altered or "played with" imaginatively, were said to have responded with a loss of distance from the inkblot. These subjects were said to have treated the inkblot as if it were something real and immutable. The tendency to lose distance from the inkblot leads the subject to attempt to discover or recognize meaning in the inkblot (instead of interpreting it). Although fabulized combinations typically exemplify such a loss of distance, Rapaport's prototypical example of a pathological loss of distance was the DW response, in which the subject bases his or her response on a single detail that is taken as an immutable reality simply because it is present.

Any discussion of Rapaport's ego psychological understanding of Rorschach thought disorder scores would be incomplete without once again mentioning Holt's PRIPRO system. Implicit in Holt's approach is a measure of ego strength, or the adaptive capacity to "regress in the service of the ego." This capacity to employ primary process ideation in a more attenuated and modulated form indicates a healthy ego that is resilient and capable of creative problem solving.

Weiner and Exner

Weiner's (1966) psychodiagnostic study of schizophrenia was based on the premise that the diagnosis of this psychotic disorder is essentially a diagnosis of impairment in ego functioning. Weiner indicated that effective secondary process thinking requires the integration of a number of ego capacities, including cognitive focusing, reasoning, concept formation, and relation to reality. Impairment in any combination of these may gain expression in different forms of Rorschach thought disorder.

COGNITIVE FOCUSING. Efficient thinking necessitates an ability to scan information selectively, to separate essential from nonessential information, and to exclude that which is irrelevant. Weiner divided cognitive focusing problems into those that he called "failure to establish a focus" and those he referred to as "failure to maintain a focus." Failure to establish a focus includes difficulties selecting for attention the most relevant aspects of the stimulus field and adjusting one's attention accordingly. Such a failure on the Rorschach may be associated with unusual location choice where the impaired capacity to identify essential details of a situation leads to choosing atypical location areas. A subject who fails to establish a cognitive focus may also produce perserverative responses. Here the subject is unable to shift attentional focus as the stimulus qualities of the different inkblots change. Without this ability to alter focus, one may be doomed to echoing previous percepts, even if these are no longer relevant to the stimulus qualities of the present inkblot.

Failure to maintain a focus consists of the intrusion of irrelevant external or internal stimuli onto a previously established set, which may lead to the overt expression of idiosyncratic associations or erratic flow and pace of associations. Idiosyncratic associations may actually reflect a deficiency in screening as the individual is unable to prevent deviant associations from intruding into the response. According to Weiner, two categories of Rorschach verbalizations may reflect a failure to maintain cognitive focus. The first he called "dissociation," which Bleuler described as a disconnect or lack of relationship between adjacent ideas. Instead of the typical process of associating ideas on the basis of contiguity or similarity, thought disordered individuals may assume an identity on the basis of this similarity or contiguity and inappropriately substitute one idea for the other. Weiner said that dissociation could also be expressed in the form of irrelevant and loosely connected thoughts. The inappropriate phrase Deviant Response (DR) category in the Comprehensive System (Exner, 1986a, 1993) (e.g., "It looks like a bat; my neighbor shot one in his backyard") and vague and looseness scores in the TDI are examples of a loss of cognitive focus, leading to a dissociation between ideas and the intrusion of irrelevant material into the response.

The other Rorschach scores that Weiner suggested reflect a failure to maintain cognitive focus are those deviant verbalizations that result from the intrusion of odd forms of expression that disturb the flow of communication. Weiner originally included peculiar and queer verbalizations under this category of cognitive focusing failure and later, with Exner, elaborated these into DV and DR categories in the Comprehensive System.

REASONING. Reasoning is a critical aspect of thinking in which one attempts to draw inferences from one's experiences and observations and look for logical connections between objects and events in the environment. Weiner organized reasoning disturbances under three subcategories, each of which is related to some extent to predicate thinking. Grouping test indices of impaired reasoning under the headings of "overgeneralized thinking," "combinative thinking," and "circumstantial thinking" lends a great deal of clarity to conceptualizing varieties of disordered reasoning.

Weiner defined "overgeneralized thinking" as overinterpreting the meaning or significance of data and then jumping to incorrect conclusions based on minimal evidence. Part of this process may involve embellishing the meaning of experiences or observations beyond what the stimulus properties in question can justify. Regarding the Rorschach, Weiner included fabulization, confabulation, and absurd Dd responses as test indices of overgeneralized thinking.

There is no better example of the primary process mechanism condensation than "combinative thinking." Weiner subsumed incongruous combinations, fabulized combinations, and contaminations under the heading of combinative thinking. When drafting the categories of Special Scores in the Comprehensive System, Weiner and Exner did away with the term "combinative thinking" and instead used the term "inappropriate combinations" to describe this group of condensation-based scores.

"Circumstantial thinking" involves inferring real relationships from coincidental aspects of the testing situation, the inkblots, or related associations to them. Circumstantial thinking is an extreme example of the broader category of predictate thinking. However, in circumstantial thinking the subject not only bases conclusions on incidental and nonessential pieces of data or evidence but makes an explicit statement to this effect. Autistic Logic, number, and position responses are all examples of circumstantial thinking.

CONCEPT FORMATION. Concept formation involves the ability to interpret experience at appropriate levels of abstraction. Impairments in conceptual thinking reveal themselves in either the extremes of concreteness or overinclusiveness. In either case, the individual has difficulty focusing on the most salient and relevant features of a given situation. Weiner suggested that two subtypes of idiosyncratic symbolism responses, symbolic interpretation of shading or color and symbolic interpretation of concrete images may represent deficits in the capacity to form concepts at appropriate levels of abstraction. Weiner also described another category of response that reflects overinclusive conceptual thinking. He called this "abstract preoccupation," in which the subject is overly focused on highly abstract ideas at the expense of attending to more relevant, and less abstract, details. These are typically highly confabulated responses in which the subject is preoccupied with vague forces or powers without specific content. Formless M responses may also reflect an impairment in level of abstraction.

It would be incorrect to assume that the Comprehensive System is formally rooted in an ego psychological model. Exner makes it clear that the Comprehensive System is atheoretical. However, the conceptual underpinning of Exner's Special Scores is anchored squarely in a model of cognitive and perceptual problem solving, which, in my view, makes it a contemporary descendant of an ego psychological model. Despite their numerous differences, Exner and Rapaport shared a conviction that the Rorschach is fundamentally a test that reveals psychological structure.

Although Exner does not employ the language of psychoanalytic ego psychology when providing an interpretive blueprint for his "cognitive triad", the concepts he uses are certainly consistent with the cognitive operations described by Weiner when he elucidated the component processes that comprise the ego functions of thought processes and relation to reality. Weiner suggested that "thought processes" consist primarily of cognitive focusing, reasoning, and concept formation. He viewed "relation to reality" as a perceptual process made up of the capacities to (1) test reality (i.e., perceptual accuracy and conventional judgment) and (2) maintain an adequate sense of reality (i.e., sensing one's inner experience of self and surrounding environment as being real). Exner's (1993) "cognitive triad" consists of three related clusters of functions, which include information processing, cognitive mediation, and ideation.

Although it is a broader category, "information processing" overlaps with Weiner's "cognitive focusing" variable. "Mediation" is heavily influenced by perceptual processes which, like "relation to reality," involve the capacity to make accurate amd conventional responses. Finally, "ideation," as a conceptual process that searches for relationships and meaning, includes both "reasoning" and "concept formation."

In terms of Rorschach thought disorder scoring, Exner's critical Special Scores and WSUM 6 make up a key component of his ideation cluster. As detailed in chapter 6, Level 1 and 2 Special Scores are organized along a continuum of cognitive dysfunction ranging from mild cognitive slippage, to more serious expressions of faulty thinking, to severe instances of cognitive impairment. Whether using the language of cognitive or psychoanalytic ego psychology, conceptually Exner's Special Scores may be viewed unequivocally as ego or cognitively-mediated indices of disordered thinking.

THOUGHT DISORDER AND OBJECT RELATIONS

There are a number of conceptual linchpins between ego psychological and object relational interpretations of thought disorder. For example, Blatt and Ritzler (1974) pointed out how overinclusive thinking could be understood as an impairment in both concept and boundary formation. The incapacity to maintain conceptual boundaries between separate events, frames of reference, and objects includes problems in distinguishing between self and others as well.

Boundary disturbances have been historically linked to psychoses, with special reference to pathology in the sphere of the ego. Tausk (1919) first used the term "ego boundary" to describe the schizophrenic phenomenon of "merging self into other" (Bleuler, 1911), a concept that presaged object relations theories. Much later, Federn (1952) elaborated on the concept of "ego boundaries" but greatly expanded its meaning. In writing about psychotherapy with psychotic patients, Bychowski (1952) introduced the term "fluidity of ego boundaries" to describe the characteristic ego weakness found in schizophrenia. Bychowski considered the lack of differentiation of the ego from the external world to account for much of the symptomatology in schizophrenia. Blatt and Wild (1976) later suggested that many of the disturbances associated with schizophrenia, such as overinclusiveness, thought insertion and broadcasting, attentional deficits, depersonalization, and hallucinations, could be explained in terms of boundary disruptions.

Early object relational theorists recognized that boundary disturbances occurring between parent and infant will gain expression in pathological ego functioning (Klein, 1930; Isaacs, 1948). These observations suggest that internalizing pathological relational paradigms has adverse impact on the organization and coherence of thought process.

Boundary Disturbances and
Rorschach Thought Disorder

Based on the ideas of Federn (1952) and Bychowski (1952), Zucker (1952) used the Rorschach and two other projective tests (Mosaic and Draw-A-Person) to operationalize and investigate the presence of ego boundary impairment in a group of inpatient and outpatient schizophrenic subjects. Zucker described five areas of boundary disturbances, including contamination, fluid and hazy contours, extension of the ego field, sensitivity to external stimuli, and disturbed body image. Despite the presence of thought disorder indicators in both groups, Zucker found that his hospitalized subjects demonstrated more severe boundary disturbance than the ambulatory group.

Jortner (1966) used the Rorschach to demonstrate that "broken boundaries of body image," and particularly those responses in which the inside and outside of a person were viewed simultaneously in a single percept (i.e., transparency responses), discriminated between a group of schizophrenic and nonschizophrenic patients. Fisher and Cleveland (1958) devised a Rorschach scoring system for two variables, which they called "barrier" and "penetration," that assessed the definiteness of the body-image boundary.

Blatt and Ritzler (1974) furthered the linkage between ego psychological and object relational approaches by conceptualizing key Rorschach thought disorder scores as different degrees of disruption in boundaries (between self and others and internal and external experiences), thus integrating both Tausk's and Federn's conceptions of "ego boundaries." The focus of their seminal study was on the diagnostic significance of different levels of boundary disturbances and the relationships between varying degrees of boundary violations, different Rorschach thought disorder scores, and level of psychopathology. They accurately predicted that levels of boundary disturbance would correlate with disruptions in reality testing, impairment in cognitive processes, interpersonal relations, and response to treatment.

Blatt and Ritzler's strategy was to define three traditional thought disorder scores as different levels of boundary disturbances. As independent percepts illogically combined because of spatial contiguity, fabulized combinations were posited to represent the process of inferring an inappropriate relationship between unrelated events, experiences, or objects. No merging or fusion of percepts takes place; each can be accurately perceived but unrealistically related to one another. In confabulation responses (Rapaport's broader definition), the boundary disruption was said to occur between external perception and internal experience. Thus, Blatt and Ritzler drew a relationship between reality testing, or the distinction between inner and outer phenomena, and confabulatory thinking. Finally, they inferred that the contamination response reflects a loss of the boundary between independent objects, concepts, or images. In object relational terms, contaminatory thinking marks a potential loss of capacity to differentiate self from others.

In their retrospective analysis of clinical records of patients treated intensively at Yale Psychiatric Institute and the Menninger Clinic, Blatt and Ritzler found that levels of thought disorder, as defined by degree of boundary disruption (represented in increasing level of severity by fabulized combinations, confabulations, and contaminations), were related to level of psychopathology. The greater the boundary disturbance, the more severe the level of psychopathology. Furthermore, the greater the boundary disturbance, the more severely cognitively and interpersonally impaired these patients were judged to be. Relatedly, more severe boundary disturbances were found to be associated with more distorted measures of object relations (in this case, human movement and human content scores on the Rorschach) and poorer response to treatment.

Lerner, Sugarman, and Barbour (1985) extended Blatt and Ritzler's paradigm to study the developmental continuum of boundary disturbances and levels of thought disorder among neurotic, borderline (outpatient and hospitalized samples), and schizophrenic patients. They found that boundary disturbances (represented by the three categories of thought disorder scores) were present in all four patient groups and that quantitatively, the hospitalized patients had a greater total of weighted boundary disturbance scores (and thought disorder scores) than the nonhospitalized patients. Their most interesting finding offered confirmation for their original hypothesis that the confabulation score distinguished the inpatient borderlines from all other groups (reflecting a disturbance in maintaining a boundary between inner and outer), whereas the contamination response characterized the schizophrenic group (reflecting a developmentally more severe disturbance in maintaining the boundary between self and other).

Blatt, Tuber, and Auerbach (1990) found one Rorschach measure of the quality of interpersonal relationships to be highly correlated with the severity of psychopathology, and thought disorder scores in particular, in a group of adolescent patients in residential treatment. The Mutuality of Autonomy Scale (MOA) (Urist, 1977) is a seven-point ordinal scale that assesses the quality of object relations by evaluating Rorschach interactions between human figures, animals, and objects. The highest MOA scores (5, 6, and 7) are scored when the interaction reflects a severe imbalance in power, envelopment and fusion, and a heightened degree of malevolence and aggression. Using the MOA, Blatt et al. found that malevolent content portrayed in interactions on the Rorschach is significantly related to fabulized combinations, confabulations, and contaminations. The correlation was highest between these malevolent interactions and confabulation scores.

In a similar study, Berg, Packer, and Nunno (1993) used the MOA to examine the relationship between pathology in thinking and object relationships in patients with schizophrenic, borderline, and narcissistic disorders. However, unlike Blatt, Berg and her colleagues looked at the relationship between scores on the MOA and critical Special Scores in the Comprehensive System. Using a composite measure of Rorschach thought disorder (WSUM 6), Berg et al. established empirical support for the observations of earlier theorists (Klein, 1930; Isaacs, 1948; Kernberg, 1967) who held that there was a relationship between pathological object relations and disturbances in thinking. Berg et al. found highly significant correlations between composite WSUM 6 scores and the most pathological scores on the MOA (MOA 5, MOA 6, and MOA 7). In terms of individual scores, the team found the highest correlation between ALOG, FABCOM 2, and INCOM 2 and MOA 5, 6, and 7 scores, which, according to Berg and her colleagues, suggests that pathological object relations are associated with defensive failures that cannot prevent primary process manifestations from intruding into secondary process thinking.

Examining the degree of overlap between MOA and the Special Scores in the Comprehensive System, Berg et al. found that, up through MOA 6, the two scales measure different facets of psychological functions. However, the severe degree of fusion and aggressive envelopment defined by MOA 7 scores indicate that there will be a significant overlap between MOA 7 and critical Special Scores.

In an earlier paper, Smith (1980) attempted to synthesize object relations theories of Klein, Mahler, Kernberg, and Rinsley with Rorschach measures of thought organization and reality testing. He used object relational concepts to delineate three levels of development within the psychotic range: autism, symbosis, and differentiation. According to Mahler's theory (Mahler, Pine, and Bergman, 1975), Smith described the autistic patient as living in an "objectless" world, without concern for external objects. He hypothesized that formal Rorschach scores such as F-responses, which signal a withdrawal of interest from external reality, and contamination scores would characterize this most primitive level of functioning. In contrast, symbiotic functioning would be characterized by Rorschach content reflecting objects that are connected, arbitrarily joined together, or by confabulatory responses, which manifest a blurring of one's internal representations with one's perceptions of external reality. Thus, Smith proposed that fabulized combinations and confabulations with merger themes would typify the symbiotic level of relatedness.

Several other research scales have been developed to assess object relation phenomena. These include Kwawer's Borderline Interpersonal Relations Scale (Kwawer, 1980) and Ipp's Developmental Object Relations Scale (1986), and Coonerty's Separation-Individuation scale (1986). Each of these demonstrates an association between the pathological points on their scales (reflecting such developmentally regressive phenomena as symbiotic merger, engulfment, enmeshment, and disintegration) and inappropriate combinatory, confabulatory, and contaminatory thinking on the Rorschach. It should be noted, however, that these scales are rooted in a developmental model that has been challenged by more contemporary infant research (Stern, 1985).

Thought Organization, Object Relations,
and Transference Enactments

In a series of intriguing papers, Athey (Athey, 1974, 1986; Athey, Fleischer, and Coyne, 1980) explored how patients' regressed thought organization, as seen on the Rorschach, parallels the way they experience object relations in the transference in psychotherapy. In attempting to conceptualize the relationship between thought organization and object relations, Athey found Blatt and Ritzler's "boundary deficit" hypothesis overly narrow and unable to adequately explain the process by which relational and ideational boundries become deficient. Furthermore, he contrasted the content and form of a patient's thinking as a way of demonstrating that representation of relational boundaries (reflected in the patient's thought content "I feel fused with you," which, by definition, implies an inherent self-other distinction) and the formal structure of conceptual boundaries (reflected in a thought disorder score such as contamination) do not always run parallel.

Athey also felt that the boundary deficit hypothesis did not go far enough in explicating the specific psychological and relational processes that underlie Rorschach thought disorder indicators. His 1974 study demonstrated the value of using these scores as indices of qualitatively different types or levels of relatedness in treatment. According to Athey, thought disorder indicators are important "in assessing the emergence of qualitatively different levels of regressed psychological processes in the stream of thought and their operation in the patient's experiences with and representations of object relations with other persons during treatment" (p. 162). In particular, Athey sought to conceptualize qualitative distinctions in the organization of thought that can help clinicians anticipate various transference paradigms that might emerge in psychotherapy.

Athey looked at detailed therapy process notes of two schizophrenic patients, one characterized by the presence of contamination responses and the other by confabulation. He also commented on the relational implications of fabulized combinations that occurred in the protocol of one of these patients. Athey suggested that the content of some fabulized combinations might reflect a preoccupation with certain kinds of self-other relationships. For example, the Card VIII response, "A weasel climbing on a butterfly," may reveal a preoccupation with sado-masochistic relational paradigms.

Athey characterized the confabulatory mode as excessive fantasy imposed on a reality that is initially perceived in an accurate manner. He described transference implications of patient B, whose Rorschach was characterized by numerous confabulation responses, as those of an individual whose perceptions of the therapist were colored by affect-laden fantasies. When this patient became angry, she reacted with an outpouring of affect-dominated fantasies of rejection by the therapist. What initially began as an accurate perception of an interpersonal event was magnified and "confabulated" into something that departed from reality but was consistent with the patient's interpersonal preoccupation.

Finally, Athey described the contaminatory mode as a loss of distinction between and condensation of different frames of reference. According to Athey, "frames of reference" are conceptual dimensions by which reality is represented internally as structures. Examples include time (past vs. present vs. future); space (here vs. there); levels of language (reference vs. referent vs. symbol); relational representations (self vs. other, object 1 vs. object 2). Athey characterized the contaminatory transference as an extreme form of fusion with the therapist in which the relationship with a separate figure is condensed and experienced as an alteration in an internal state. He gave the example of a patient who was terrified that she had physically harmed her therapist because she had condensed the *internal fantasy* with the *external reality* of injuring the therapist.

Athey pointed out that different levels of psychotic experience may occur in the "confabulatory" and "contaminatory" modes. However, he also indicated that the same patient may fluctuate between different levels of experience, with different relational implications associated with different levels of thought (dis)organization. For example, progression from the contaminatory to the confabulatory mode may signal the capacity to differentiate internal self from other representations. The diagnostician should pay attention to the conditions which facilitate this kind of progressive shift. On the other hand, regression from a fabulized combinatory to confabulatory mode of experience involves losing the reality basis for representing relationships and replacing reality with idiosyncratic affect-laden fantasies. The diagnostic understanding of the conditions that make an individual vulnerable to such a regression in functioning has important treatment implications.

Athey's 1986 article is a sophisticated and abstruse extension of his earlier efforts to capture the interface between structural and object relational aspects of thought organization. In his later elaboration, Athey proposed a developmental continuum of five superordinate levels of thought organization through which individuals could represent object relations and enact patterns of transference in psychotherapy (reviewed later in this chapter).

Disordered Thinking and Self-Experience

A useful way to conceptualize the psychology of the self is in terms of a number of related dimensions or continua of self-experience. Kohut and Wolf (1978) suggested several self-related dimensions which distinguished

different syndromes of self pathology, including "cohesion" vs. "fragmentation"; "vitality" vs. "enfeeblement"; and "order" vs. "chaos."
Likewise, Stern (1985) proposed a tentative list of experiences available to
the nascent self in infancy and necessary for the formation of a sense of
core self which included (1) "self-agency," (2) "self-coherence," (3) "self-
affectivity," and (4) "self-history."

These lists and dimensions can be combined to form a more comprehensive list of dimensions of self-experience that provide a structural
framework for understanding healthy and pathological expressions of
the self. For example, the self can be conceptualized along the dimensions of (1) "cohesion" vs. "fragmentation," (2) "integration" vs. "splitting," (3) "authenticity/realness" vs. "inauthenticity/ falseness," (4)
"vitality" vs. "depletion," (5) "internal agency" vs. "external locus of
control," (6) "differentiation" vs. "fusion," and (7) "continuity" vs.
"discontinuity." This list of dimensions is by no means exhaustive, but
I believe that it captures essential structural components of self-experience
that may be reflected in some prominent Rorschach thought disorder
categories.

Arnow and Cooper (1988) explored the Rorschach psychology of the
self but did not specifically address the interface between disordered
thinking and disordered self-experiences. Instead, they conceptualized
some of the Rorschach features associated with the self-pathological
syndromes described by Kohut and Wolf (1978). For example, they
referred to the "overstimulated self" in which the selfobject may have
excessive needs for self-display and admiration and may end up using
the self as an extension. Arnow and Cooper suggested that the grandiose
fantasies of these patients may be seen in both the content and structure
of the response. Structurally, these individuals may feel the need to provide original and distinct responses that exceed their integrative or synthetic capacities. Again, we may view this as another juncture between
an "ego" capacity and some aspect of "self-" or, as described in the previous section, "relational" experience. Arnow and Cooper hypothesize
that these grandiose individuals may overstrive to produce unsuccessful
combinative responses that are not well justified by the realities of the
inkblot. Thus W+ confabulations and fabulized combinations, with
poor or unconvincing form level, may reflect the needs of an overstriv-
ing grandiose self that is unable to harness or deploy these needs for
adaptive purposes.

Arnow and Cooper suggest that Kohut and Wolf's "fragmenting self"
may reveal itself in a psychotic confabulatory response such as "It's a
person blowing into pieces before my eyes" (Arnow and Cooper, 1988,
p. 65). Other expressions of "fragmentation" may be embedded in various incongruous combinations such as "A person without a head" or

Rapaport's "oligophrenic" response, where the subject sees only a portion of an object that is normally seen as a whole entity. Finally, the fragmentation response, as scored in the TDI, may reveal the language equivalent of a fragmented core self-experience, in which the splintered form of linguistic expression itself mirrors one's subjective sense of incoherence or disintegration.

The hypothesized dimension of "integration" vs. "splitting" addresses the degree to which discrepant self-experiences (or, for that matter, object representations) are cognitively woven together and affectively tolerated as opposed to walled off and unintegrated. Certain kinds of inappropriate combination responses may reflect splits or a lack of integration in the self. Schafer (1954) listed "integratedness of scores, images, and attitudes" as one of six criteria for judging the overall success or failure of defensive and adaptive operations reflected by an individual Rorschach response. Schafer indicated that the dramatic opposition of images in a single response signals a failure in the individual's adaptive and defensive functioning. He gave as examples of such a lack of integratedness the Rorschach responses "A pink polar bear," "A horrible monster with shriveled arms," and "An infant with a fang" (Schafer, 1954, pp. 180–181). Although Schafer approached his analysis from a classical impulse-defense tradition, a self-psychological interpretation of these incongruous combinations, as they would be scored in the TDI and Comprehensive System, might suggest a lack of integration between disparate aspects of self-experience.

The dimension of "differentiation" vs. "fusion" reflects an inherent overlap between this key dimension of self-experience and a structural component of relational representation. Internal representations of merger, engulfment, enmeshment, and fusion capture both the gestalt of a paradigmatic object relational experience, and, at the same time, an irreducible subjective sense of self. Thus, as seen in the last chapter, any of the thought disorder scores that have condensation as a base may represent not only relational paradigms but also an ambience of self-experience.

Lerner (1988) conceptualized Rorschach manifestations of the dimension of "authenticity" vs. "inauthenticity" when he wrote about the "false self." Drawing on the work of Winnicott (1961) and Schachtel (1966), and his earlier work (Lerner and Lerner, 1980), Lerner theorized that the passive compliance with, and accommodation to, environmental demands, that is so characteristic of the false self, may be reflected by the FCarb response (the Rapaportian subtype of the incongruous combination response), in which the subject clings to the inappropriate inclusion of color, simply because the environment has presented it. Winnicott (1961) suggested that the development of the self is stifled when the individual is unable to maintain a distance from the environment and becomes, instead, overly dependent on it. Lerner viewed FCarb responses as a loss of adaptive detachment or perspective in which the individual has abandoned a more objective, critical, judgmental attitude. Events in one's life or the dictates of significant objects are not critically examined but accepted as so, based on their most obvious, surface qualities. The compliant self passively goes along with the implicit demand to accept an external world that is in some ways incongruous with internal perceptual experience, and is left with a sense of unreality or falseness. Thus the response "A pink polar bear" may simultaneously reflect a lack of critical thinking and a subjective sense of falseness or unreality.

Mayman (1977) teased out different nuances of meaning of human movement responses on the Rorschach. In addition to explicating the fantasy-ideational, kinesthetic, and relational aspects of M responses, Mayman suggested that certain kinds of human movement responses may reveal something about an individual's capacity for empathy. Mayman distinguished between empathic and narcissistic relatedness based on identification. Mayman stated that empathy implies a two-way process in which self-other boundaries are maintained, while identification suggests that the separate existence of the object is not respected. Based on an active identification with others, narcissistic relatedness involves the attribution, or projection, of characteristics of the self on to the other. Thus, based on theory and clinical observations, Mayman reasoned that individuals who relate to others on a narcissistic level tend to produce M responses that are infused with aspects of the individuals themselves. Furthermore, Mayman suggested that these M responses are largely fabulized and described with vividness and conviction. The subject may become absorbed in these M's, enlivening them with attributes quite distant from the reality of the inkblot. This process was dramatically portrayed by an envious and self-absorbed woman, quite dissatisfied with her life, who responded to Card VII:

> Could be two matrons having a talk over coffee at 10:00 in the morning, and I suppose the bottom is symbolic of the thread that binds them together as homemakers, wives. They're in the same bridge club, bound together by all those ties. Kinda haughty and pretentious with their hands out. They're wealthy too. Pigtails up makes me think of uppity society women.

Projective identification is a concept that bridges object relations and self psychology. Lerner and Lerner (1980) and Cooper (1983) reviewed the Rorschach manifestations of this defensive process in borderline patients. The Lerners suggested that confabulatory responses involving human figures with poor form level indicated the tendency to blur boundaries between self and other, which permitted the placement of disowned aspects of the self into the other. Lerner (1988) elaborated on this theme when writing about narcissistic and self-pathology, by proposing that the confabulated human response, scored at an F– or Fw– level, indicates a severe self-other blurring with a defensive aim to control the other.

Thought Disorder and Developmental Processes

Werner's (1948) orthogenetic principle provides a basis for understanding the developmental unfolding of all mental and behavioral phenomena from diffuse and global to increasingly differentiated and integrated levels of functioning. With this principle in mind, developmental perspectives of Rorschach thought disorder scores cannot be separated from the various conceptual foundations reviewed in the last sections. Whether viewed from the interlocking lenses of the shift from primary to secondary process, adaptive regression in the service of the ego, levels of object representation, or aspects of self-experience, the contrast between pathological and reality-based thinking typically implies developmental processes. Although Peterfreund (1978) pointed out the problems in assuming an isomorphic relationship between adult psychopathology and earlier stages of normal development, the concepts of progression and regression have historically played important roles in understanding various forms of pathology and adaptation.

Three conceptual models of thought organization, based on traditional Rorschach thought disorder scoring concepts, have attempted to integrate psychoanalytic and developmental perspectives in order to form a coherent basis for understanding the progression from immature to more mature levels of cognitive structure formation. Lerner and Lerner (1982, 1986; Lerner, 1996) proposed a developmental object relations model of thinking by integrating Piagetian theory of cognitive development (Piaget, 1959) with Mahler's theory of separation-individuation (Mahler et al., 1975). Athey's (1986) developmental continuum of modes of thought organization was an attempt to expand on his earlier work, correlating level of thought organization with object relational manifestations in the transference. Finally, Leichtman's comprehensive analysis of the Rorschach (Leichtman, 1988, 1996) examined all aspects of the Rorschach situation, including thought disorder scores, from a developmental perspective which proposes that children pass through different stages in their abilities to take and master the test. By specifically employing a developmental framework, each of these models contributes to a broader understanding of Rorschach thought disorder scores.

Lerners' Rorschach Model of Cognitive Impairment

Using the developmental theories of Piaget and Mahler, the Lerners (1986) hypothesized three "interdigitated" stages in the development of thought processes. Later, Paul Lerner (1996) applied Rorschach indices of thought disorder and other variables to describe this three-stage developmental progression, focusing specifically on the roles of the caregiving object in either facilitating or hindering the unfolding of cognitive structures in infants and young children.

STAGE I: EARLY SENSORIMOTOR. The Lerners conceptualized this first stage as including the first two phases of Piaget's sensorimotor period. Piaget described the nascent awareness of external objects during these phases, which overlap with Mahler's shift from infantile autism into the phase of normal symbiosis. According to both theorists, during these first few months of life the infant begins to sense that satisfaction of needs emanates from something in the outside world. A failure to provide adequate holding and containing during this period results in a derailed separation-individuation process, characterized by emotional detachment from the interpersonal world, use of primitive defenses, and difficulties conceptualizing the world in human terms.

In addition to a lack of human content or differentiated color responses, Lerner (1996) suggested that the Rorschachs of these individuals would include "boundaryless" responses in which two or more percepts are arbitrarily combined. Thus, Lerner surmised that both contaminations and Level 2 fabulized combinations may appear in the records of these individuals, signaling structural problems and experiential themes reflective of failures in preseparation-individuation stages of caregiver and infant interaction.

STAGE II: MIDSENSORIMOTOR. Stage II integrates the third, fourth, and fifth phases of Piaget's sensorimotor period with Mahler's differentiaton and practicing subphases of separation-individuation. According to the Lerners, Piaget viewed the main cognitive task during these latter phases of sensorimotor functioning as one of distinguishing objects from their environmental surroundings and then representing them symbolically. Mahler's first two subphases of separation-individuation describe the process by which the infant "hatches" from the symbiotic orb and begins to move progressively farther away from the primary caregiver.

Lerner (1996) stated that an overdependence on the environment would result in a lack of critical objectivity and a tendency to accept passively the demands of the external world. Lerner inferred that arbitrary Form-Color responses (Rapaport's FCarb or Exner's more familiar INCOM response), mildly incongruent combinations (Exner's Level 1 FABCOMs and INCOMs), or uncritically accepted peculiar verbalizations (Exner's DV1) would all be characteristic of stage II functioning.

STAGE III: EARLY PREOPERATIONAL. The Lerners described Piaget's early preoperational period as a time in which the infant begins to internalize and symbolically represent external experiences. They pointed out how the transition to preoperational thinking coincides with Mahler's rapprochement subphase of separation-individuation. The infant-toddler becomes increasingly aware of its separateness, which leads to an oscillation between attempts to reestablish symbiotic union, on the one hand, and push toward further autonomy, on the other. Parental failure to maintain emotional availability may result in impairment in the ability to achieve object constancy characteristic of borderline-level pathology.

Lerner (1996) suggested a number of Rorschach scores that he thought would characterize the third stage. Most of his examples reflect the process of splitting, in which percepts abruptly shift from one qualitative extreme to the other. In an effort to identify Rorschach manifestations of splitting, Grala (1980) identified the combination of incompatible percepts as a test equivalent of this primitive process. As the capacity to integrate affectively contrasting object and self-representations increases, the individual can either screen out or integrate disparate details in a logical or benign manner.

Athey's Developmental Continuum of Modes of Thought Organization

Athey (1986) attempted to expand upon his earlier integration of structural and object relational paradigms by proposing a developmental continuum of five different modes of thought organization. Athey intended his developmental model to provide a continuum of thought organization, ranging from more primitive modes of primary process thinking to normal levels of secondary process experience.

Athey based his continuum on Rapaport's (Rapaport et al., 1968) view of the Rorschach response process and Werner's (Werner, 1948; Werner and Kaplan, 1963) developmental theory of differentiation and integration. Athey viewed Rapaport's "closeness-distance" dimension as a dialectic between subjective experience and objective reality. Following Rapaport, Athey referred to Werner's two coordinated vectors of development, differentiation and integration, as critical components of both the perceptual organization of the objective reality of the inkblot and one's subjective's association on the Rorschach. Thus, perceptual differentiation and reintegration go together as do associative elaboration and conceptual specification.

Athey suggested that the normal, healthy manner of integrating one's internal, subjective experience with adherence to external reality is based on the processes of "fabulation" and "combination" or "construction." On the Rorschach, healthy fabulation enriches perception in ways that are consistent with the reality and perceived identity of the inkblot. Successful combination and construction responses integrate differentiated parts of the inkblot in a manner that is consistent both with the contour-reality of the blot and with logical-reality in general. According to Athey, fabulation responses are the successful counterpart of displacement and combination/construction responses the healthy counterpart of condensation. Put differently, the pathological expression of fabulation is found in confabulation and absurd responses, while the pathological extension of combination/construction occurs in fabulized combinations and contamination responses.

In addition to describing both normal and creative modes of organization (adaptive regression), Athey conceived of four pathological modes of thought organization as extensions of normal fabulation and combination and regressions to developmentally earlier ways of integrating objective and subjective reality. Regressive phenomena can occur primarily in the domain of representational processes, or what Athey referred to as "percept identity and combination." Likewise, regression in any one response can be manifested chiefly in associational processes (or in the "affective and ideational specificity and elaboration" of the percept, as Athey termed them).

Arranged from the least developmentally primitive to the most, Athey's four primary process modes of thought organization included the following.

LEVEL 1: INSULATED IDIOSYNCRACY. At this first level of primary process organization, associational processes begin to have an odd quality, as manifested in peculiar and inappropriate specificity of thought content; or they may reveal overly personalized preoccupations. Perceptual combinations that reflect this level of organization do not violate reality; they just play with it. Image combinations are not impossible but generally improbable. Although the level 1 thinker may appreciate reality, his or her associational and representational processes are overly influenced by internal experience. Athey suggested that Rorschach thought disorder scores reflecting this level of thought organization would include peculiar verbalizations and milder fabulized combinations (and incongruous combinations or composite figures) in which the subject acknowledges the unrealistic nature of the combination.

LEVEL 2: CIRCUMSCRIBED REALITY REJECTION. Thought at this level involves an unresolved clash between fantasy and certain aspects of objective reality. Whereas the level 1 subject recognizes the unrealistic basis for his or her response, the subject at level 2 does not attend to the inappropriate nature of the response. Even though reality may provide the basis for fantasy, thoughts and feelings here may have gained sufficient valence to allow for a circumscribed dismissal of reality at the moment the subject allows private experience to impinge on external and interpersonal reality. Athey included impossible and bizarre fabulized, incongruous, and object-action combinations, as well as logical and affective contradictions at this level of organization. It also seems that milder or playful confabulations may occur at this level as well.

LEVEL 3: REALITY REPLACEMENT. Level 3 thought reflects the building of subjective associative processes with a progressive loss of anchoring in the referents of objective reality. Objective reality (in the case of the Rorschach, the reality contours of the inkblot) no longer serves as an initial basis for the response. Instead, the subject assigns meaning on the basis of private associations. Unlike the attenuated loss of reality that occurs at level 2, the fantasy process of level 3 is not circumscribed but becomes the essence of the response. Scores at this level include confabulations, absurd responses, fluid associations, bizarre symbolism responses, and autistic logic. Athey indicated that in his earlier study (Athey, 1974) he had found evidence of this level of functioning in affectively disordered schizophrenic patients.

LEVEL 4: CONDENSATION. A loss of distinction between different frames of reference characterizes the most primitive level of regression. Here, the subject loses the distinction between the processes of thought and perception; between self and nonself, object 1 and object 2; past and present; and so on. In essence, there is no distinction between external referents or between internal experience and external reality. Classic Rorschach thought disorder scores representative of this level are contaminations and neologisms (verbal condensations).

Athey completed his study by presenting rich clinical examples of functioning at each level. By qualitatively correlating "Rorschach events" (specific types of thought disorder scores) with "clinical events" (interpersonal aspects of the patient-examiner relationship), Athey attempted to demonstrate the parallel processes that emerged in the patients' thinking and their object relations, with specific reference to treatment and transference implications for each patient.

Leichtman's Developmental Theory of Rorschach Thought Disorder Signs

Leichtman (1988, 1996) proposed a developmental theory to explain Rorschach thought disorder scores. Although youngsters typically produce a number of thought disorder scores on the Rorschach, Leichtman stated that developmental normalcy should not be equated with adult psychopathology. Leichtman believed that the developmental theory of Heinz Werner (Werner, 1948, 1957; Werner and Kaplan, 1963) illuminates the Rorschach response process. According to Werner's theory, primitive states of mental functioning tend to be less complex, undifferentiated, diffuse, rigid, and labile. By contrast, more mature states reflect greater differentiation, articulation, integration, flexibility, and stability.

Leichtman conceived of the Rorschach situation as three vectors radiating outward, one to the subject, one to the examiner, and one to the Rorschach task itself. At the most primitive stage of Rorschach development, all three are blurred together. The young subject cannot effectively separate the task from the examiner or from him or herself. With each progressive stage, the subject, the examiner, and the task become more distinct and clearly defined.

Leichtman also highlighted Werner and Kaplan's (1963) model of symbol formation as a framework for understanding the development of the child's capacity for representation. Symbol formation is viewed within an interpersonal coordinate system, including an addressor-addressee axis and a symbol-referent coordinate. Consistent with the orthogenetic principle, addressor-addressee and symbol-referent axes are experienced in global, undifferentiated, and unstable ways during the earliest stages of development. With maturation, the subject is increasingly capable of differentiating and integrating each of these four components.

Leichtman examined perceptual theories of the Rorschach and concluded, like Blatt (1990), that the test is best understood as a representational task in which the subject imaginatively creates responses, as opposed to perceptually recognizing them. According to Leichtman, a representational theory of the Rorschach subsumes both perceptual and associational processes but goes beyond these by positing that Rorschach responses are symbolic creations that interpretively shape the blots into meaningful images that represent something in the real world.

Leichtman (1988) originally proposed a developmental progression of three stages to explain how young children come to be able to take the Rorschach. According to Leichtman, each stage is characterized by shifts in how the Rorschach is given and taken. Each stage is also associated with different test-taking behavior and test responses. Finally, each progressive stage incorporates aspects of the earlier stages. Leichtman called his three stages: I. Perseverative approaches to the Rorschach; II. Confabulatory approaches to the Rorschach; and III. "The Rorschach." His stages are defined by specific patterns, not ages per se.

STAGE I: PERSEVERATIVE APPROACHES TO THE RORSCHACH. Leichtman pointed out that when one is bold enough to attempt to get two-year-olds to focus on the Rorschach, their responses tend to be characterized by perseveration and absurdity. Leichtman noted that researchers have long observed that toddlers respond to the 10 cards as if there is little difference between them (Klopfer and Margulies, 1941). Additionally, examiners have concluded that the basis for the toddlers' response is frequently unclear (Klopfer and Margulies, 1941; Ford, 1946).

Leichtman elaborated upon the views of Klopfer and Margulies by pointing out that this perseverative pattern may be an adaptive problem-solving solution for the toddler. Presented with a difficult and unfamiliar task such as the Rorschach, the youngster may arbitrarily seize upon the first response and then stick, for the remainder of the test, with what apparently seemed to work for them in the beginning.

Just before turning three, the toddler may exhibit a bit of a shift in his or her perseverative pattern. Although absurd perseverations may still prevail, the two-and-a-half-year-old may either try to refuse some of the cards or give new responses to others.

STAGE II: CONFABULATORY APPROACHES TO THE RORSCHACH. Three- and four-year-olds take the Rorschach in a qualitatively different manner. Now the youngster may give different responses to each blot, which serves as a springboard for often idiosyncratic fantasy. The child's Rorschach may take a more familiar form and may even reveal something about the child's personality functioning. Although the form level of most responses is better than that of the perseverating toddler, most of the three- to four-year-olds' responses are confabulatory wholes. The child has become enamored of ideas, which take precedence over perceptual reality. The boundary between reality and fantasy is permeable, and affect states tend to influence perception.

As children make the transition from stage II to III, there is an increase in the number of responses and large detail responses (as opposed to wholes). Klopfer, Spiegelman, and Fox (1956) believed that this transition period was also marked by the introduction of "confabulatory combinations," which they defined as essentially thematically embellished incongruous combinations. Other researchers (Ames et al., 1952) noted that the Rorschachs of five-year-olds are characterized less by confabulations and more by incongruous combinations.

STAGE III: "THE RORSCHACH." At the age of seven, the child is able to move from DWs to Ds and to exclude incongruous details that would spoil an otherwise adequate response. At this point, Leichtman noted that the Rorschach has become a reliable test for the subject and can be taken in the same way as adults take the test. The child is now capable of more successful integration between perceptual and associative components of the response process. Leichtman stated that confabulations are more uncommon at this age and can be taken as a sign of ideational disturbance.

Leichtman integrated his developmental stage model with Werner and Kaplan's orthogenetic principle and their concept of symbol formation to explain several of the common Rorschach thought disorder signs. First, he observed how many of the scores found in children's Rorschachs are commonly associated with disordered thinking in adults. However, as suggested before, he was careful to view these responses in the records of children as developmentally normative and not pathological or "primitive."

In keeping with his representational model, Leichtman indicated that the response process is an act of shaping the inkblots into a symbol that stands for something and is simultaneously shared with or communicated to someone. Thought disorder scores can be understood in terms of something that has gone awry in some aspect of the symbol situation, between addressee and addressor or between referent and symbol. Leichtman used this model as a basis for explaining certain aspects of thought disordered responses, including poor form level, DWs, perseverations, disturbances in the choice of referents, disturbances in the coordination of vehicle and referent, atypical color responses, and disturbances in language and logic.

In Leichtman's view, form level is more than simply a measure of reality testing based on visuo-perceptual accuracy. Adequate form level requires: (1) choosing relevant details on which to focus; along with (2) sufficient details to serve as a good basis for representation; (3) parts are correctly articulated in order to make a whole; and (4) that irrelevant details are excluded. Leichtman pointed out that the first two criteria rest on Werner's principle of differentiation, while the latter two are based on his principle of integration of parts into a coherent whole.

Similarly, DW responses indicate that the subjects have based their responses on too few details, while ignoring incongruous or poorly fitting details. In such cases, individuals may have trouble separating qualities of the referent from their feelings about it.

In conclusion, Leichtman noted that good form level is an indication of the capacity to represent experience in coherent and integrated ways that are stable, remain faithful to the external world, and can be readily shared with others. On the other hand, primitive modes of representation, which are based on too few or poorly integrated details, lead to experiencing the world in diffuse, inflexible, and labile ways. Leichtman suggested that such individuals may have difficulty separating their moods from their experience of themselves and the external world, communicating their experience to others, and sharing in a consensual sense of reality with them.

If poor form level involves misuse in the handling of the symbolic medium (i.e., the inkblots), scores such as inappropriate combinations, contaminations, and confabulations typically reflect a bizarre choice of referents that the subject tries to represent. In such responses, the subject either combines ideas unrealistically or embellishes them with inappropriate fantasy material. Leichtman states that odd and socially inappropriate responses indicate strange thinking but also poor social judgment or, as Harrow and Quinlan (1985) termed it, "impaired perspective."

According to Leichtman, perseveration responses indicate problems with the referent dimension of the symbol situation, namely a restriction in the range of content of responses. However, he indicated that this is the case specifically for what Exner (1986a, 1993) labeled "mechanical perseveration," in which the subject does little more than repeat the same response over and over again. Mechanical perseveration serves similar adaptive and defensive functions for toddlers and neurologically or intellectually impaired adults, who find the inkblots too complex to produce a range of responses. Instead, these subjects stick with a limited set of responses, which provide them with a strategy for managing the complexity of the task. Leichtman distinguished "content perseveration" as a developmentally more advanced form of perseveration, found in children transitioning to Stage II. In adults, content perseveration might be more suggestive of the intrusion of overvalent, conflict-based ideas as opposed to intellectual or organic impairment.

Leichtman believed that the most distinctive Rorschach thought disorder scores are indications of disturbances in the coordination of the symbolic vehicle and the referent object. In other words, in the symbol situation of the Rorschach, there is some discontinuity between the object or concept, itself, and the way in which it gets mentally represented. The outcome of such lack of coordination between object/concept and symbolic representation includes familiar scores such as incongruous combinations, fabulized combinations, confabulations, and contaminations.

Leichtman observed that a comparative-developmental perspective lends support to the ways in which researchers have ordered these four scores along a continuum of psychopathology. Recall that most thought disorder researchers viewed the contamination response as the most severe thought disorder score, followed by confabulations, and then by fabulized combinations (Blatt and Ritzler, 1974; Johnston and Holzman, 1979). Similarly, normative data demonstrate that these scores occur in a developmental sequence in children's Rorschachs, with scores at the lower end of the continuum (except for contamination responses) occurring at earlier stages and more differentiated and better integrated scores occurring later on. Thus, while Leichtman conceived of the typical Rorschach thought disorder scores as part of a normal developmental progression of increased differentiation and integration in the records of youngsters, he considered them signs of a regressive "de-differentiation and dis-integration" in the records of adults.

Leichtman noted that three atypical color responses have implications for understanding thought organization from both developmental and pathological perspectives. Color naming responses are the most developmentally primitive way of handling the inkblots. Typical of Stage I functioning, youngsters who give this kind of response have adopted a concrete, stimulus-bounded approach to the task which they find too complex. Color projection, on the other hand, reflects a primitive, but somewhat more advanced, response strategy to the Rorschach, in which the subject merges perception of the inkblot with ideas and feelings about it. Associative material overshadows perceptual reality resulting in a confabulatory process in which fantasy impinges on reality. Finally, arbitrary color responses (i.e., Rapaport's FCarb or Exner's INCOM) reflect developmentally higher responses consistent with late Stage II thinking which is characterized by confabulatory combinations.

Leichtman ended his developmental analysis of disordered thinking by discussing disturbances in language and logic, which occur in the process attempting to communicate and justify responses to the examiner. According to Leichtman's model, both language and logic are representational processes that can be understood from both a developmental/progressive and a pathological/regressive understanding of the symbol situation. For example, he pointed out that subjects in

Stage III reason and use words in a conventional manner and maintain a clear distinction between addressor and addressee. Stage II subjects, by contrast, may exhibit a more egocentric approach in which the addressee is treated almost as an extension of the self, as the subject may reason and speak in personalized and increasingly private ways which tend to alienate and confuse the listener. Peculiar, queer, and deviant verbalizations are typical responses of children at Stage II of development or adults who have regressed to this level of thinking. Autistic logic, confusion, and vague responses may characterize the reasoning processes of the Stage II youngsters or the strained logic of the moderately thought disordered adult. Finally, Stage I subjects demonstrate a more extreme lack of distinction between addressor and addressee. In such cases, words are no longer used to denote objects but are used in bizarre and autistic ways that cannot be explained to the listener. Absurd and incoherent responses, word salads, and neologisms are normal occurrences during this earliest developmental phase of Rorschach test-taking and reflective of the most severe level of regression in adult thought disordered patients.

Leichtman's model represents a shift in thinking about development and psychopathology. Instead of viewing thought pathology as regressive phenomena, Leichtman explains Rorschach thought disorder signs in a progressive and adaptive manner. Understanding thought disorder progressively helps one avoid the inference-making problem that Peterfreund (1978) described. Both Athey and the Lerners may be vulnerable to Peterfreund's criticism of developmental approaches to psychopathology that rely more on reconstructive theorizing than prospective study of infants and children. Furthermore, despite their eloquent theoretical synthesis, the model put forth by the Lerners is rooted in the developmental theory of Mahler which, has been subjected to increased criticism over the last 10 years (Stern, 1985).

Despite these criticisms, each of these models demonstrates sophisticated integration of developmental theories and disordered thinking, as measured by the Rorschach. Whether viewed as progressive or regressive phenomena, these researchers have shown how static Rorschach thought disorder signs can be linked to developmental experiences, both normative and pathological. Such a linkage contributes to both a broader understanding of psychological development and a more incisive grasp of the meaning of Rorschach thought disorder scores.

CHAPTER

9

CONFABULATORY THINKING

Confabulatory thinking is generally taken as an indication of cognitive impairment or thought disorder, regardless of whether one's frame of reference is neurology, psychiatry, or psychodiagnostic testing. Verbal confabulation implies a filling in of gaps or erroneous overgeneralization from part to whole, leading subjects to form sometimes far-reaching conclusions based on inadequate data. However, a number of conceptual and semantic issues have made the term more complex and difficult to understand and have contributed to confusion, controversy, and a lack of clarity when attempting to discover the meaning and clinical implications of the term. In this chapter, I review and attempt to deconstruct the term "confabulation" so that its clinical roots, dimensionality, and nuances of meaning can become clearer and hopefully more diagnostically useful.

PROBLEMS IN SEMANTICS AND TERMINOLOGY

One cannot understand the multiple meanings of the term "confabulation" without also examining the concept of "fabulation" or "fabulization." However, the terms "fabulation" and "confabulation" have a variety of meanings in different contexts. For instance, *Webster's New Universal Unabridged Dictionary* (1983) defines "fabulize" as "to fable" and the related term "fabulous" as "legendary, imaginary, devised, and fictitious" (p. 654). The same source defines "confabulation" as "familiar talk; easy, unrestrained, unceremonious conversation"

(p. 381). Taken together, both terms imply spontaneous acts of speech that may involve imagination and story telling.

Although Adolf Meyer originally used the terms to describe a process of fabrication, "fabulation" or "fabulize" have since dropped out of contemporary psychiatric usage. "Confabulation," however, has continued to endure as a part of the neuropsychiatric lexicon. The neuropsychiatric definition of "confabulation" has historically involved a pathological filling in of memory gaps with imagined experiences, usually characteristic of organic brain syndromes (Freeman, Kaplan, and Saddock, 1976). Others in this field have defined it as a falsification of memory occurring in a state of clear consciousness (Berlyne, 1972); an extreme form of lying or deception (Joseph, 1986); or "honest lying" (Moscovitch, 1989).

Studies from behavioral neurology suggest that confabulation may be a specific clinical syndrome found in brain-damaged and schizophrenic patients (Nathaniel-James and Frith, 1996). Confabulation may express itself in different ways depending on the nature of the underlying problem. Most interestingly, confabulation may express the subject's efforts to somehow adapt to and compensate for some latently perceived deficit or vulnerability (Weinstein, Kahn, and Malitz, 1956; Weinstein, 1996). These findings may help broaden our understanding of the types of confabulatory thinking commonly encountered in the Rorschachs of some thought disordered subjects.

CONFABULATION ON THE RORSCHACH

Rorschach (1921) introduced the term "confabulation" into the psychodiagnostic literature when describing the types of perceptual overgeneralizations that schizophrenic, unintelligent, and organically impaired subjects made when responding to the inkblots. He used the term in two related ways. First, when discussing the scoring of Whole responses (W), Rorschach referred to the "confabulated" whole response (or DW) as "a single detail, more or less clearly perceived, [which] is used as the basis for the interpretation of the whole picture, giving very little consideration to the other parts of the figure" (p. 37). Secondly, Rorschach talked about "confabulating" subjects, whom he distinguished from subjects who used their imaginations in more successful and adaptive ways. In his analysis, Rorschach seemed to relate confabulation to the processes of contamination and combinative thinking.

The meaning of confabulation in Rorschach parlance remained unchanged until Rapaport broadened the definition and introduced the concept of fabulation. While he retained Rorschach's original perceptual definition of confabulation (DW), Rapaport placed confabulation in relation to the concept of fabulation and elaborated on the ideational processes that underlie many of these types of responses. Rapaport defined fabulation as associative and affective elaboration that tends to be overly subjective but not so unrealistic as to suggest psychoses. Rapaport was careful to point out that fabulized responses can be given by creative and artistic subjects but that an abundance of these responses may signal difficulties. According to Rapaport, confabulations carried to an extreme the tendencies present in fabulized responses, but that the degree of elaboration or overspecificity suggested maladaptive immersion in fantasy and the presence of autistic trends in the person's thinking.

In his broader definition of confabulation, Rapaport implicitedly described four distinct subtypes. These include (1) the familiar DW response; (2) the associatively embellished response that takes the fabulizing process beyond what the inkblot can justify (the extreme increase-of-distance, associationally based confabulation); (3) the overly specific response, in which the confabulation is based on attributing a degree of specificity to the inkblot that is unwarranted; and (4) the autistic logic confabulation, which reflects the subject's loss of distance from the blot and idiosyncratic reasoning based on concrete spatial or positional features of the inkblot.

Schafer (1946, 1954) viewed confabulations in the broader ideational-story telling context that Rapaport had introduced. A number of other analytically oriented Rorschachers also followed Rapaport and Schafer's broader use of the term "confabulation" (Allison et al., 1968; Appelbaum, 1975; Mayman, 1982; Lerner et al., 1985; Lerner, 1991). Schafer believed that confabulations represented a breakthrough of primary process thinking reflective of a problem in distinguishing fantasy from reality. Lerner et al. (1985) suggested that confabulations are a Rorschach manifestation of the primary process mechanism of displacement.

As indicated in chapter 4, Holt objected to Rapaport's use of the term "confabulation" which he felt was too easily confused with the DW response. Instead, Holt (Holt and Havel, 1960) introduced the term "autistic elaborations" (Au El 1) to refer to the presence of thematically unrealistic and fantasy-ridden elaboration of a response, as if the instructions had been to make up a story to fit the inkblot.

Weiner's (1966) category of impaired reasoning that he called "overgeneralized thinking" is characterized by "jumping to erroneous conclusions on the basis of minimal evidence and investing experiences with elaborate meanings not justified by their actual stimulus properties" (p. 64). According to Weiner, three types of Rorschach responses that reflect overgeneralized thinking include fabulizations, confabulations, and absurd Dds. Like Holt, Weiner retained the term confabulation only for DW responses and felt that all associatively embellished responses should be subsumed under the heading of "fabulized responses." Weiner believed in a continuum of fabulized responses, ranging from those responses that consist of minimally elaborative words or phrases to those that weave the response into a thematic narrative. Weiner referred to this latter type of fabulization as "extended fabulations," similar to Holt's "autistic elaboration."

Weiner's "absurd Dd" response was essentially an extended fabulization to a tiny Dd area of the blot. Here the tiny detail is imbued with elaborate or specific meaning that leaves behind the reality of the inkblot to such a great degree that the response takes on an absurd quality.

It was observed in chapter 5 that much of Weiner's thinking laid the foundation for Exner's (1986a, 1993) Special Scores in the Comprehensive System. Thus, it is no surprise to find that Exner, too, restricted the use of the term "confabulation" to DW and DDd responses. In keeping the confabulation a perceptually versus associatively based overgeneralization, Exner subsumed CONFAB responses under a heading of "perseveration and integration failures" in order to distinguish them from either deviant verbalizations or inappropriate logic. Exner introduced the DR score in an effort to capture the extended types of fabulizations that Weiner had written about two decades earlier.

It is clear that confabulation is not a unitary concept. The different definitions and conceptual nuances make it a slippery term that is difficult to pin down. In the section that follows, I examine the various dimensions that are subsumed by the broader concept of confabulation.

DIMENSIONS OF CONFABULATION

Confabulation responses can be examined along a number of dimensions that capture many of the aspects discussed by past and present researchers. Below is a list of possible dimensions which distinguish among the various interpretive nuances that might be useful for clinicians to consider in their efforts to better understand their patients.

Confabulatory Distance from the Inkblot

As indicated previously, Rapaport used the term confabulation primarily to describe a variety of associative, as opposed to perceptual, elaborations. Generally, the confabulations to which he referred were examples of pathological increases of distance from the inkblot in which the subject either tells a story or becomes excessively tangential, circumstantial, inappropriately abstract, or symbolic. However,

Rapaport also pointed out that confabulations could also reflect either a pathological loss of distance from the inkblot, or a mixture of both types of inappropriate distance. For example, a subject could respond to the blot in an overly literal manner—demonstrating loss of distance—and then overly embellish the response—demonstrating an increase of distance.

There is another meaning of the term "distance" that can be applied to the concept of confabulatory thinking. As indicated above, in the Rapaportian sense, one's associations are either anchored "too much" (loss of distance) or "too little" (increase of distance) in the perceptual reality of the inkblot. However, by thinking of distance in terms of "immersion in" versus "departure or alienation from" the inkblot, one may shift the connotation from a perceptual to an emotional dimension. For example, consider the following response to Card II:

> These look like two angry women. I can see anger in their eyes and you can see by the way they're standing that they are upset. The way they are dressed, they probably have just gotten back from some dance and I'd guess from the way they're looking at each other that they're not too happy with each other.

Does this represent a pathological loss or increase of distance from the inkblot? On the one hand, the subject clearly makes attributions that are not anchored in consensually perceived aspects of the blot, suggesting too much distance has been taken. However, the term "distant" does not quite capture the manner in which the subject has become immersed in the inkblot. His cathexis of interest and emotional investment in this particular card is intense. Contrary to viewing this as a typical example of a pathological increase of distance, the subject has lost himself in the card, falling into the blot. But this response does not typify the usual example of a pathological loss of distance either, where some concrete detail forms the basis of an inappropriate perceptual overgeneralization. Instead, one might conceive of this process as an emotional, as opposed to concrete perceptual (DW), loss of distance. Not only is the subject taking the inkblot too seriously, but it is almost as if he is emotionally consumed by a need to find meaning in it.

The opposite of emotional immersion in the inkblot would be something like a tangential departure or alienation from the inkblot, response proper, or general task set. Here the subject demonstrates less interest in the card itself or in its interpretation of meaning. Instead, something about the card or its associations prompts a tangential departure from the field. Exner (1993) gave the following example of this type of response, which he referred to as a circumstantial response, scored as a DR2: "It could be part of a crab, I'm just trying to think of the angle we're looking at it from, maybe it's a stone crab, I really like those. If you are ever in Maine try them, the only thing you ever get is the leg cause they're only allowed to harvest the legs" (p. 167). This response not only becomes extremely distant and strays from the inkblot, but the subject giving this response has departed from the task set, which calls upon subjects to say what the inkblots look like. The subject in the first example has almost taken this instruction too seriously and has gotten caught up in it emotionally. It is as if some immediately present stimulus has captured his attention in an emotionally absorbing and mesmerizing fashion. However, the second subject has trouble sticking to the basic instruction and becomes emotionally distant from what is placed in front of him. Instead of becoming immersed in discovering or ascribing meaning in the card, the second subject shows a relative indifference or inattentiveness to the inkblot, as if he has become alienated from further involvement with what is immediately present.

Continuum of Confabulatory Activity

Fabulation (representing less extreme enlivenment of the inkblot) and confabulation responses represent two ends of a continuum of elaborative associational activity. Rapaport et al. (1968) indicated that confabulation responses carried "to the extreme those tendencies which are already present in both fabulized responses and fabulized combinations" (pp. 434–435). Putting aside fabulized combinations for the moment, we can see that Rapaport viewed fabulized responses as milder, perhaps adaptive, versions of the elaborative (or overspecific) associative process that go astray in confabulation responses. Despite his emphasis on identifying deviant Rorschach verbalizations, Rapaport believed that even healthy and sensitive subjects could give a few fabulized responses, which they may verbalize with a playful and appropriate sense of distance. Athey (1986), too, suggested that fabulation responses are the successful counterpart of confabulation and that healthy fabulation enriches perception in ways that are consistent with the reality and perceived identity of the inkblot. However, Rapaport also believed that more disturbed subjects will give a greater number of fabulations, which they deliver with an air of certainty, absent the playful, "as if" quality seen in healthier subjects. Weiner (1966) indicated that when many fabulized responses are given with an air of seriousness, without any justification, and in a distorted (F–) manner, it is likely that these reflect disordered thinking.

Believing that Rapaport overemphasized the primary process, pathological implications of "fabs," Mayman (1960) developed an elaborate scale to measure degrees of fabulization on the Rorschach. Mayman viewed fabs as an index of introversiveness, or the subject's capacity to detach him- or herself from external stimuli in order to access ideas and fantasies with which to enliven perceptual images. Put simply, fabs are indicators of ideation. Mayman related fabs to Rorschach's (1921) original formulation of "experience types." In particular, Mayman believed that fabs were similar to human movement responses (Ms), which were seen as a measure of an individual's interest in ideation and inner life. However, he stated that fabs without Ms suggested a store-house of ideas not available to consciousness (interfered with by excessive repression).

Mayman constructed a five-point scale to assess the degree to which the subject's responses were determined by objective versus subjective factors. Mayman's interest was in determining how much the subject was either bound to reality or immersed in fantasy when associating to the ambiguous inkblots. His scale, described below, was an attempt to measure this response variable.

Fab 1: Minimal Fabulizing. These are unelaborated or popular movement responses with minimal fantasy development. An example would be the Card VIII response of "Animals climbing up a hill." Nonmovement responses that convey vividness and liveliness, such as "an ugly face" or a "beautiful butterfly," would also be scored at this level. Phillips and Smith (1953) also suggested that the mildest fabulizations included single words (usually adjectives or verbs, such as a "fearful" man or a "screaming" face) or phrases that introduced some affectively descriptive quality into the response.

Fab 2: Attenuated Fabulizing. Passive movement responses or those in which some lifelike activity is caught or arrested are scored at the level of Fab 2. For example, "A monster about to pounce" reflects this kind of arrested or potential movement.

Fab 3: Moderate Fabulizing. Here the subject elaborates the response in a rich and fanciful manner but without becoming too immersed in the content. The subject can dip into a fantasy, enjoy the process, but not get lost in it. Mayman believed that most animal and human movement responses are usually sufficiently enlivened to belong to this category. An example of a Fab 3 would be the Card VII response of "Two girls with pony tails doing a fun dance together."

Fab 4: Fabulizing, Loss of "Distance" from the Response Process. The subject becomes increasingly absorbed in the response content so that he or she loses optimal distance. Unseen characters may be introduced and emotional states and motivations may be attributed to the characters, who are treated with an air of realism. Although Mayman did not indicate this, responses of the Fab 4 variety are already in the confabulation range. Examples would include the Card II response

"Two Chinese warriors fighting fiercely, each wanting to win. They've probably killed several other guys before this final fight."

Fab 5: Fantasy with Extreme Loss of Distance. Mayman's concept of an "extreme loss of distance" seems similar to Rapaport's concept of a "pathological increase of distance" from the inkblot. I believe that they were using different terms to describe a similar phenomenon. In any case, Mayman's "extreme loss of distance" Fab 5 response is an example of the type of emotional "loss of distance" to which I referred above. Subjects who give these responses demonstrate intense fantasy immersion. The subject takes the inkblot as a piece of reality and gets lost in the content of the response. How do Fab 5 responses differ from confabulations proper? Mayman did not make a distinction between them. However, the examples he gave seem to be grounded in accurate form. For example, he said that the following Card II response shows the degree of fantasy absorption characteristic of a Fab 5 response.

> The bodies look like they could be bears with paws up together warming their feet at a bonfire left by campers. But the heads don't look like bears. Well, except that being red there might show it's reflecting heat from the bonfire. . . . That's it, unless the paws being up there could signify their being happy to have found some warmth. Sort of mutual feeling [Mayman, 1960, p. 13].

Mayman's Fabulization Scale was an interesting effort to define a continuum of fabulation-confabulation in Rorschach responses. However, I know of no published reliability data on Mayman's scale, nor any studies that have attempted to relate it to different psychological processes or diagnostic entities.

Schafer (1948, 1954) introduced a gradation of severity into confabulatory responses by suggesting that subthreshold confabulations should be scored as "confabulation-tendencies." According to Schafer, these confabulation-tendencies represented mild or uncrystalized propensities for pathological projection that may signal a potential cause for concern. Unfortunately, the distinction between these lesser forms of confabulation and the real thing was not made very clear.

Two 1985 studies, which followed Blatt and Ritzler's (1974) thought disorder-boundary deficit paradigm, proposed scales that depicted varying degrees of confabulation severity. Lerner et al. (1985) developed a Rorschach Boundary Disturbance Scale that distinguished between confabulation tendency and confabulation proper (similar to Schafer's distinction and that found in the TDI). Lerner and his colleagues indicated that the affective component in confabulation tendency responses was stronger than that in the fabulized response and less well justified, whereas affect elaboration (or overspecificity) completely overshadows form in the confabulation response.

Wilson (1985) delineated further subtypes of thought disorder scores in an attempt to measure boundary disturbances in psychotic and borderline patients. His mildest type was the "Fabulation-Confabulation" response, which he defined as a response that begins with a mild associative elaboration that eventually begins to take over the response. However, it is unclear what distinguishes this from confabulation tendency response. His second level of severity was the "Confabulation Tendency" response which he described as an associative tendency that threatens to overpower the perceptual accuracy of the response. However, the idiosyncratic nature of the response never quite overrides the perceptual requirements of the blot. As an example of the confabulation tendency response, Wilson gave something nearly identical to one of Rapaport's confabulation examples: Card IV, "The white streak in here reminds me of the wide and powerful Mississippi River" (Wilson, 1985, p. 350). Finally, Wilson's "Confabulation" response takes associative embellishment to the extreme so that the perceptual features of the blot are all but ignored and the idea expressed is often unrealistic.

The distinctions between these different levels of confabulation are somewhat fuzzy and subjective. For example, Wilson leaves it up to the examiner to determine when the associations begin to "overpower" the perceptual accuracy of the response.

Saunders (1991) attempted to add operational clarity to Wilson's confabulatory continuum by adding the following measurable criteria to each level. Fabulation-Confabulation: Mild elaborations that go beyond fabulized responses. The elaboration has a narrative quality depicted by either an implicit time sequence (e.g., "Looks like someone has gotten run over") or the attribution of a psychological state—motivation or affect—to the characters (e.g., "They look hungry"; "They are angry"). Confabulation-Tendency: The response has all the features of a fabulation-confabulation response, except that the subject has introduced unseen characters that have no perceptual basis in the card. The example, "Looks like two angry bears were stabbed by someone," not only reflects a psychological state but implies influence by some unseen figure. Confabulation: Only a single or subsidiary feature of the inkblot is identified as the basis for the extreme elaboration, while the rest arises from fulminating associative activity. With so little in the blot to justify the response, Saunders implies that the perceptual accuracy of the full confabulation response will be poor.

The concept of a continuum of confabulation of thought disorder scores was an inherent feature of the Menninger Thought Disturbance Scales (Athey et al., 1992, 1993). Here the Menninger researchers attempted to define objectively the criteria for each level of confabulatory severity. Instead of basing the discriminations only on perceptual accuracy, the introduction of psychological variables, or unseen characters, Athey et al. tried to define each level on the basis of the number of associations that exceed that which can be justified by the blot and by whether or not there is a "qualitative shift" in the subject's attitude toward increased immersion in fantasy. However, scorers might subjectively differ in what they count as associations that exceed what the blot can justify. Furthermore, it might be difficult for scorers to agree on whether a "qualitative shift" has occurred in the subject's attitude toward the response.

Table 9-1 may help lend some coherence and cohesion to various efforts to describe a continuum of confabulation by attempting to create a kind of concordance of the different ratings.

Reality Testing and Confabulation

How do different types of confabulation responses relate to the concept of reality testing? To explore this relationship, it is useful to understand the components of reality testing first and then apply this understanding to the Rorschach.

In his early theory development, Freud (1895) discussed the distinction between ideas and perceptions as a core aspect of reality testing; Hartmann (1953) elaborated that this essential capacity formed the basic layer of reality testing. However, reality testing was never viewed as an unitary concept. Balint (1942) and Hartmann stated that the capacity to distinguish ideas (internal) from perceptions (external) was only one component of reality testing. To this most basic component, they added the capacity to attach meaning to or discover the significance of an accurately perceived stimulus. Introducing this aspect of reality testing moved the level of discourse into the realm of interpretation and assignment of meaning to a stimulus, as opposed to the more basic realm of visual recognition of it. Interpretation of meaning of a stimulus may be related to, or independent from, one's ability to perceive accurately an external stimulus. This is reminiscent of Rapaport's essential belief that the successful Rorschach response entailed the "cogwheeling" of perceptual and associative processes.

Reality testing has usually been associated with form level on the Rorschach. Inaccurate perception of the inkblots (F–) typically suggests that either a subject's internal states have overwhelmed or impinged on his or her ability to perceive accurately (or consensually) external reality, or that visual perceptual capabilities are somehow inherently defective, regardless of the influence of the person's inner states on perception (Korchin, 1960). Difficulties of the former type usually point to a

Table 9-1 Continuum of Confabulatory Responses

Rapaport (Rapaport et al., 1968)	Fabulization				Confabulation
Schafer (Schafer, 1948, 1954)	Fabulization		Confabulation tendency		Confabulation
Holt (Holt, 1960)				Au El 1	Au El 2
Weiner (Weiner, 1966)	Fabulization			Extended Fab. Confabulation (DW)	
Mayman (Mayman, 1960)	Fab 1	Fab 2	Fab 3	Fab 4	Fab 5
TDI (Johnston & Holzman, 1979)			Confab tend & Playful Cfb (.5 level)		Confabulation (.75 level)
Lerner (Lerner et al., 1985)	Fabulization		Confabulation tendency		Confabulation
Wilson (Wilson, 1985)		Fab–Confab	Confabulation tendency		Confabulation
Saunders (Saunders, 1991)		Fab–Confab	Confabulation tendency		Confabulation
Athey (Athey et al., 1992)	Fab.	Mild Confabulation	Moderate Confabulation		Severe Confabulation

psychological origin, whereas those of the latter type might suggest an organic one.

Problems in reality testing, associated with F– responses, are typically linked to difficulties in distinguishing between ideas and images (reflecting internal states), on the one hand, from perceptions of external consensual reality, on the other. In other words, the subject fails to distinguish some idiosyncratic internal image, aroused by the inkblot, from the "external reality" of the inkblot stimulus. A secondary failure in critical, evaluative appraisal of the adequacy or appropriateness of the image to the stimulus (related, perhaps, to Harrow and Quinlan's concept of "impaired perspective") results in the subject's distorted, minus form level response.

Kleiger and Peebles-Kleiger (1993) discussed how confabulation responses can be associated with different levels of reality testing problems. Varying degrees of confabulation responses can occur at different levels of perceptual accuracy, suggesting differential diagnostic and interpretative implications (Table 9-2). In some severe cases, misinter-

Table 9-2 Possible Diagnostic Implications of Different Levels of Confabulation

	Severity of Confabulation	
Form Level	Confab Tend	Confab Severe
Plus/Ordinary (+/o)	Hypervigilant Narcissism	Paranoid Style
Unusual (u)	Borderline	Delusional Disorder
Minus (–)	Manic Psychosis Schizoaffective Schizophrenia	Manic Psychosis Schizoaffective

From Kleiger and Peebles-Kleiger (1993).

pretation can adversely affect perceptual accuracy, whereas in others it may not. For example, an external stimulus may be accurately perceived but interpreted in an overly subjective or, worse yet, idiosyncratic manner, giving rise to prejudice, the impingement of past ideas on current perceptions, and, in extreme cases, delusional convictions (Waelder, 1949). The following example, from chapter 8, of an accurately perceived, confabulated response reveals how idiosyncratic meaning has been ascribed to (projected onto) the stimulus situation, without doing violence to the perceptual accuracy of the basic stimulus situation.

> Card VII: Could be two matrons having a talk over coffee at 10:00 in the morning, and I suppose the bottom is symbolic of the thread that binds them together as homemakers, wives. They're in the same bridge club, bound together by all those ties. Kinda haughty and pretentious with their hands out. They're wealthy too. Pigtails up makes me think of uppity society women.

Here, overvalent, preconceived ideas direct the interpretation of an event. The basic elements of the event are accurately perceived, but the subject's reality testing has been significantly diminished by her excessively egocentric subjectivity. It is as if the subject has correctly perceived an external event, two women interacting with one another; however, she misinterprets (by virtue of her idiosyncratic overinterpretation) the meaning, significance, or causality of the interaction. At its worst, misinterpretation in the context of crisp and accurate perception might suggest a capacity for delusional thinking.

In another situation, idiosyncratic (mis)interpretation of a stimulus may obliterate perceptual accuracy, implying a more severe level of reality impairment, in which perception cannot be distinguished from ideas and images. Consider the following confabulated response that is scored at a minus form level: "Card VII: Looks like a woman split in half, with an empty space where someone has scooped out her insides. She was all alone and met with an untimely fate." Here, the interpretation not only goes beyond what the inkblot can justify, but, more important, the subject has distorted a piece of external reality. It is as if the subject had seen a stimulus and misperceived it based on his idiosyncratic interpretation. Hallucinatory experiences accompanied by delusional thinking reflect the simultaneous presence of misinterpretation and misperception.

Confabulatory Span

Rorschach confabulations can be excessively broad or narrow in scope. They might involve the unfolding of a dramatic elaboration or a lengthy tangential or circumstantial commentary, on the one hand; or they may be crisply overspecific, on the other. Subjects may tell stories, with a beginning, middle, and end, or they may leap to one- or two-word conclusions that are absurd in their degree of specificity.

The overly specific confabulation is characterized by the inappropriately precise identity assigned to the image. In this sense, the overly specific confabulation may be a brief response, quite different from the typically longer and more verbose ideationally embellished responses. For example, the Card VII response of "A Schnauzer, looks to be a female about three years old" doesn't reflect excessive thematic, affective, or fantasy embellishment. The content is unremarkable and rather prosaic in nature, but it is inappropriate because the subject has provided specificity far beyond what the blot could justify. Overspecific confabulations with ordinary form level may reflect a situation in which an obsessional subject's internal press for exactitude leads him or her to read inappropriate meaning into an event, revealing a need to be right and overly precise. On the other hand, overly specific confabulations with poor form level become absurd responses, as exemplified by the following psychotic-level Card III response, "This here looks a lot like my grandfather, like part of his stomach." (We will return shortly to this point—and this response—in our discussion of diagnostic implications.)

Rapaport considered both the story-telling and the overspecific responses to be confabulations. Johnston and Holzman (1979), however, separated these in their scoring system for the TDI. Overspecific responses are scored at the mildest level of severity (.25), whereas story-telling (and DW) confabulations are scored at the .75 level. Poor form overspecific responses would be scored as absurd responses (.75) in the TDI.

In the Comprehensive System, both the thematic story-telling and tangential commentary responses would be scored as a Deviant Response (DR), Level 1 or 2 depending upon one's judgment of severity. However, the inappropriately specific response really does not have a scoring equivalent in the Comprehensive System. Some have considered DR an equivalent category for Rapaport's confabulation responses (Meloy and Singer, 1991). As I indicated in chapter 6, the two categories (DR and confabulation) do not neatly overlap. Even if they did, however, the overly specific response would probably not be scored as a DR in the Comprehensive System. Consider the overly specific response given above, "A Schnauzer, looks to be a female about three years old." It certainly does not fulfill the criterion of a "fluid or rambling" elaboration necessary for a "circumstantial" DR. On the other hand, "inappropriate phrase" DRs involve the inclusion of inappropriate or irrelevant phrases like "A bird, but I was hoping for a butterfly." The Schnauzer response is neither inappropriate in its phraseology nor is it rambling or fluid. "Dog" is adequate form D2 on Card VII, so chances are that the Comprehensive System would not assign this response a Special Score for its inappropriate specificity.

Confabulatory Content and Tone

Confabulation is associated with formal thought disorder because it reveals something about the process of thinking. However, independent of the elaborative or inappropriately specific process of confabulatory thinking are a myriad of content variables. These can be classified several ways, either in terms of whether the elaboration involves primarily thematic, affective, or fantasy material (or some combination of these) or in terms of the specific tone or theme of the content (e.g., morbid, fusion, malevolent, magical, playful).

Ideationally embellished confabulations may reflect the unwarranted infusion of either thematic, affective, or fantasy material into the response (or, of course, some mixture of each). For example, the response to Card III of "Two women who have just finished doing the wash together; they're tired but will probably plan to rest awhile before going out to get something to eat" tells a story. There is little explicit affect and the story is grounded in realistic events (women may do wash and may be tired afterwards). On the other hand, the Card II response "It looks like two fighters, really pissed off at each other, fighting to the death, bloody, pummeling each other into the ground until the loser cries out in agony. God what a mess!" exudes highly charged sadistic aggression. Although interpretatively inappropriate given the stimulus, the response content itself is anchored in realistic concepts (fighters can engage in a fight to the death). In contrast, although the following confabulation example from the revised TDI scoring manual (Solovay et al., 1986) is excessively thematic and carries an implicit affective charge, it is characterized primarily by its departure from reality and immersion in fantasy. "It looks like the meeting of two, um . . . dragons who are comparing swords . . . or who are each so self-absorbed in themselves they're ignoring each other and doing a hell-like, hellish . . . demonic . . . dance of the underworld . . . or they're just staring at each other on rollers or standing on clouds, kind of pink clouds" (p. 495). Whether affect or fantasy is driving the confabulation may provide diagnostic information about whether disordered thinking occurs when the subject is affectively aroused or when he or she withdraws into fantasy.

The specific content of the confabulation can reflect a theme or tone of malevolence, symbiosis, magic, or playful humor. Obviously, each of these, together with the degree of confabulation (mild, moderate, or severe) and the form level (–, u, o/+), may provide further interpretive and diagnostic clues about the nature of the confabulations found on a particular record. For example, a severe confabulation with poor form and malevolent thematic content might suggest a psychotic process associated with both misperception and misinterpretation of a paranoid nature. One might also infer that this individual will exhibit marked perceptual impairment along with overly inferential thinking in the context of situations in which some external threat is identified. Hallucinations and paranoid delusions might be suggested by this type of confabulation. Similarly, a moderate level confabulation anchored in adequate form and associated with merger fantasies might indicate heightened oversubjectivity in the context of symbiotic wishes.

Although not diagnostically specific, considering confabulatory content along with form level and extent of confabulation helps provide a more complete picture of the psychological processes represented by a particular confabulation response. Knowing something about the circumstances under which the subject's thinking becomes confabulatory and the degree to which ego functioning is affected are necessary if one wishes to achieve a deeper understanding of the person producing the test responses.

CONFABULATION AND DR IN THE COMPREHENSIVE SYSTEM

In chapter 6, I argued that the two categories are different; and that DR is not "slightly more expansive" than Rapaport's concept of confabulation, as Meloy and Singer (1991) suggested, but a much broader and conceptually looser category. Meloy and Singer suggested that Exner's "inappropriate phrase" DRs would probably be scored as confabulation tendencies in the analytic literature and cited Wilson (1985) as their source. A closer look at Wilson's "confabulation tendency" category indicates that this is quite different from Exner's "inappropriate phrase" DR. Wilson defined "confabulation tendency" as an idiosyncratic elaboration that threatens to overpower the perceptual accuracy of the response. His examples are similar to Rapaport's sample confabulation responses, not to the "inappropriate phrase" DR best typified by Exner's example, "A bird, but I was hoping for a butterfly" (Exner, 1993, p. 167). I have argued elsewhere (Kleiger and Peebles-Kleiger, 1993) that Exner's "inappropriate phrase" DR involves focusing and filtering problems, similar to the Deviant Verbalization category.

Exner's other category of DR, the "circumstantial response," seems heavily tilted in the direction of a tangential departure from, as opposed to an immersion in, the blot. As argued above, this type of personalized associative straying from the response to the blot (as most of Exner's examples of circumstantial DRs demonstrate) is only one type of confabulation response. I also noted above that there is no adequate equivalent score in the Comprehensive System for the overly specific confabulation. Thus in some ways, DR may be an overly broad category, but in other ways, it seems rather narrow, de-emphasizing many of the types of confabulation responses that Rapaport first presented.

As I have tried to show above and in chapter 6, comparisons between the traditional scoring concept of confabulation and Exner's DR special score may be overstated. Although the overlap may exist, I do not think that there is sufficient evidence to assume an isomorphic relationship between these scoring categories.

Diagnostic Considerations

Although chapters 13 through 16 review specific differential diagnostic issues concerning all indices of disordered thinking, a brief summary of some of the diagnostic implications of confabulatory responses follows. In order to think about the diagnostic implications of confabulatory thinking on the Rorschach, it is important to consider the multiple dimensions discussed above. The following diagnostically based categories of confabulatory thinking are conceptually based and informed by empirical findings.

Schizophrenic Confabulations

Rapaport considered confabulations to be clearly within the realm of schizophrenic thinking. They were certainly common in Johnston and Holzman's (1979) TDI sample of recently hospitalized schizophrenic patients (45%) and more recently in Koistinen's Finnish schizophrenic sample (59%). However, we know that confabulations can occur in a variety of syndromes. Given this, what might qualitatively distinguish a typical schizophrenic Rorschach confabulation (if there is such a thing)? First, we would certainly expect either full confabulations (Wilson, 1985) or confabulation tendencies (Lerner et al., 1985) which do not have playful or humorous content. Thematically, there may be primitive, alien, or magical content. On the other hand, the content may be quite ordinary or banal. In either case, there may be something strange and confusing about the manner in which it is delivered. The associated form level would likely be poor, reflecting a disturbance in perception along with bizarre interpretation of the meaning of the inkblot. The other defining characteristic of the schizophrenic confabulation is its absurd degree of overspecificity. Here, the response might be extremely brief and notably peculiar in its overspecificity. Example: Card III (side detail), "This here looks a lot like my grandfather, like part of his stomach."

Manic Confabulations

A number of researchers have associated confabulatory thinking with affective disturbances. Weiner (1966) described the expansive emotional style of manic patients who tend to embellish their responses with fanciful details, symbolism, and fabulized injection of personal feelings. Athey (1974) found that severe confabulation responses were prominent among affect-disordered schizophrenic patients. In their principal component factor analysis of the TDI, Solovay et al. (1987) found that playful confabulations loaded most highly on their combinatory thinking factor, and that manic patients scored significantly higher on this factor than did schizophrenics. Schuldberg and Boster (1985) considered confabulations among the responses found on their fluid dimension and stated that "expansive manics" would likely score high on this dimension.

Although I've cautioned against drawing too many parallels between Exner's DR score and traditional confabulation responses, Exner (1986a) did state that DRs occur frequently in the records of patients with affective problems. Exner defined DR2 as an ideational impulse control problem, which he said occurred frequently "in the records of hypomanic subjects whose affective disorganization impairs their ability to stay on target" (Exner, 1993, p. 480).

Two characteristics seem to distinguish the manic confabulation. First, its humorous, flippant, or playful quality places it apart from the schizophrenic or schizoaffective manics (Holzman et al., 1986). Playful confabulations may not be long and overly thematic but express an affectively evocative quality, sometimes in only a few words. Secondly, we might expect an expansive, narrative quality in which the subject overreaches in his or her comfabulatory activity. The response itself might not have the peculiar or confusing quality, as with schizophrenic and schizoaffective patients. Instead, the thematic imagery may be dramatic, colorful, and infused with symbolism. Example, Card II: "Two creatures huggin'. Holdin' hands. An' they have two heads. An' looks like they're prayin' together sayin' it's all right, an' they're dancin'. Sort of like ALL RIGHT! Know what I mean? Bet you never heard that one before."

Borderline Confabulations

How might we detect a confabulation of borderline severity? The research reviewed above suggests that embellished responses may either be confabulation tendencies or full confabulations. Affect-laden fantasies reflecting themes of malevolence, aggression, loss, and reunion or merger might characterize the confabulations of classically borderline patients (see chapter 15). Immersion in the response, as opposed to tangential departure from it, may also capture the borderline patient's difficulty regulating affect. Finally, form level may be unusual or even adequate, reflecting an intact capacity to distinguish internal images from external percepts (self from other). Example, Card III: "Looks like two lovers whose hearts are one. They've been apart so long that they felt ripped apart. Now they have joined together and are in blissful happiness."

Posttraumatic Confabulations

What seems to characterize the traumatic confabulation is its affectively-driven loss of distance, as the subject becomes immersed in the blot characteristics and the response that follows. There may be a striking loss of reality testing that goes beyond misinterpretation. The intensity of the imagery that is aroused by the inkblot may overtake the subject's critical capacity to perceive reality accurately, resulting in a response of poor form quality. Finally, graphically violent, aggressive, morbid, or sexual content may permeate the embellishment in which the subject loses him/herself. Examples:

Card II: "The first thing I see is my art which tends to be black and covered in blood!" (Inquiry) "That's what I did before; I cut myself and had a black marker which I wrote with. I cut myself and covered the black with blood." (Circumstantial DR revealing a simultaneous loss of perceptual and emotional distance and also a departure from the bolt.)

Card IV: "Looks like a long dark road where there's been an explosion. Something's gotten killed, blown to bits. Blood and bodies all over, people yelling for help, crying and screaming to get 'em." (Having lost emotional distance, subject is immersed in the blot.)

One might consider a confabulated response that includes (1) an emotional loss of distance, (2) minus form level, (3) inanimate movement, (4) CF or C, (5) contents consisting of blood or anatomy, and (6) themes that reveal the aftermath of aggression to represent the test equivalent of a reality-distorting flashback. Thus, in one such response, we would see the breakthrough of traumatic imagery and the sudden loss of reality testing, emotional distance, and affect regulation capacities.

CHAPTER
10

COMBINATIVE THINKING

Starting with Rorschach, researchers have paid attention to the ways in which subjects go about organizing their responses to the inkblots. Whether taken as a discrete whole or broken into separate elements described individually, subjects are faced with the task of deciding how to deal with part-whole relationships among the elements that make up each blot. Between these two extremes of global whole responses, on the one hand, and simple details, on the other, subjects have the opportunity to link together individual details in order to form a more complex response made up of a combination of details. The resulting "combinative" response will, of course, involve the whole inkblot, substantial portions of it, or two smaller details organized together by some linking idea.

This chapter concerns the anomalies that occur when subjects attempt to link parts of the inkblot in ways that are illogical and unrealistic. Commonly referred to as "combinatory" or "combinative" thinking, these responses typically include those indicators of disordered thinking referred to as incongruous and fabulized combinations and contaminations. Before studying the various meanings of these familiar thought disorder scores, however, it is useful to begin with a review of the broader category of integrative and organizational activity on the Rorschach. Understanding the psychological underpinnings of nonpathological combinative thinking will thus set the stage for a closer examination of the conceptual moorings of deviant combinatory activity.

Integrative and Organizational Activity

As we have seen so often, all roads lead back to Rorschach himself. Although he did not refer directly to organizational activity, he addressed it indirectly when talking about the scoring of whole (W) responses. In describing the "mode of apperception," or cognitive-perceptual strategy for choosing where to focus, Rorschach indicated that the subject may choose to respond to the whole inkblot or parts of it. Wholes are of either the "primary" or the "secondary" type. Primary whole responses are global and cannot be broken down into smaller elements. A bat on Card V is the most obvious example of a response that takes the inkblot as a gestalt. Rorschach described secondary whole responses as those that are made up of smaller details that are either *confabulated* into a whole response ("confabulated whole answer") or *combined* with other details to form a whole response. Rorschach identified two types of combinative responses, which he called "successive-combinatory answers" and "simultaneous-combinatory answers." Successive-combinatory responses were those in which the subject identifies a few details, then combines them into a whole response. Rorschach gave the Card I example of "Two men (sides) and a woman (middle). . . . The men are quarreling about the woman" (Rorschach, 1921, p. 38). Simultaneous-combinatory responses differed only in the rapidity of the associative-combinatory process. If the above Card I example had been stated as "Two men who are arguing over a woman in the middle," then Rorschach would have called this a simultaneous-combinatory answer and considered it a primary whole response. Rorschach found both types of combinatory responses to be characteristic of imaginative normal subjects, but added that successive-combinatory responses were also found in the records of manic and Korsakoff patients.

Rapaport et al. (1968) used the terms "combination" and "construction" to describe the ways in which subjects might associatively link parts of the inkblot in order to form larger composite or whole responses. Combination responses, designated as "comb," were somewhat similar to Rorschach's "simultaneous-combinatory answers," whereas construction responses ("constr") were essentially the same as "successive-combinatory answers." If the link is spontaneously stated in the whole response, then this would qualify as a combination response. Rapaport considered the Card I response of a "winged man" to be a combination response since the wings are conceptually separate from the body of the man. In contrast, the response of "a bat" to the same card would not be viewed as a combination response because all of the parts (wings, body, etc.) are interdependent.

According to Rapaport, combination responses result from a subject's associative elaboration of spatially contiguous details that transcends what is perceptually contained in the inkblot. Thus, well-integrated and accurately perceived combinations suggest an intelligent, ideationally oriented subject who can look at the inkblot in a novel manner. Although Rapaport felt that the incidence of combination responses was less frequent in more pathological conditions, his group found that obsessive-compulsives, overideational preschizophrenics, and acute unclassified schizophrenics were likely to have at least one combination response. In contrast, inhibited, ideationally constricted individuals were the least likely to give any.

Others recognized the interpretative significance of combination responses. Beck (1933) was the first to introduce a formal way of scoring organizational activity (Z score). By assigning different weights to responses depending on the degree of complexity of the organizational activity, Beck sought to measure a subject's capacity to grasp relationships and organize stimuli in a meaningful way. Over the years, he conceptualized his Z score to be an index of the amount of energy available for intellectual activity.

Vernon (1933) made an early study of organizational activity by introducing a g score to assess combinative and integrative capacity. Hertz (1938, 1942) used an approach to scoring organizational activity that also employed a g score ("g" taken from the word "organization"). As indicated in chapter 2, Hertz suggested that the qualitative differentiations of the g score reflected the quality and efficiency of an individual's analytic, synthetic, and integrative capacity. She rated highly successful, realistic, logical, and well-integrated combinatory responses g O+ comb, weighted 1.5.

Coming at organizational activity from a different direction, another group of Rorschachers (Friedman, 1952, 1953; Phillips, Kaden, and Waldman, 1959) applied Werner's (1948, 1957) theory of cognitive development to the Rorschach. Using Werner's orthogenetic principle, both Friedman and Phillips and colleagues devised scoring systems to assess a subject's level of cognitive maturity. Developmentally mature responses are those in which the subject accurately perceives individual components of the inkblot in an articulated manner which he or she then reintegrates into a well-differentiated unifying whole. These are successful combinative responses that involve breaking the inkblot down into smaller parts and then combining them into a unified whole.

Exner's (1993) study determined that some sort of score for organizational activity scoring was important for the Comprehensive System. His review of the empirical literature led him to incorporate Beck's organizational scoring method into the Comprehensive System. Exner agreed that organizational activity scores correlate positively with some aspects of intelligence but that this relationship is more complex and varies according to the subject's response style.

PATHOLOGICAL COMBINATORY ACTIVITY

Rorschach (1921) described "confabulatory-combined whole answers" as "amalgamations of confabulations and combination in which the forms are vaguely seen and the individual objects interpreted are combined without any real consideration for their relative positions in the picture" (p. 38). As an example of a confabulatory-combination, Rorschach gave a fairly conventional Card VIII response in which the forms of the animals were perceived accurately but the positions of the various objects were neglected. Curiously, he indicated that these responses are common among psychotic patients but later stated that they are seen less frequently in schizophrenia and mania. Rorschach said that confabulatory-combinations are seen frequently in the records of normal individuals with subnormal intelligence, delirious patients, and a condition which he referred to as "confabulatory morons."

Rapaport coined the term "fabulized combination" to describe combinatory responses in which the basis of the relationship between blot elements was essentially illogical and unrealistic. He concluded that the final formulation of the response could reflect either an increase or loss of distance from the inkblot; however, he believed that the fabulized combination was primarily the product of a perceptual loss of distance. Schafer (1948) added that fabulized combinations occur when an "accidental" spatial relationship is taken to indicate a real connection which results in an absurd combination that is essentially impossible. Neither Rapaport nor Schafer distinguished between absurd combinations that occurred between two or more different objects or within the features of a single object in the inkblot.

In their organizational and developmental scoring systems, both Hertz and Friedman included scores for fabulized combinations. Hertz's score for fabulized combinations was "g O- comb," reflecting thinking that was irrational and bizarre and dictated by internal conflicts. Friedman's category was designated by the symbol "FabC."

Despite his tutelage under Rapaport, Holt broke with him in two ways in the scoring of illogical combinations. First, he wanted to label the scores in his PRIPRO system in such a way as to reduce confusion that he felt existed in Rapaport's scoring of deviant verbalizations and to remain close to the psychological process underlying each score. As a result, Holt called fabulized combinations "arbitrary combinations of separate percepts" (C-c-a). He specified that these were impossible combinations in which the incongruity was based either on a discrepancy in size, a combination of things that do not occur in nature, or a mixture of natural and supernatural frames of reference. Second, Holt distinguished between "impossible combinations" involving two separate but contiguous percepts and impossible combinations or "fusions" within a single percept. He referred to the latter type of illogical combinatory response as "composition" responses (scored at either Level 1 or 2). Holt included a separate category that he called "arbitrary combinations of color and form (C-arb) to describe the inappropriate integration of color with a particular form.

Weiner's (1966) view, as presented in chapter 8, was that combinative thinking was one of the major manifestations of disturbed reasoning and especially the primary process mechanism of condensation. Like Holt, Weiner separated inappropriate combinations that occurred *within* a single blot element from those that occurred *between* two or more elements. While retaining Rapaport's term "fabulized combination" for the latter type, he introduced the term "incongruous combination" to describe four subtypes of inappropriate combinations occurring within a single blot element (composite responses, arbitrary form-color responses, inappropriate activity responses, and external-internal responses). Weiner stuck closely to Holt's system in describing the varieties of fabulized combinations. Finally, Weiner classified the contamination response as the most severe example of combinative thinking.

Johnston and Holzman (1979) borrowed Weiner's categories and terminology for classifying combinative thinking on the TDI; and of course, Weiner's influence is clearly present in the scoring of inappropriate combinations in the Comprehensive System. Probably stated more explicitly in the Comprehensive System than elsewhere, Exner (1986a, 1993) classified INCOMs, FABCOMs, and CONTAMs as increasing points of severity along a dimension of inappropriate combinations.

A CONTINUUM OF PATHOLOGICAL COMBINATIONS

A number of authors reviewed thus far have attempted to study varying degrees of severity among deviant combinations (Holt, 1956, 1977; Weiner, 1966; Lerner et al., 1985; Wilson, 1985; Exner, 1986a, 1993; Athey et al., 1992, 1993). Leaving aside contamination responses for the moment, we have seen how both incongruous and fabulized combinations can be conceptualized along a dimension ranging from benign or unlikely to impossible or malignant. Klopfer and Spiegelman (1956) observed that even blatantly inappropriate combinations may differ in the degree to which they deviate from reality. In this regard, they noted that the more a subject is unable to justify the inappropriate combination by means of realistic, artistic, or aesthetic referents, the more this becomes indicative of severely pathological reasoning.

In their efforts to link Rorschach thought disorder scores to boundary disturbances in borderlines and psychotics, both Wilson (1985) and Lerner et al. (1985) distinguished between mild and severe degrees of boundary disturbances represented by different types of fabulized combinations. In keeping with Blatt and Ritzler's (1974) original boundary/thought disorder hypothesis, Lerner and his colleagues classified "fabulized combination (regular)" responses under the heading of "Boundary Laxness" (the mildest form of boundary disturbance). Under the heading of "Self-Other Boundary" disturbance, they listed a more severe subtype as "Fabulized Combination-Serious (blends)," which they defined as

> two percepts combined to make an incongruous percept with disparate parts. Conceptual boundaries maintained but combined within the percept in an arbitrary way (e.g., "A person with a bird's beak for a nose"). Blends can be along the lines of human/animal, animate/inanimate, or within categories (e.g., "An elephant with a lion's tail"). Idiosyncratic means of joining two percepts (e.g., "Siamese twins," "two girls attached together at the stomach") [p. 54].

In this definition, Lerner was including Weiner and Exner's more benign category of incongruous combinations and what Holt, Weiner, and Exner would all consider as unusual but not impossible combinations (e.g., "Siamese twins").

Wilson, too, identified two subtypes of fabulized combination, which he labeled "benign" and "malignant." Wilson was a bit clearer in his distinction, mentioning that the "malignant" subtype reflects a threat to one or both of the boundaries. He included internal-external responses and bodies that have had boundaries violated as examples of this more severe subtype that he considered to be one step away from contamination. His two examples of malignant fabulized combinations were "A lion with eggs inside it" and "A butterfly with a man's leg coming out of it" (p. 350).

Athey et al. (1992, 1993) took the notion of a continuum farther than other researchers by positing a range of combinative thinking extending from mild to moderate to severe subtypes. Differentiating *improbable* from *impossible* combinations, intact versus violated boundaries, and animate versus animate/inanimate combinations formed the basis for defining three different levels of severity for both composite figures and fabulized combinations.

MILD (IMPROBABLE OR UNLIKELY): Combinations which are *improbable* in reality but can occur in a publicly shared context without violation of body boundaries or the boundary between animate and inanimate objects. A subtle incongruity that spoils an otherwise acceptable image in a minor way. Mild combinations (both incongruous and fabulized) are operationally defined as follows: (1) Questionable mislabeling of body parts. VII. "A dog and these are its hands." CPF mld. (2) Questionable misplacement of body parts. V. "A bug with two stingers on top of its head." CPF mld. (3) Unusual view of an otherwise acceptable composite figure. I. "An angel with wings coming out of the lower part of its back." CPF mld. (4) Unusual clothing transparency without violation of body boundaries. I. "A woman with a skirt, you can see her legs and her vagina." CPF mld. (5) Marginal size discrepancy. VIII. "Animals climbing a tree." FBC mld. (6) Improbable spatial arrangements. VII. "A duck standing on another duck." FBC mld. (7) Natural/supernatural combinations appropriate to a publicly shared context. I. "Angels carrying a person to heaven." FBC mld. (8) Object combinations unlikely to be found in nature. II. "A dog and a lion rubbing noses." FBC mld. (9) Improbable animate/inanimate contact without boundary violation. II. "A man tied to a watermelon." FBC mld.

MODERATE (IMPOSSIBLE): Inappropriate combinations which are *impossible* in reality but without violation of body boundaries or the boundary between animate and inanimate objects. Specific criteria and examples include: (1) Definite size discrepancy. VIII. "A weasel stepping on a butterfly." FBC mod. (2) Impossible or extremely unlikely spatial arrangements. VII. "Heads stacked on top of each other." FBC mod. (3) Natural/supernatural combinations inappropriate to or without a shared social context. I. "Angels carrying a dressmaker's dummy." FBC mod. (4) Object combinations impossible or extremely unlikely to be found in nature. III. "Monkeys fighting over a bow tie." FBC mod. (5) Impossible animate/inanimate contact without boundary violations. III. "People holding a cloud." FBC mod. (6) Hybrids without inanimate parts and appropriate placement of body parts. V. "A rabbit with wings." CPF mod. (7) Internal-external view rationalized as an X ray with appropriate structure. CPF mod.

SEVERE (ABSURD OR BIZARRE): Impossible combinations in which there is a violation of either body boundaries or the boundary between an animate and inanimate object. Blatant composite figure, inappropriate placement of parts, or a combination of animate and inanimate parts into one hybrid figure. Criteria and examples include: (1) Hybrids with inanimate parts or parts inappropriately placed. V. "A bat with a landing gear." CPF sev. (2) Internal-external view without X ray rationalization or with inappropriate structure regardless of X ray rationalization. V. "A bat, you can see its heart inside." CPF sev. (3) Marginal size discrepancy. VIII. "Bears on a mountain peak." FBC sev. (4) Improbable spatial arrangements. VII "A duck standing on another duck." FBC sev. (5) Partial transparency of one figure in front of another. (6) Partial fusion between animate figures. VII. "Women melting together at the waist." FBC sev. (7) Impossible animate/inanimate attachment. VIII. "A bear joined with a rock." FBC sev. (8) Boundary violations of a figure by an inanimate object. II. "A man with a pole up his spine." FBC sev.

Theoretical Underpinnings

Finding relationships between theoretical constructs and the process of combinative thinking on the Rorschach is an interesting exercise that can potentially breathe clinical life into otherwise static test scores. The process of searching for conceptual links with traditional Rorschach thought disorder scores is, in itself, inherently combinatory, although, one hopes, integrative and helpful in expanding our standard understanding of these scores. Borrowing from Hertz, it is hoped that the following hypothesized relationships between pathological combinations and various theoretical constructs fall in the range of a "g O+ comb!"

Fabulized and incongruous combinations (or composite figures) are widely understood to occur when the subject posits an unrealistic relationship between blot elements on the basis of spatial contiguity. Here the subject assumes that because the details are adjacent, there must be some explicable connection between them. The perceptual relationships concretely present on the card are taken as real relationships without being subjected to critical evaluative appraisal. We can see a mixture of concrete loss of perceptual distance from the inkblot, together with implicit autistic logic and failure of critical thinking as the subject reasons that because two things are touching, they must belong together, no matter how unusual, unrealistic, or absurd the relationship may seem.

Are there constructs that exist in the developmental and psychoanalytic literature that can further buttress our understanding of the kinds of psychological processes underlying fabulized and incongruous combinations? I believe there are a number of interesting "connections," some of which have already been mentioned.

Condensation

Describing the psychology of dreaming, Freud (1900) suggested that latent elements of separate ideas or images that have something in common are combined into a single entity in the manifest content. Holt was the first to link combinative thinking to Freud's primary process mechanism of condensation. Holt believed that the condensation of ideas and images was represented by Rorschach scores that reflected arbitrary and inappropriate combinations (fabulized and incongruous combinations, or "composition" responses) and contaminations.

Meloy related von Domarus's (1944) concept of "predicate thinking" to the mechanism of condensation. According to Meloy, condensation involves a horizontal condensing of representations, on the basis of having one element in common, that ends up violating the conceptual boundaries of Aristotelian logic. In the case of pathological combinations, only one common element, spatial contiguity, becomes the principal focus of attention, while other relevant characteristics of the objects are ignored.

Boundary Disturbances

Blatt and Ritzler (1974) defined the boundary disturbance represented by fabulized combinations as a form of "boundary laxness." More specifically, each separate element in the response is kept intact and may be perceived accurately, but the conceptual boundary between elements is breached. The implication is that for boundaries to be maintained, conceptually distinct entities, regardless of spatial proximity with one another, *should* be kept separate.

Blatt and his followers, Lerner and Wilson, originally considered incongruous combinations to be a more malignant form of combinative activity, closer to the process of contamination, because the boundaries between separate elements were more severely ruptured. However, this hypothesis has not been supported by research (Lerner et al., 1985) or by normative data (Exner, 1986a, 1993). This issue is examined in more detail in the next chapter.

The Magic of Contiguity

In his study of primitive and magical thought, Werner (1948) introduced the term "magic of contiguity" to describe the belief that the properties of one thing, when brought into contact with another entity, can pervade that entity. He described rituals in the primitive Papuan culture wherein an individual rubbed his back and legs against rocks in order to partake of their strength. Contact, or tactile-mediated spatial connection, between the subject's body and a hard substance implies that the desired qualities of hardness are transferred to the body. The combinative activity inherent in this type of thought process would speak to a greater degree of permeability of boundaries (of a near contaminatory quality) than is typically associated with fabulized combinative thinking. If we were to assign a score to this magic ritual, it probably merits a FBC sev (fabcom-severe), in that a spatial connection between an animate and an inanimate object occurs with an implicit rupture of boundaries between them.

Werner pointed out that the magic of contiguity characterizes the reasoning of both the young child and psychotic individual. It is developmentally appropriate for the youngster to assume that temporal or spatial proximity to magically potent objects will result in the acquisition of the desired or undesired quality. Thus, the two-year-old who combs his hair with a black comb with the hope that it will make his hair black reveals this form of magical combinative thinking.

Parataxic Distortion and Preoperational Thought

Friedman (1952) believed that fabulized combinations and contaminations are products of the "magic of contiguity." Goldfried et al. (1971) expanded this connection by bringing in Sullivan's concept of the parataxic mode of functioning. According to Sullivan (1953), parataxic thought occurs in late infancy and involves primitive and erroneous logic that relies on signs, symbols, and signals. Hall and Lindzey (1957) described the parataxic mode as "quasilogical thought." They brought Sullivan's concept of "parataxic distortion" even closer to the Rorschach concept of pathological combinations by stating that the parataxic mode of thinking "consists of seeing causal relationships between events that occur at about the same time but are not logically related" (pp. 140–141).

Although the timing of Piaget's preoperational period (Piaget, 1959) does not coincide with Sullivan's parataxic mode, both of these developmental constructs are characterized by magically contiguous thinking. During the early preoperational period, from ages two to four, children view the world egocentrically. They think according to their immediate perceptions which are processed through an egocentric view of the world. Typically, preoperational youngsters focus on only one attribute of an object at a time. Thus, an event that is spatially or temporally contiguous to a feeling state within the child becomes the most salient feature of a complex event and can become paired with the child's feelings in a causally meaningful way.[1] For example, a scared three-year-old who hears a stranger raise his voice may conclude that the stranger is trying to scare him. As children move beyond preoperational thinking and begin to develop more sophisticated ways of representing the world, they become capable of "decentering" and varying the focus of their attention. Instead of remaining concretely fixated on only one perceptually salient aspect of a situation (e.g., contiguity) they become capable of considering more than one attribute at a time.

By summoning the concepts of parataxic and preoperational thinking, we can begin to view pathological Rorschach combinations as having something in common with superstitious, egocentric, and correlational thinking. Most superstitious beliefs are based on positing a special, meaningful connection between two inherently unrelated events based on temporal or spatial proximity. The hat a player is wearing when he hits a homer becomes a talisman and is forever imbued with special power. In egocentric thinking, the youngster assumes that if mother is upset and in close proximity, then he must have caused her upset. In more scientific circles, correlational thinking erroneously assumes that two things that are *correlated* (or occur together) have a *causal* relationship.

Superstitious beliefs and egocentric and correlational thinking are clear, experience-near examples of inappropriate combinative thinking. Each is based on an immature level of cognition and an overly subjective, egocentric orientation toward the world. It comes as no surprise to find that Exner's normative data (1986a, 1993) reveal that both FABCOMs and INCOMs occur more frequently in young children and decrease with age. In fact, children at the age of 14 typically give one INCOM, whereas FABCOMs are found more frequently in the records of younger, latency age children. The norms clearly suggest that FABCOMs are the more serious of the two types of combinative responses.

Despite his view that parataxic thinking occurs in late infancy, Sullivan held that much adult thinking does not extend beyond this more primitive level where causality is assumed to exist between experiences that have nothing to do with each other. Egocentric and correlational thinking are characteristic in individuals whose conviction about the immediacy of their own perceptual experience supersedes

---

1. We are essentially referring to the phenomenon of a conditioned stimulus (perhaps one that is neutral but spatially or temporally contiguous to an unconditioned stimulus) that becomes capable of evoking an emotional response (conditioned response). Neutral stimuli that are contiguous with traumatic events can become associated with and may actually bring about traumatic reactions.

their capacity to "decenter" or objectify and consider an event from more than one viewpoint. Combinatory thinking may reflect this form of cognitive rigidity, in which conclusions are based on immediate and obvious perceptions without engaging in thoughtful, reflective activity. Broadly speaking, we are describing an immature cognitive style characteristic of what David Shapiro (1965) called "impulsive styles." In describing the cognitive style of impulsive individuals (diagnostically considered as action-oriented character disorders), Shapiro wrote:

> First, if we say that the impulsive person's attention does not search actively and analytically, we may add that his attention is quite easily and completely captured; he sees what strikes him, and what strikes him is not only the starting point of a cognitive integrative process, but also, substantially, it is its conclusion. In this sense, his cognition may be called *passive*. Second, if he does not search—critically examine this aspect and that aspect—he does not perceive things in their potential and logical significance, but sees them only in their most obvious, immediately personally relevant qualities. In this sense, the impulsive mode of cognition is relatively *concrete* [pp. 150–151].

In linking this immature form of passive combinative thinking with impulsive character disorders, one might wonder about the prevalence of inappropriate combinations in the Rorschach of these patients. Exner's (1986a, 1993) norms for 180 outpatients with character problems reveal high mean INCOM and FABCOM scores similar to the scores that occur in the records of preadolescents, thus adding support to the notion that character disordered individuals tend to exhibit a more developmentally immature cognitive style.

This kind of passive reactivity to the environment is also reflected by a greater frequency of pure color (Pure C) responses in the records of character disordered patients and younger nonpsychiatric subjects. In fact, character disordered patients have a mean number of Pure C responses roughly equivalent to the number found in the records of eight- and nine-year-olds. Rapaport et al. (1968) suggested that pure C responses represented emotional reactivity that short-circuits the capacity to delay, while Shapiro (1960) stated that C responses involve perceptual passivity in relation to the stimulus and a relaxing of cognitive controls. Although Exner (1993) indicated that pure C responses should not be equated with impulsivity, per se, he stated that these formless color responses represent a more intense and poorly managed style of emotional expression. In essence, the subject expresses emotion first, then sees how the environment responds. Thus, we might infer that the concurrence of pure C responses with INCOMs and FABCOMs would increase the likelihood that the subject has an immature cognitive style, characterized by the tendency to react immediately and uncritically to environmental stimuli without sufficient delay or thoughtful consideration of the appropriateness of the reaction.

False Connections and Transference

One can think of transference as a combinative process, in which something from the past becomes inappropriately and erroneously linked to someone in the present. Freud (Breuer and Freud, 1893) originally conceived of transference as a "false connection" between a wish from the past (connected to a particular object) and a person in the present. Freud wrote, "Transference on to the physician takes place though a *false connection*" (p. 302). The linking factor is some internal psychological variable such as a wish or affect which becomes "falsely connected" to the wrong object who happens to be in the "right place at the right time."

Singer (1993) discriminated between two levels of "false connections" that occur in transferences of preneurotic and neurotic patients. According to Singer, transference in more intact patients reflects a higher developmental level where the subject can recognize, discriminate, and differentiate between his and her affects and those of others. In this form of transference, the engagement is with the sought-after object. In other words, the false connection is made with the object, recognized as a separate person. Hypothetically, we may consider that fabulized combinations between two separate and accurately perceived objects, which happen to be falsely connected, are conceptually representative of this higher level transference displacement. In more developmentally primitive patients, on the other hand, where there is less complete separation between one's affects and those of another person, transference may reflect greater permeability of boundaries (like Werner's example of the primitive ritual mentioned earlier). For example, the subject's internal feeling state may become erroneously linked in a causal manner with an object who just happens to be present at the time. This would be another example of parataxic distortion. The subject may then falsely assume that his bad feeling is being caused by this other person, just as he had believed bad feelings were always caused by significant figures from the past. In this case, the false connection is between the subject's internal state and the contiguous object, not between a past object and a present one. More severely pathological combinatory responses, in which the boundaries of the separate objects are somehow breached, could represent this more primitive level of transference projection.

Athey (1986) elaborated on a similar distinction in his description of transference phenomena in patients who produced different levels of combinatory responses on the Rorschach. Recall that Athey's interest was to understand the relationship between pathological modes of thought organization and object relations as expressed through transference. One patient gave benign inappropriate combinations that were given in a fantasy context. In these responses, this patient maintained the distinction between separate ideas/images and recognized the incongruity of the combinations. An example of one playful incongruous combination (perhaps scored as "playful confabulation" in the TDI) was his response to Card X: "This looks like a very unlikely family argument being arbitrated by a piece of celery" (indicates upper gray detail). "Everybody's arguing, not listening. I was fantasizing, making up a Disney character, something that can't talk but does. Everything was focused up to him, sitting there like a judge, squatty feet, very comical" (p. 40). As can be seen from the structure of this response, the patient placed his inappropriate combination in a fantasy context that he clearly recognized as unrealistic. Nonetheless, he chose to stick with this incongruous response. Athey presented a clinical vignette to describe how this patient had devalued a formerly idealized father who had been a critical taskmaster before he died. Athey went on to demonstrate how the individual reacted to the examiner as an ineffectual judge, reminiscent of his father, and failed to integrate this transference reaction with some actual aspects of the working relationship. Although he was able to see the unrealistic "as if" nature of his false connection, his particular view of the examiner persisted.

Athey then presented impossible Rorschach combinations of a more primitively organized patient followed by clinical material to demonstrate how this patient's more primitive transference was mediated by the structure of his thought.

Card I. Well, could be two animals on something that rotates 360 degrees, head, feet, tail, feet attached to the 360 degree rotating thing . . . (Animals?) Nose, ears, head, tail, and their feet, body. (Alive?) Yes. (Rotating thing?) Like a teddy bear or something, bearcub or something like that. (How relate to the teddy bear?) Well, there is something central there, like a pole, and naturally I assumed it would be able to rotate 360 degrees if it was cylindrical. (Were the bear and the pole the same thing?) Well, it was attached in some fashion, but being in dark colors it's difficult to discern the nature of the attachment. Like a merry-go-round, something you'd find in a park, amusement park, or something. They're holding on, attached to it, could be bear cubs. (Attached?) Like a ride in an amusement park, so they certainly wouldn't be alive, it would be like horses on a merry-go-round, carved [pp. 41–42].

Although the patient ultimately attempted to cast the combination in an acceptable context (an amusement park ride), his spontaneous response was an impossible combination that revealed an arbitrary connection between something animate and inanimate (live bears attached to something mechanical). The bizarre connection between these two objects also reveals a tendency towards fusion in which the boundaries of each become somewhat diffuse. Athey described a similar permeability in the patient's ego boundaries when he combined an internal feeling state ("I feel I'm looking silly") with the examiner's behavior (conducting the inquiry by asking a series of questions) and concluded that he must have done something wrong for the examiner to have been asking these questions. At the end of the testing, the patient commented that he felt that the examiner had invaded his privacy and robbed him of his self-respect. Athey related how this patient had had an invasive father who dominated him throughout his childhood. The examiner's questioning evoked an internal state of being critically intruded upon, and this became the dominant experience of the relationship with the examiner. There was no "as if" quality to these feelings; the patient had essentially falsely combined his painful internal state with the examiner's neutral questions.

A final link between transference phenomena and combinatory thinking harkens back to chapter 8, in which I discussed the object relational implications of thought disorder scores. Unlike the foregoing discussion of transference and combinative thinking, which focused on the process of making false connections between separate entities (a present and past object or between one's feeling state and the presence or actions of another person), the following linkage between combinative thinking and transference focuses more on the content or paradigmatic nature of the transference phenomenon. A particular object-relational paradigm may lead a subject preemptively to perceive relationships in a particular manner consistent with this internal template. In his earlier work, Athey (1974) stated that the fabulized combination "A weasel climbing on a butterfly" may suggest a propensity to view relationships in a sadomasochistic manner. Athey defined fabulized combinations as the interpretation of a relationship that disregards whether the fit is consistent with reality. Meloy and Singer (1991) also considered that fabulized combinations could signal possible problems in object relationships. Although the object percepts themselves are unimpaired, the subject posits a faulty relationship between them.

DIAGNOSTIC CONSIDERATIONS

Combinative thinking occurs in a range of clinical and normal subjects. The norms of the Comprehensive System indicate that it is not unusual for Level 1 INCOMs and FABCOMs to occur on the Rorschachs of nonpatient adults and children. For example, 46% have at least one INCOM and 16% one FABCOM, whereas 84% of nonpatient 5-year-olds have INCOMs and 80% have FABCOMs. The frequency of both scores remains relatively high up to the age of 16 when 65% have one INCOM and 20% one FABCOM. However, Level 2 INCOMs and FABCOMs are extremely rare in the records of nonpatients, with a frequency of 0.4% INCOM2 and 1.7% FABCOM2. Even 5-year-old subjects produce much lower numbers of these more severe combinative responses, with roughly 9% giving one INCOM2 and 22% one FABCOM2.

A variety of clinical groups have been found to produce combinative responses. A great deal of research has investigated the relative frequency of combinative thinking among schizophrenic, manic, borderline, and obsessional subjects. A number of these differential diagnostic issues concerning combinative responses will be reviewed in chapters 13 through 16.

Because of the ubiquity of combinative thinking across the diagnostic spectrum, it is important to avoid a rigid sign approach when considering diagnostic implications of fabulized and incongruous combinations. With the possible exception of manic conditions, the diagnostic specificity of both combinative scores is suspect. Several additional factors must be weighed before making premature links from combinative scores to diagnostic conclusions. Form level, intactness versus impairment of boundaries between adjacent objects, absurdity/bizarreness of the combination, thematic content of the combination (morbid, violent, sexual, neutral, fusion/merger), and distance taken from one's response are all critical factors that need to be considered when evaluating the diagnostic significance of a pathological combination.

Aside from questions about psychopathology and differential diagnosis, are there some general conclusions of a psychological nature that can be drawn about inappropriate combinative responses? Is there some irreducible meaning or interpretation that can be attached to these responses? If we return to the beginning of the chapter, I believe that we can find a general psychological principle that subsumes most every combinative response. Recall that combinative thinking is related to organizational activity or attempts to integrate observations and experiences. Here the organizational efforts go awry, however, resulting in a combination that flies in the face of reality. Nonetheless, it is important to remember that the subject is trying to organize and account for his or her observations. Perhaps, as in the case of the manic patient, the subject is simply attempting to make sense out of a flight of ideas or manage an expansive perceptual style that makes it difficult to ignore or screen out any detail within his or her perceptual grasp. Unfortunately this attempt to organize perceptions and attach meaning eventually outstrips critical evaluative functions and leaves the subject with a failed organization. Thus, the problem for the manic patient (and some others who give combinative responses) may be less one of "disorganization" and more one of "misorganization." In contrast, the relatively lower frequency of combinative thinking among schizophrenic patients may reflect their difficulties in organizing perceptual stimuli in the first place or their "disorganization." Meissner (1981) addressed this issue when he characterized the schizophrenic process as a deficiency in the capacity to organize perceptual material into conceptual categories We return to this issue in chapter 13 when the conceptual deficits associated with schizophrenia will be explored.

CHAPTER
11

CONTAMINATED THINKING

"The Liver of a Respectable Statesman." Hermann Rorschach's first example of a "contaminated whole answer" is almost as amusing as it is bizarre. Indeed, if we guess that the respondent was a physician, and that he saw the liver as diseased, then we could almost imagine him as making an ironic joke, betraying his suspicions about statesmen in general. But, alas, this is not a joke but a kind of psychotic confusion—as would become readily clear if we asked the man, "which is which?" In general, contaminations are often so outrageously strange that they are difficult to forget.

Virtually all major systematizers of the Rorschach have included a contamination score for these bizarre responses that merge two or more overlapping images into a single percept using the same inkblot location. In the "liver of a respectable statesman" response (Rorschach, 1921, p. 38), Rorschach pointed out how his catatonic patient interpreted the same blot area twice, once as a liver and *simultaneously* as a man, followed by an absurd association to the concepts of "respectable" and "statesman." Likewise, Rapaport indicated that his well-known "bloody island" response was the product of the fusion of the images of a bloody spot and an island, both of which occupy the same blot area.

Viewed by Holt (1977) as the waking analog of dream condensation (Schwartz and Lazar, 1984), contamination responses are simultaneously seen as the most pathological of all Rorschach thought disorder scores. Although most would agree that this statement is largely correct, it contains some problematic assumptions that may be misleading. For example, the statement may imply that contamination is synonymous with condensation and, relatedly, that condensation, like contamination, is a pathological process. The relationship between the concept of condensation and the Rorschach score of contamination is more complex than the statement suggests. Condensation is a concept that originated in a theory of mental functioning (Freud, 1900) and is quite broad in scope, while contamination has a narrower purview, pertaining to a discrete response category. Additionally, condensation, as a central mechanism of primary process thinking, reflects not only pathological, but adaptive functioning and creativity as well.

In the following sections, I examine the nature of the relationship between contamination and condensation in more detail. Then I suggest a classification of contamination responses, followed by a discussion of diagnostic implications. Finally, I attempt to clarify some of the areas of conceptual confusion that surround the contamination response.

CONDENSATION

Regardless of whether or not one subscribes to an economic theory of drive energies (as described in chapter 8), primary process thinking is characterized by the fluid shifting of images and ideas. Unlike secondary process thinking, primary process-mediated ideas and their referents lack orderliness and stability. As a result, images and ideas can intermingle with one another and become condensed in ways that are incompatible with external reality. Separate images can become fused resulting in bizarre hybrids that represent several images or ideas simultaneously.

The conventional definition of condensation is based on the concept of "compacting" or "compressing" ideas or information. The *American Heritage Dictionary* (1981) defines "condense" as "to reduce the volume of; compress . . . to become more compact . . . to make dense" (p. 277). The same source defines "contaminate" as "to make impure or corrupt by contact or mixture" (p. 287). Similarly, condensation implies a more neutral process that serves a particular function (the act of compressing), whereas contamination suggests a mixture that has become tainted or polluted. However, the traditional psychoanalytic definition of condensation also includes the notion of "intermingling" or "merging" as well. Images and ideas are not merely "compressed"; they may also undergo a process of interpenetration, fusion, or merger. In developmental psychology, themes of fusion and merger typically suggest less well differentiated or pathological states. However, even though condensation is a primary process mechanism that is characterized by intermingling or merging, we must be careful not to pathologize automatically this process. Condensation can be separated into two broad categories: those that reflect pathology and those that reflect adaptation. The two categories of condensation and their relationship to contamination responses are described below (see Table 11-1).

Pathological Condensations

As a pathological process, condensation may reflect either a regressive wish for merger or a deficit in the ability to suppress the intermingling of incompatible or conflicting impressions (Schwartz and Lazar, 1984). Additionally, pathological condensations involve the unintentional collapse of boundaries between different frames of reference, such as time (past, present, and future); space (here and there); personal identity (self and other); and sensory events (actions, thoughts, and feelings). Such perceptual and conceptual condensations are typically the result of a passive and unreflective, as opposed to consciously motivated, process. The key question in distinguishing pathological from adaptive (in particular, creative) condensations concerns the attitude and intentionality of the person employing the mechanism of condensation.

Holt and Havel (1960) were the first to translate this primary process mechanism into the language of Rorschach thought disorder. They initially included seven varieties of Rorschach responses that reflect varying degrees of image fusion.[1] The first four varieties represented different degrees of fusion or merger between images, in which more than one image was simultaneously assigned to the same blot area. The last three represented fusion between adjacent, versus single, blot areas, or pathological combinations of discrete blot elements (see chapters 4 and 8). In essence, Holt and Havel were suggesting a continuum of pathological condensation responses, a precursor to the continuum concept elaborated on by the Menninger group.

Holt described the most extreme example of image-fusion as the contamination response in which overlapping images are fused into a single percept. Holt and Havel originally included internal-external responses on this continuum, followed by two scores that reflected the subject's difficulty distinguishing or choosing between two percepts for the same blot area. Holt (1977) later introduced the term "interpenetration" to capture this partial fusion process (which could be considered a contamination-tendency).

---

1. Holt (1977) later revised this category by adding several scores including Arbitrary combinations of color and form (C-arb), Contagion (C-ctgn), and Interpenetration (C-int). Holt's formal PRIPRO scoring for condensation is presented in chapter 4.

Table 11-1 Categories of Condensation

I. Pathological Condensation: Ego deficit
  A. Contamination
    1. Full contamination
    2. Contamination-Tendency
  B. Composition
    1. Composite Responses
    2. INCOM Levels 1 & 2
  C. Combination
    1. Arbitrary Combinations
    2. Fabulized Combinations

II. Creative and Adaptive Condensations: R.I.S.E. (Regression in the service of the ego)
  A. Creative Condensations
    1. Janusian Thinking
    2. Homospatial Perception
    3. Metaphor
    4. Puns and Jokes
  B. Adaptive Condensations
    1. Dreams
    2. Symptom formation

Creative and Adaptive Condensations

If pathological condensations occur without conscious design and in the context of an impaired perspective, most adaptive condensations are fully intended and consciously motivated. In an adaptive sense, condensation is used as a mechanism to express a particular thought, feeling, or experience. In essence, by secondary process design, a primary process mechanism is employed for a specific purpose, whether to convey meaning, solve a problem, make one laugh, or sell a product.

Adaptive condensation is germane to the topic of creativity (see chapter 17) and occurs most frequently in works of art and literature. In writing about the creative process, Rothenberg (1971, 1976) coined the term "Janusian thinking" to describe the conscious capacity to conceive and utilize simultaneously two or more opposite or contradictory ideas, concepts, or images. Rothenberg believed that this cognitive process, which defies conventional logic, lies at the heart of creative breakthroughs. Rothenberg also introduced another related term reflecting adaptive condensation which he called "homospatial process." He used this term to describe the simultaneous placing of two discrete entities in the same perceptual-cognitive space. Rothenberg first described Janusian thinking in the context of his study (Rothenberg, 1969) of Eugene O'Neill's play *The Iceman Cometh*. In his original work, Rothenberg presented evidence that the central iceman symbol simultaneously represented several opposite concepts, or a condensation of seemingly incompatible connotations. According to Rothenberg, the iceman symbol had at least three meanings: (1) death; (2) Christ; and (3) a sexually potent adulterer. If one substitutes these meanings in the play, the notion of the "iceman coming" produces a number of logically opposite ideas.

Surrealistic artists such as Dali and Magritte frequently merged incompatible images to create disturbing, dreamlike scenes. Dali, in particular, was influenced by Freud's writings on the mechanisms of dreams and unconscious mental processes. Typical of Dali was his technique of using commonplace objects to set up a chain of metamorphoses that are gradually or suddenly condensed and transformed into a nightmarish image.

Creative condensations abound in poetry, as the poet sees similarities in things that are inherently dissimilar. Condensation underlies the creation of metaphor, and metaphorical language is one of the essential components of poetry. Humor and comedy make liberal use of condensation. Freud (1905) wrote about the psychology of wit and humor after he noticed that certain dreams resembled jokes. In particular, he observed how witticisms often contain word condensations (or creative neologisms) in order to achieve comic effect. For example, the word "shy-chologist" condenses the meanings of the words "shy" and "psychologist" and can be applied to either psychologists who study "shyness," psychologists who themselves are shy, or both.

Nowhere is creative condensation more apparent than in puns and plays on words. Freud noted that the double meanings found in puns were a preferred technique in jokes. A senior analyst offered this play on words when kidded by colleagues about his new luxury sedan: "It's a case of pure auto-eroticism!"[2] One word "auto-eroticism," conveys two distinct meanings that blend synergistically to make this a clever and amusing verbal condensation.

Creative condensations are also found in commercial and technological products. In recent years, toy manufacturers marketed "Transformers" and "Gobots" to youngsters, who were intrigued by these toys that could be two things at once. However, in most of these toys, the two objects (car versus robot, for example) could each retain their separate identities in a non-overlapping fashion. Technological developments have led to the merging of seemingly incompatible business and service enterprises resulting in such condensations as "Telepsychiatry" and

---

2. I am grateful to Irwin Rosen, Ph.D. for providing this example.

"Agribusiness." The defense department popularized the term "war bird" to describe a particular type of combat aircraft.

Chief among adaptive condensations are dreams themselves. Freud (1900) identified three varieties of condensation in dreams: (1) the formation of "collective figures," (2) "composite figures," and (3) "intermediate common entities." Collective figures referred to those dream figures that represented two or more different people at the same time. Usually the identity of one figure is concealed behind the other (e.g., the figure may be recognizable as A but act like B). In Freud's Irma dream (Freud, 1900), Dr. M. reflected such a collective figure. "He bore the name Dr. M., he spoke and acted like him; but his physical characteristics and his malady belonged to someone else, namely my eldest brother. One single feature, his pale appearance, was doubly determined, since it was common to both of them in real life" (p. 293).

Composite figures reflect the combination or condensation of aspects of two or more figures into a new gestalt. By superimposing two or more images upon one another, the dreamer condenses features of several figures, resulting in a final hybridized image that the subject may not recognize. In his Dr. R. dream about his uncle, Freud indicated that Dr. R.'s yellow beard actually represented more than two separate people: Freud's friend R., his uncle Josef, his father, and himself (Freud, 1900).

Finally, in Freud's intermediate common entities variety, a new gestalt is formed from the ideational content of several independent trains of thought. Unlike collective and composite figures, ideas here are combined without regard to their conceptual fit. Any physical or associative relationship may serve as the basis for the condensation. Again from his Irma dream, Freud gave an example of a single word ("Propyl") which, by associative connection, represented two very different constellations of meaning.

From a psychoanalytic perspective, symptom formation may be viewed as a form of adaptive condensation. Unlike creative condensations, symptoms are not the product of conscious intention to convey meaning. However, as compromises between opposite forces, a single symptom can simultaneously represent a defense against an impulse and the expression of that same impulse. The resulting compromise is a condensation of opposing forces that emerges in the form of a symptom.

Creative condensations may appear on the Rorschach in the form of milder varieties of incongruous and fabulized combinations. However, one might ask if is it possible to have creative contaminations as well, or whether these scores are always associated with severe thought pathology. If it is possible, we would expect creative contamination responses to have good form level (indicating adequate perceptual reality testing) and to reflect sufficient defense effectiveness (Holt's DE). The presence of adequate form level, sufficient control and defense features, and an attitude of playfulness (or maintaining an "appropriate" versus "impaired" perspective) would significantly soften the usually malignant implications of such a response.

Having addressed the broader meanings of condensation, we can focus more narrowly on the pathological varieties that are represented on the Rorschach by the contamination response. In the following section, I present a classification of contamination responses and then discuss some of the diagnostic implications of this score.

CLASSIFICATION OF CONTAMINATION RESPONSES

If one accepts that contaminated responses are not unitary phenomena, there are a number of ways that these responses can be broken down and categorized. Understanding the different ways in which contaminatory thinking can occur on the Rorschach can help diagnosticians better attune to the subtle, less easily recognized manifestations. I present three ways to classify contamination responses beginning with a simple levels approach, followed by classifications based on cognitive domains and a theoretically derived taxonomy, respectively.

Levels of Severity

Historically, most Rorschachers viewed contamination responses as all or none phenomena. As we have seen throughout this book, however, most thought disorder scores can exist along a continuum of severity. For example, Lerner et al. (1985) constructed a six-point boundary disturbance scale that included two levels of contamination, thought to reflect degrees of impairment in the boundary between self and others (see chapter 8). Their most severe referent was the contamination response, followed by a contamination-tendency score, which they defined as a response in which the "conceptual boundaries between two ideas referring to the same area of the blot are maintained with difficulty" (p. 52). Included among their examples of contamination-tendency were fluid responses in which the subject could not commit to one of several different percepts (e.g., "Here's the Liberty Bell; it could be one bell or it could be three bells. I'm not sure which; it keeps changing" [p. 52]). Another example of this milder form of contamination was transparency responses involving unrealistic, simultaneous views of external and internal percepts (e.g., "External female genitalia, here are the fallopian tubes" [p. 52]).

Three levels of contamination were defined on the Menninger Thought Disturbance Scales (mild, moderate, and severe). The mild subtype was analogous to Lerner et al.'s contamination-tendency. Both moderate and severe varieties included full-fledged contaminations. What distinguishes the moderate from the severe level was the adequacy of the form level and the coherence of the relationship between the condensed images in the moderate subtype. In the severe variety, at least one of the images cannot be seen (F– form level) and the relationship stated or implied between the images is not stable or coherent.

Cognitive-Perceptual Domains

Contaminations may be primarily verbal, conceptual, or perceptual in nature, or they may involve several or all of these domains together.

VERBAL CONTAMINATIONS. Responses containing an element of verbal condensation always announce themselves dramatically with bizarre sounding neologisms. For example, idiosyncratic responses such as "bug-ox," "pig-people," "butter-flowers," and "intesticles" all signal the presence of a contamination process.

Verbally-based contaminations rarely occur on the Rorschach without some other associated form of contamination (conceptual or perceptual). In fact, it is difficult to think of an example of a Rorschach contamination that is purely verbal in nature. One possible example may be the response of a psychotic adolescent who looked at Card VIII and said "This looks like all of the inner organs of the body. You got your lungs, liver, the heart, and the *intesticles.*" The neologism "intesticles" condenses, of course, intestines and testicles, both of which belong to the same broad conceptual domain (internal organs of the body). Although it is possible to think of this neologism as a conceptual condensation, as well, (i.e., testicles and intestines are distinct concepts representing different organ systems), the subject really was focusing on a broader conceptual class of internal organs, of which both intestines and testicles are members. There was also no evidence of perceptual condensation. The subject did not see the small blot detail in question first as intestines, *then* as as testicles, only to condense them both. He simply saw one blot area as some sort of bodily organ, which he referred to with the neologistic term "intesticles."

PERCEPTUAL CONTAMINATIONS. Perceptual contaminations that result from the fusion of two separate images (e.g., the "bug-ox" variety) are quite easy to spot. However, perceptual contaminations that do not reflect the fusion of images from different conceptual categories or involve word condensation may, at first, sound quite conventional. This is especially true when the contamination comes about as a result of the simultaneous presence of two incompatible views of the same object.

Consider the Card I example from the Comprehensive System Workbook (Exner et al., 1995) "It's a butterfly" (p. 67). At first blush, this sounds like a well-perceived popular response. Certainly there is nothing to suggest the presence of contamination. In response to the examiner's inquiry, however, the subject reasoned that "These are his wings (D2) and his body (D2) and here are his eyes (Dd26) and mouth (DdS29) and ears (Dd28)" (p. 67). Two separate views of the butterfly (one using the whole card as the popular response of "bat" or "butterfly" and the other using many of the same details as the insect's head and facial features) were merged into one absurd image. The final response "butterfly" forms a coherent concept that does not include the tell-tale merging of verbal referents. The contaminatory process is only apparent as the examiner queries the subject about the response. Examples such as this indicate the importance of conducting a careful inquiry so that one is able to understand the reasoning process that lies behind the subject's responses, even those that sound quite conventional.

CONCEPTUAL CONTAMINATIONS. Contaminations that are based primarily on the merging or simultaneity of conceptual categories (without perceptual fusion or verbal condensation) may also be rare and difficult to envision. Here only the boundaries between conceptual domains are breached without accompanying perceptual image fusion. The Card V response "A dead bat that was flying like this before it got killed," reflects only a collapse of the boundaries between past and present. In a single percept, we can observe the loss of temporal boundaries, resulting in two incompatible concepts—"dead" and "flying/alive"—that are merged into one bizarre-sounding response. Instead of separate objects or images being fused into one blot area, we have here a unitary object/image (a bat) that essentially looks the same, dead or alive. The resulting contamination is purely conceptual.

Theoretical Taxonomy

In their empirical and conceptual study of contamination responses, Schwartz and Lazar (1984) proposed three types of contaminations based on Freud's classification of dream condensation, which included (1) simultaneous contaminations, (2) fusion contaminations, and (3) contamination by means of influence.

SIMULTANEOUS CONTAMINATIONS. Like the perceptual category described above, simultaneous contaminations are typically not accompanied by neologisms and can be missed if not inquired into carefully. Schwartz and Lazar gave the Card VII example of "Women eating shrimp" (p. 322) to illustrate the simultaneous presence of two separate images.

In this benign-sounding response, the women and the shrimp are simultaneously represented by the same blot detail (D2 or Dd22). Each image by itself would be adequate, but the activity (in this case "eating") links the two in an unrealistic manner. Schwartz and Lazar proposed that simultaneous contaminations reflect Freud's dream condensation category of "collective figures."

In their earlier study of 100 contamination responses (Lazar and Schwartz, 1982), the researchers found that 24% of the contamination responses in their sample were of this variety. More than half involved popular elements, and 88% had accurate form level. The researchers stated that these responses reflect a preservation in the attunement to perceptual reality but an impairment in their understanding of reality. I think that a clearer interpretation of this finding is that the subjects are able to accurately perceive the details in the world around them but falter psychotically in their efforts to organize or meaningfully integrate these individual elements.

Finally, 42% of these simultaneous contaminations included content reflecting merger or incorporation fantasies. Their examples included contaminations such as "A cat eating a woman" and "A rocket, and this could be drawing it into its mouth, drinking it, eating it" (Schwartz and Lazar, 1984, p. 323). Schwartz and Lazar concluded that these responses may be expressive of the subject's wishes for merger.

FUSION CONTAMINATIONS. Analogous to Freud's composite figure dream condensation, fusion contaminations blend together two or more images that can be seen separately. Responses such as on Card VII, "Rabbit maidens," Card X, "Lunganimals," and Card VIII, "mantree" (from Wilson, 1994, p. 29) include elements of separate images that are condensed in a way that changes the meaning of one or both of the perceptual images.

In their earlier study, Lazar and Schwartz found that a quarter of their sample contaminations were fusion responses. Of these, 80% of these fusions consisted of images that would have been accurately perceived had they been seen separately and not condensed. The researchers again made the point that contact with external perceptual reality is maintained whereas the individual's interpretation of reality is impaired.

CONTAMINATION BY MEANS OF INFLUENCE. Unlike the fusion contamination, this last category includes images that overlap in time but not space. The result is a change in the meaning of one percept under the influence of some extraneous impression. Schwartz and Lazar (p. 328) gave the example of "A storm. A bleeding storm. The whole thing is a storm (points to the black area) and there's bleeding this way (points to red in the upper corner). That shows how violent I am" (Card II). The authors suggested that this type of response provided an example of Freud's immediate common entities category of dream condensation. Here the common associative element (presumably, "violence") lead to the thoughts that "storms are violent" and "bleeding is the result of violence." The result is the contamination that "the storm is bleeding." A third element in the contamination may have included the subject's loss of boundary between his response and himself ("That shows how violent I am").

Schwartz and Lazar pointed out that the main source of influence in these responses was an unmodulated response to color, which was found in 77% of these types of contaminations. Unlike the generally accurate form level associated with the other types of contamination, only 45% of these contaminations were associated with accurate form. The authors concluded that the affect generated by the color in the inkblot undermined the accuracy of the subject's perception and may have contributed to the resulting contaminatory process.

FREQUENCY AND DIAGNOSTIC SPECIFICITY

Contaminations have long been viewed as a pathognomic sign of schizophrenia (Rorschach, 1921; Klopfer and Kelly, 1942; Piotrowski and Lewis, 1950; Bohm, 1958; Weiner, 1966; Rapaport et al., 1968; Harrow and Quinlan, 1985). However, clinicians may overlook the fact that contaminations are such rarely occurring responses that their diagnostic sensitivity is extremely low, while their specificity remains quite high. Meloy and Singer (1991) compared the frequencies of contamination responses in the records of schizophrenic subjects from five different studies (Rapaport et al., 1968; Johnston and Holzman, 1979; Edell, 1987; Exner, 1986a,b). They demonstrated that contaminations occurred at an average frequency of 15.9%, or in only one of every six or seven schizophrenic Rorschach protocols! For example, Rapaport et al. found contaminations in 17% of their combined schizophrenic sample, while Johnston and Holzman (1979) scored contaminations in only 13% of their acute and chronic schizophrenic patients.

Exner's (1993) normative data revealed a frequency of 36 CONTAMs in the records of 3345 normal and psychiatric subjects between the ages of 5 and 65+. Of the 36 CONTAMs, 35 occurred in the records of inpatient schizophrenics (N = 320) and the remaining CONTAM showed up in the record of a 7-year-old (7-year-old N = 120). Only three (0.27%) of Exner's 1095 other psychiatric subjects (borderlines, schizotypals, inpatient depressives, outpatients, and character disorders) had CONTAMs. Interestingly, all three of these occurred in the records of subjects diagnosed with borderline personality disorder (N = 84) and none were found in the protocols of schizotypal subjects (N = 76) (Exner, 1986b). Furthermore , none of the subjects with depressive or character disorders produced CONTAMs. In sum, Exner demonstrated that CONTAMs occurred at a total normative and reference sample frequency of 1% and in the records of 10.9% of his 1993 inpatient schizophrenic sample (or in 18% or his 1986a sample)[3]; 3.8% of his borderlines; 0% of his other psychiatric subjects; 0% of his adult normals; and 0.07% of nonpsychiatric subjects ages 5 to 16.

Koistinen's Finnish adoption data (Koistinen, 1995) offered similar findings regarding both the rarity and diagnostic specificity of contamination responses. Of the 44 subjects diagnosed with schizophrenia (including disorganized, catatonic, residual, undifferentiated, and paranoid subtypes), 15.9% had contamination responses (slightly greater than the frequency of 10.9% found in Exner's schizophrenic sample). One (3.8%) of the 26 subjects with a schizophrenia spectrum disorder (defined as schizophreniform disorder; schizoaffective disorder; schizotypal personality disorder; paranoid personality disorder; psychotic disorder, not otherwise specified; and delusional disorder) had a contamination response. When these two groups are combined, 8 of 70, or 11.4%, of schizophrenic and schizophrenic-spectrum subjects produced contaminations. However, Koistinen's data yielded a total of three contaminations (1.3%) in the records of 226 other psychiatric subjects in the following diagnostic groups: affective disorders (3.2%), nonspectrum personality disorders, including borderline personality (2.7%), neurotic disorders, and other psychiatric disorders (0.0%). Of the 246 "healthy," nonpsychiatric subjects, one (0.46%) gave a contamination response.

Both Lerner et al.'s (1985) and Wilson's (1985) schizophrenic subjects produced more contaminations than either preschizophrenic or depressed subjects. Edell (1987) demonstrated that 16.7% of his "early schizophrenics" gave contaminations, while none of his borderline, schizotypal, or normals produced any.

Thus, empirical data support the claim that a single contamination response is pathognomic of schizophrenia. Taken together, the combined data from a variety of studies demonstrate the *extreme* rarity, low diag-

---

3. Exner's 1986a data on 320 inpatient schizophrenics showed a CONTAM frequency of 18% and in another study on 80 inpatient schizophrenics (Exner, 1986b) a frequency of 15%. His 1993 psychiatric reference data include the same number of inpatient schizophrenic subjects (N = 320) but with a lower frequency of CONTAMs (10.9%).

nostic sensitivity, and high specificity of contamination responses. Roughly, contamination responses can be expected to yield a false positive rate for the diagnosis of schizophrenia of less than 1%, but a false negative rate for the diagnosis of closer to 85%. Aronow et al. (1994) stated that one should be extremely careful in scoring contamination responses, suggesting that it is better to err on the side of assuming that one has made an error in scoring or administration.

The near total absence of contaminations in Exner's normative data for children and adolescents supports Leichtman's (1996) contention that, unlike other forms of combinative thinking, contaminations should not be expected to occur in the records of normal youngsters. One "carefully scored" contamination in the record of the youngest of subjects (if it is possible to score any response carefully and with confidence in the records of young subjects!) can be taken as a pathological sign.

Controversial Issues

Some lingering questions regarding the nature of contaminated thinking may now be resolved. These questions include specifying the relationship between contaminatory and combinative thinking. Should the contamination response be grouped under the heading of combinative thinking or inappropriate combinations, or does it reflect a different process? Another question involves the relationship between form level scoring and contamination responses. In the past, the presence of a contamination response would automatically mean that the form level was poor. Finally, are incongruous combinations more closely related to contaminations as some (Blatt and Ritzler, 1974; Lerner et al., 1985; Wilson, 1985) have suggested? In the final section, I review briefly each of these issues and offer some conclusions that are consistent with the empirical literature.

Contamination and Combinative Thinking

Like Weiner (1966) and Exner (1986a, 1993), Johnston and Holzman (1979) viewed contaminations as the most severe variant (1.0 level of severity) of their combinatory factor (.25: incongruous combination; .50: fabulized combination; .75: confabulation). Similarly, Solovay et al. (1987) grouped contaminations under their a priori factor of combinative thinking. However, subsuming contamination under a combinatory category is consistent with neither theory nor empirical findings. Table 11-1 shows that both contaminatory and combinative thinking are conceptually organized under a superordinate category of condensation.

Viewed this way, contamination and combination are different processes by which the primary process mechanism of condensation expresses itself.

Empirical and normative data also suggest a more complex relationship between combinative and contaminatory thinking. Solovay et al.'s factor analytic classification of TDI scores indicated that contamination responses do not load on an empirically derived Combinatory Thinking factor (that includes such scores as playful confabulations, incongruous combinations, flippant responses, and fabulized combinations). Instead, contaminations load heavily on a Fluid Thinking factor that includes only one other TDI score, Fluidity.

The absence of contaminations in the records of even the youngest of normal subjects (unlike the developmentally normative presence of incongruous and fabulized combinations) further supports the contention that contaminations are conceptually separate from other combinative scores. Finally, as we shall see, incongruous and fabulized combinations are more characteristic of affective and borderline disorders, whereas contaminations are generally pathognomic of schizophrenia.

Ideational Versus Perceptual Impairment

As alluded to earlier, Lazar and Schwartz (1982) challenged Rorschach literature that held that contaminations should automatically be scored F–. They examined the formal characteristics of 100 contamination responses from the Rorschachs of psychiatric inpatients. The only responses they included in their sample were those on which two scoring judges agreed. Any contamination given in a playful, rationalized, or hesitant manner was also discarded. The majority of the subjects in the sample carried the diagnosis of schizophrenia, while very few were diagnosed as borderline personality. Lazar and Schwartz looked at the other formal scoring features of these responses and found some surprising results. Seventy percent of the contaminations involved percepts with form level of F+; 39% of them involved popular content; and 50% contained human movement and some form of human content. The researchers noted that they had not expected to find such conventional variables associated with contaminations and thought disorder. They wondered if contaminations are a psychotic solution to dealing with interpersonal anxiety and conflict. Furthermore, the presence of color in 30% and human movement in 50% of the responses suggested that contaminations occur in the context of ideational and affect-arousing experience.

Exner (1993) also corrected his previous practice of assigning all CONTAMs a minus form level, regardless of whether the form was appropriate to the blot area. He concluded that CONTAM represents an ideational failure that may or may not involve perceptual distortion.

Incongruous Combination and Contamination

Rapaport and his colleagues' failure to distinguish between fabulized and incongruous combinations led some later researchers to wonder about the nature of incongruous combinations and, specifically, to question their relationship to contaminations and fabulized combinations. Holt (1956, 1977) was the first to note the distinction between incongruous (composite) and fabulized combinations (arbitrary combination). Although Holt never made this distinction explicit, I believe he would have considered composition responses (or incongruous combinations) to be more closely related to the process of contaminatory rather than combinative thinking. The implication of this association would be that composition responses signal greater pathology than arbitrary combinations. Holt's emphasis on the term "fusion" in his definitions of composition, contamination, and interpenetration; and the absence of this term in his definition of arbitrary combinations (in which he used the term "combination" vs. "fusion") suggests that he would view composition as a close cousin to contamination.

Following Holt's classification, Blatt and Ritzler (1974) observed that, unlike fabulized combinations, composition or incongruous combinations involve a violation of the basic boundary of a single object. On this basis, they concluded that incongruous combinations, which they did not have a specific term for, were more similar to contaminations than fabulized combinations. Lerner et al. (1985) called incongruous combinations "Fabulized Combinations Serious (blends)" in their six-point Boundary Deficit Scale, placing it right under Contamination in degree of severity (Contamination = 6; Fabulized Combination Serious = 5). In contrast, they called combinations involving two separate percepts "Fabulized Combination Regular" and assigned these a more modest score of 1.

The Lerner group predicted that schizophrenic patients would demonstrate greater self-other boundary impairment, as measured by a greater number of contaminations, contamination-tendencies, and fabulized combinations-serious scores. However, they found that schizophrenics differed from borderlines and neurotics in their mean number of contamination and contamination-tendency scores. There were no significant differences in fabulized combination-serious scores between any of the groups, leading the Lerner group to conclude that "this response is not as related to the contamination and contamination-tendency response as is thought" (p. 59).

Equally convincing are the normative data on the Special Scores in the Comprehensive System, which clearly indicate that INCOMs occur more commonly in the records of nonpatient adults and children than do FABCOMs. This normative finding refutes Blatt and Ritzler's hypothesis that regular incongruous combinations are more serious signs of thought disorder, closer to contamination, than fabulized combinations.

Meloy and Singer (1991) raised an interesting point that may offer some support for Blatt's hypothesis. Meloy and Singer note that, while INCOMs occur at a frequency of 46% and FABCOMs at a frequency of 16% in Exner's (1993) nonpatient adults, Level 2 INCOMs are four times as rare as Level 2 FABCOMs in the records of normals. Although both are rare among nonpatients (INCOM2: .4% and FABCOM2: 1.7%), Level 2 INCOMs are second only to CONTAMs in their rarity among nonpatient adults. Thus, the more bizarre incongruous combinations, as Blatt and Ritzler suggested, may be more closely related to contaminatory versus combinative activity.

Contamination: A Continuous or Discontinuous Variable

In this chapter, and throughout the book, I have argued that each Rorschach thought disorder score can be conceived along a continuum of severity. Even such extreme manifestations of thought disorder as contamination responses may be understood as points along a continuum of contaminatory thinking, with milder versions of this process occurring as well. However, it is important to consider another perspective that views the contamination score as a discontinuous variable. This perspective would hold that contaminatory thinking is qualitatively (not simply quantitatively) different from anything that occurs within the normal range, that it goes beyond the pale of normal experience. If we agree that contamination responses on the Rorschach, though rare, are pathognomic of schizophrenia, then we must also entertain the possibility that the contamination response reflects a manner of thought organization that is phenomenologically distinct from anything that occurs in the normal range of experience.

CHAPTER

12

PALEOLOGIC THINKING

Before launching into the world of primitive logic, a clarification of terminology is useful. As a critical cognitive function, "reasoning" involves the ability to ascertain relationships between objects and events in the world. One of the primary aims of everyday reasoning and scientific reasoning alike is to discover the causes of events. Observers often want to know whether two events simply occur together in time or space, or whether there is a causal relationship between them. Reasoning is a way of organizing observations or sensory information to reach conclusions, often about causality. A "conclusion" is generally the endpoint of a reasoning process, whereas an "inference" involves the use of reasoning to reach a conclusion. "Logic" may be regarded as the science of correct, or conventional, reasoning (Ruchlis and Oddo, 1990). "Paleologic thinking," a term coined by Arieti (1967), is a primitive form of reasoning that runs contrary to the rules of formal logic.

It is axiomatic to state that reasoning plays a key role in almost every higher cognitive operation, and similarly, that impaired reasoning, or illogicality, is present in almost every form of disordered thinking on the Rorschach. Weiner (1966) noted that illogical reasoning may be expressed in three of the major categories of disturbed thinking ("overgeneralized," "combinative," and "circumstantial" reasoning). In the last three chapters, we looked closely at the impairments in reasoning that underlie confabulatory, combinatory, and contaminatory thought processes, which can be understood in terms of Weiner's first two categories. But what about Weiner's third type of illogical reasoning, "circumstantial thinking," or what is commonly referred to as "autistic logic" on the Rorschach?

In this chapter, I begin with a brief overview of the concept of autistic or "paleo"-logic in the psychiatric literature, followed by a review of its development in the field of Rorschach assessment. Then I examine the conceptual underpinnings of autistic logic and attempt to flesh out the pathological, as well as the normative, manifestations of primitive forms of logic.

PRELOGICAL, PARALOGICAL, AND PALEOLOGICAL THOUGHT

Although there are other forms of disturbed logic, the psychiatric literature has traditionally focused on a particular form of illogical reasoning, found in schizophrenia, primitive cultures, and children. Referred to by a number of names, this process was first called "paralogical thinking" by the German psychiatrist and philosopher Eilhard von Domarus (1944). Von Domarus devoted his studies to the application of logic and anthropology to psychiatry. Based on his studies of schizophrenia, von Domarus formulated a principle that assumes that two objects are identical if they share a common predicate. Thus, the schizophrenic subject may reason that if "A has/is a B and C has/is a B, then A must be C." The classic example given by Arieti (1974) was the patient who thought she was the Virgin Mary based on the following paralogical reasoning: "The Virgin Mary was a virgin; I am a virgin; therefore I am the Virgin Mary" (Arieti, pp. 231–232). The subject creates a false belief, of delusional proportions, based on equating two distinct subjects (the Virgin Mary and the subject herself) simply because they share the same predicate (being a virgin).

Arieti (1967, 1974) fine-tuned and elaborated this concept in his detailed studies of schizophrenic cognition. He coined the term "paleologic" (from the Greek *palaios*, which means "ancient and old") to describe a stage in the development of logical thinking which precedes the stage or level of Aristotelian logic. Arieti argued that paleologic may appear illogical according to Aristotelian standards but that it is simply a primitive form of logic that conforms to a different set of rules than those employed in conventional forms of logic. As support for his thesis, he referenced Werner (1957) who discussed this form of logic and magical thinking in the rituals of primitive cultures. Werner cited French anthropologist Levy-Bruhl (1910) who described paleologic thinking in the following African allegory:

A Congo native says to a European: "During the day you drank palm wine with a man, unaware that in him there was an evil spirit. In the evening you heard a crocodile devouring some poor fellow. A wildcat, during the night, ate up all your chickens. Now, the man with whom you drank, the crocodile who ate the man and the wildcat are all one and the same person" [Werner, 1957, p. 16].

Werner also made the point that this form of primitive logic, which holds that a thing can simultaneously have two different identities (i.e., a thing can be "a" and "b" at the same time), is neither illogical nor "prelogical," in a cross-cultural sense. "It is simply logical in another, self-contained sense" (p. 16), qualitatively different from the scientific thinking of civilized societies.

Werner also introduced the idea that young children engage in this form of logic in the course of normal development. For example, a two-year-old will often say something like "doggy" when shown a picture of a four-legged animal. Likewise, "Daddy" is often the term used to greet all adult men, by virtue of the fact that they, like daddy, are men. If one considers the ALOG response to be the Rorschach expression of paleo-logic cognition, then Exner's developmental norms (1993) support this ontological perspective. For example, only 4% of Exner's nonpatient adults give ALOGs, whereas 63% of 5-years-olds do. This percentage remains at a similar level up to the ages of 10–11, at which time the frequency of ALOGs drops to roughly 43%. At the age of 16, the frequency approximates that of the adult nonpatient normative value. Thus, from a developmental perspective, paleologic thinking can be thought of as a manifestation of preoperational and parataxic experience, in which magic pervades the youngster's world view and two things can be the same based on their sharing common properties.

Although, terms like "paleologic" or "paralogical" thinking have never really been parts of psychodiagnostic nomenclature, there is a clear linkage between the concepts introduced by von Domarus and Arieti and Rorschach indices of disordered reasoning. Let us now review briefly the development of the Rorschach concept of autistic logic.

PALEOLOGIC THINKING AND AUTISTIC LOGIC

As indicated in chapter 3, Rapaport, Gill, and Schafer introduced the term "autistic logic" to characterize the types of fallacious logic that von Domarus and Arieti described. However, the reader may remember that Hermann Rorschach originally had a similar score, which he called the "position-determined response" (Po) to depict one type of paleological thinking on the Rorschach. Here, the subject reaches an erroneous conclusion based simply on concrete spatial relationships between, or the relative position of, the blot elements. Most of the early Rorschach pioneers retained a score for the position response, which they felt was pathognomic of schizophrenia (Rickers-Ovsiankina, 1938; Piotrowski, 1957; Beck, Leavitt, and Molish, 1961).

Rapaport saw the Po response as an explicit example of autistic logic. Typically, the listener is cued to the subject's autistic reasoning when the subject announces his or her reasoning error with the word "because." Thus, the subject who gives the position response to Card IX of "the North Pole" goes on to justify this response, "*because* it is at the top." Although Rapaport thought that these types of responses were rare, he too believed that they almost always suggest schizophrenia.

In discussing forms of impaired reasoning on the Rorschach, Weiner (1966) introduced the concept of "circumstantial thinking" which he said occurred when a subject inferred real relationships from coincidental or nonessential aspects of the inkblot or from one's associations to them. Weiner believed that circumstantial thinking was implicit in both overgeneralized and combinatory thinking, which he felt were indirect expressions of predicate logic. Like Rapaport, Weiner separated his category of circumstantial thinking into two Rorschach scores, autistic logic and position/number responses.

Although most would agree that autistic logic marks a severe degree of thought disturbance, several researchers have suggested that autistic logic may exist in milder forms (Weiner, 1966; Athey et al., 1992, 1993). Weiner described mild instances of autistic logic that may be expressed only in relation to size coincidences. For example, the lower detail on Card III may be seen as a "big beetle (Big?) It's big in proportion to these two men here" (p. 83). Although this clearly sounds strained and overly concrete, there is some blot support for the subject's inference. The Menninger system included a moderate level in the "Disturbed Logic" category. This level was defined on the basis of whether the idea expressed is coherent and, like Weiner, whether there is some element of blot support for the subject's strained logic. Examples of a moderate level of disturbed logic include the following responses: IV. "A huge monster *because* it takes up almost all the space." VII. "These two things next to the rabbits *must be* lettuce *since* that's what rabbits eat."

In contrast, responses were rated at a "severe" level whenever there was no blot support for the illogical inference or when the conclusion was extremely idiosyncratic. Examples of responses scored as Disturbed Logic, Severe, include: I. "It has to be a tree since it has two branches coming out." I. "A man and a woman embracing" (Inq) "Because they are together and men and women belong together."

Apart from concluding that the autistic logic response indicates an explicit expression of disturbed thinking, or more precisely, predicate thinking, is there more we can say about the conceptual underpinnings of this phenomenon? Can "autistic logic" and the psychiatric concept of "paleological thinking" be broadened so that the various nuances of psychological meaning can be better understood?

Conceptual Underpinnings of Paleologic Thinking: Normative and Pathological Forms

If paleologic is the obverse of Aristotelian Logic, then exactly how do the two systems of logical inference differ? We know that Aristotelian logic is a product of secondary process thinking, whereas paleologic is associated with primary process, but how else do these forms of reasoning differ?

Aristotelian logic is a deductive method of formal logic, best respresented by syllogistic reasoning. A "syllogism" is a simple form of deductive reasoning that involves two premises, one major and one minor, from which a logical conclusion is deduced. "Premises" may be facts, speculative statements, or hypotheses. The syllogism "All men are mortal" (major premise); "Jones is a man" (minor premise); "therefore Jones is mortal" (conclusion) reflects this form of reasoning, in which the subjects of both premises ("all men" and "Jones") are related. Some conclusions, such as Descartes' statement, "I think, therefore I am," if closely examined, implicitly follow this same syllogistic pattern (i.e., "Thinking people exist"; "I am a thinking person"; "Therefore, I exist").

Aristotelian logic is based on three fundamental laws (Arieti, 1974): (1) law of identity, meaning A is always A and never B; (2) law of contradiction, that states A cannot be A and not A at the same time and place; and (3) law of excluded middle, which holds that A must be A or not A; it cannot be an intermediate state. In paleologic thinking, these three laws are annulled. Two premises are equated on the basis of their sharing the same predicate, whereas the properties of the subjects are largely ignored. Regarding the law of identity in paleologic, A may be B, provided that B shares a common quality with A (e.g., "I am a *virgin*; Mary was a *virgin*; therefore I'm the Virgin Mary"). Likewise, A can be both A and B at the same time. Finally, by condensing several subjects, paleologic thinking neglects the law of excluded middle in that things are often seen as composites of both A and B. In paleologic, Descartes's pronouncement becomes "I am, therefore I think" based on the implicit reasoning "Thinking people are (exist); I am (exist); therefore, I think." One can quickly see how fallacious this conclusion is given the fact that not everything that exists is a sentient being.

Arieti (1974) identified three characteristics of the predicates involved in paleologic thinking, and Weiner (1966) elaborated these in terms of the Rorschach. "Predicates of quality" describe attributes that are intrinsic to an object, such as thinking or being a virgin are qualities of being human. "Predicates of spatial contiguity" are based on two objects or events sharing a common space." Weiner gave the example of a man seeing several people standing in front of a police station and concluding that they are all policemen *because* of their spatial contiguity to the police station. Likewise "predicates of temporal contiguity" lead the paleologician to assume identity between two objects on the basis of their sharing a similar place in time.

There are other general characteristics of paleologic, predicate, or autistic thinking that are useful to consider. Paleologic thinking has an *immediate* quality. The subject "jumps" to conclusions, quickly seizing on one element of a situation on which to base a conclusion, while prematurely foreclosing and excluding other elements. Naturally, it follows that paleologic reasoning is also *reductionistic*, in that it ignores complexity and bases conclusions on simple, one-dimensional, observations. Pars pro toto thinking, in which a part comes to stand for the whole, is an essential aspect of paleologic thought. *Selectivity* is another characteristic. Discrepancies, contradictions, or discontinuities are screened out or ignored, and only those qualities that are consistent with one's conclusion are selected. Finally, paleologic thinking is usually accompanied by a high degree of *certainty*. The paleologician has great conviction in his or her conclusions. There is little room for doubt.

Arieti's concept of teleologic causality in paleologic thinking is related to this high degree of certainty that the paleologician has in forming conclusions. According to Arieti, paleologicians base their conclusions on the belief that *every* act or event has a cause that was either willed or wished by someone. Conclusions are reached *because* one believes that things are predetermined or destined to occur, and this lends a degree of conviction or certainty to one's conclusions. To elaborate this point, Arieti distinguished the different meanings of the word "because" in secondary process and paleologic spheres. For the secondary process thinker, "because" generally means "on account of," whereas, for the paleologic thinker, "because" takes on a slightly different meaning of "for the purpose of." This slight difference in meaning is significant in that it suggests that the paleologician assumes a different basis of causality, one that is predetermined. Belief in predetermined causality increases one's certainty about one's conclusions.

Shifting to a discussion of the psychological implications of paleologic thinking, it is natural to link paleologic thought with the process of delusion formation. Arieti certainly believed that this primitive type of reasoning formed the substrata of delusional thinking. The example of the patient who reasoned that she was the Virgin Mary is inherently delusional. However, the hypothesis that links paleologic reasoning to the formation of delusions is controversial and will be examined more closely in chapter 16 when disordered thinking in delusional disorders is explored. For now, we can assume that severe forms of paleologic thinking, or autistic logic on the Rorschach, are associated with more serious forms of thought disorder. For example, 44% of Exner's (1993) inpatient schizophrenic subjects gave ALOGs, compared to 12 to 14% of his inpatient depressives, outpatients, and character disordered patients.

The issue to consider at this time is whether all degrees of paleologic or autistic-like thinking are indicative of such serious disturbances in thinking and reality testing. Are there psychological correlates of the milder forms of autistic logic that Weiner and my colleagues and I at Menninger have discussed? If we assume that not all paleologic thought is necessarily psychotic, then what are the implications of the nonpsychotic varieties?

Normative Paleologic Thinking: "Benign Paralogia"

It is my contention that all forms of disordered thinking can occur across a range of severity, from the most severe psychotic manifestations to those that are relatively benign and nonpsychotic. Clearly, at its worst, paleologic thinking may form the cognitive substrata for psychotic delusions, but how are the milder forms of paleological thought expressed?

Glasner (1966) introduced the term "benign paralogical thinking" or "benign paralogia" to describe a nonschizophrenic syndrome characterized by paralogical thinking, tangentiality, circumstantiality, pars pro toto thinking, and other manifestations of primary process activity. According to Glasner, individuals who demonstrate benign paralogia are not psychotic. The kind of individual that Glasner described might today be considered borderline; however, Glasner made the point that these individuals are not preschizophrenic. Instead, they are people with intact reality testing, adequate relationships, and adaptive personality functioning. Their only anomalous feature is their blend of primary and secondary process thinking. Glasner concluded that benign paralogia was a nonpsychotic thinking disorder that could express itself in one of four different subtypes. Although his subtypes seem somewhat elusive and unrelated to the subject at hand, the concept of benign paralogia, as a class of mild deficits in logical reasoning, is itself appealing.

I think there are a number of examples of benign paralogia from common experience that, while clearly nonpsychotic, are nonetheless rooted in fallacious logic. The examples of benign paralogia that follow are encountered daily. Each subtype defines a subtle, normative reasoning fallacy that has the potential to lead to interpersonal conflicts and foment social injustice.

STEREOTYPED THINKING. The formation of stereotypes is a common example of benign paralogia. Here, one trait or characteristic of a group is automatically attributed to an individual member of that group, ignoring individual uniqueness and differences. For example, how common is it to see a tall man and assume that he plays basketball. The inherent predicate logic expressing this stereotype is "Basketball players are tall; he is tall; therefore he is a basketball player." There is clearly nothing psychotic about this conclusion, which may actually be correct. However, structurally, it is based on fallacious reasoning, not unlike the kind we have been discussing above. Although ubiquitous, succumbing to stereotypic thinking reflects a less differentiated and less mature form of reasoning.

At its worst, stereotypes beget prejudice that spawns hatred and injustice. Arieti (1974) made this point when he discussed the transmission of irrationality in Nazi Germany. Almost every society engages in stereotyping that ostracizes individuals based on their sharing features in common with a larger group. At the heart of every injustice of this kind is a form of nonpsychotic predicate thinking that focuses on single features, reduces complexity to stereotypes, and reaches immediate affective-laden judgments.

COINCIDENTAL THINKING. Coincidental logic is present whenever we base our conclusions on circumstantial factors. In legal settings, cases based on circumstantial evidence are considered "weaker" and in most cases fall short of legal standards of acceptable proof. An example of the inherent predicate logic in a circumstantial evidence case would be something like "Murderers leave fingerprints at the scene of a crime; your fingerprints are at the scene of the crime; therefore you must be the murderer." Though convincing to many because of its emotional appeal, the evidence above is circumstantial and not conclusive. Again, complexity and alternative explanations are minimized, while simplicity is highlighted. At worst, circumstantial logic can lead to a rush to judgment as a group of citizens, possibly succumbing to regressive forces within the group, engages in a form of socially-sanctioned paralogia.

Coincidental thinking can be even more benign and commonplace. Consider the saying "Where there's smoke there's fire." Related to the issue of circumstantial evidence, this adage also has more general applicability to the paralogia of jumping to conclusions. Unlike the more malignant forms of paralogical thought, jumping to conclusions may pay off in correct and efficient judgments. Whenever the reasoning contains an element of predicate logic, however, we may jump to the wrong conclusions just as easily.

In his delightful novel *There Must Be a Pony*, James Kirkwood (1960) relates a vignette of a psychiatrist who performed an experiment on his twin sons, one an incurable pessimist and the other an optimist. Filling the pessimist's room with every toy he had ever wished for and the optimist's room with horse manure, the father sat back to observe his sons' reactions. His pessimistic son eyed his windfall suspiciously, trying to ascertain the "catch," while the optimist dug into the manure with great glee and enthusiasm. The puzzled father finally asked his manure-covered son what he was so happy about, to which the boy replied, "Gee, Dad, I figure with all this horse shit—there must be a pony!" (p. 201).

Are there Rorschach features that may help to distinguish benign forms of paralogia from the more malignant types, those that may, in fact, be associated with delusional thinking? We might expect that both types of paralogia would be expressed by autistic logic responses, which would vary in terms of reality attunement, bizarreness, and adequacy of form level.

Some ALOGs are not only based on an accurate perception of the inkblots but on details that are more or less relevant to the conclusions that the subject draws. For example, seeing the large details on Card II as rabbits and the top red details as lettuce "because it's next to the rabbits and rabbits eat lettuce," clearly reveals a strain of predicate logic. However, the form level is adequate, and the inference is suggestive of leaping to conclusions. In any case, what we may have here (barring other signs of deviant thinking) is a style of reasoning that is rigid and immature. Even seeing blood on a colored card, "because it is red," reflects a tendency to base conclusions on single features, characteristic of this type of reasoning.

On the other hand, who wouldn't begin to wonder about a psychotic-level thought disorder in the following responses:

> Card VIII. Rabbits climbing on garbage. I imagine that where rabbits are, there's garbage (Wilson, 1994, p. 30).
>
> Card IV. Giant tree, a dead tree, a dead tree, its leaves falling off. (What made it look like that?) Looked like something was dead. So something that towers over you and is dead to me follows it would be a dead tree (Solovay et al., 1986, p. 495).
>
> Card VIII. An animal or a bug. (What made it look like that?) The colors, the way they were in order . . . I associate color with moving around and animals aren't very stationary usually; anything that is colorful is movable . . . like a wall would be of one color and that was a series of colors and therefore movable and animals are usually very active (Rapaport et al., 1968, p. 440).

Each of these ALOGs (especially the last two) reflects a weakening of perceptual accuracy along with increasingly strained logical inference. The second example even becomes slightly incoherent, revealing confused syntax ("So something that towers over you and is dead to me follows it would be a dead tree"). Even the usual formula for predicate logic is difficult to apply to these responses, which reflect a bizarre, almost absurd, reasoning process. Such responses clearly reveal severely impaired thinking, in which even the fallacious trail of reasoning is difficult to follow.

PART
4

DIFFERENTIAL DIAGNOSIS
OF RORSCHACH
THOUGHT DISORDER

The lack of specificity between thought disorder phenomena and clinical diagnosis can make the psychodiagnostic assessment of thought disorder a tricky undertaking. In addition to schizophrenic conditions, Rorschach indices of disordered thinking have been found in affective psychoses, borderline disorders, traumatic and dissociative conditions, and neurological disorders, to mention a few. Furthermore, the continuum of thought disorder manifestations, ranging from mild idiosyncrasies of speech to severely impaired reasoning, may make differential diagnostic decisions more complex than was once thought.

Is thought disorder a final common pathway for the general expression of severe forms of psychological disturbance? Do all patients with disturbances in their thought organization manifest the same degree and kind of pathological verbalizations on the Rorschach? The chapters in this section review the quantitative and qualitative distinctions in Rorschach thought disorder manifestations in patients with a variety of diagnoses.

Chapter 13 reviews Rorschach indices of disordered thinking associated with schizophrenic spectrum conditions. Chapter 14 contrasts forms of schizophrenic thought disorder with those found among patients with affective psychoses. In chapter 15, the contrast will be with borderline disorders, and in chapter 16, miscellaneous clinical syndromes including posttraumatic stress and dissociative disorders, obsessive compulsive and delusional disorders, and, finally, selected neurological conditions. Finally, chapter 17 will review the issue of creativity and disordered thinking on the Rorschach.

CHAPTER

13

SCHIZOPHRENIA-SPECTRUM

DISORDERS

The historical lens used in this book has already revealed that the search for Rorschach indices of schizophrenia is as old as the Rorschach Test itself. In earlier chapters, however, we saw how this search was marred by conceptual confusion and diagnostic misunderstanding. In the past, thought disorder was considered to be a monolithic, noncontinuous construct, synonymous with schizophrenia. A thought disorder was either present or absent; and the existence of a disturbance in thinking was assumed to be diagnostic of a schizophrenic illness (a mild form of diagnostic paralogia).

Not only were there conceptual difficulties in defining the scope and nature of thought disorder and its relationship to schizophrenia, but the diagnostic criteria for schizophrenia were traditionally quite broad and unreliable, leading to a trend in North America to overclassify patients as schizophrenic. Patients with affective psychoses and borderline disorders were often misdiagnosed and given labels such as "latent or borderline schizophrenia."

Thought disorder is no longer considered pathognomic of schizophrenia. The presence of pathological thought processes is known to occur among a range of psychiatric conditions. Diagnostic criteria for schizophrenia are now more narrowly defined, making the patients who meet these more rigorous criteria generally more homogeneous and more disturbed. However, despite the narrowing of this diagnostic population, schizophrenia is generally considered to be a relatively heterogeneous group or spectrum of illnesses without a common etiology.

Following the recognition that Rorschach thought disorder scores were not at all specific to schizophrenia, many concluded that the test was less useful in making differential diagnostic distinctions (Harrow et al., 1982; Harrow and Quinlan, 1985; Marengo and Harrow, 1985; Simpson and Davis, 1985; Carter, 1986). Rorschach manifestations of disturbed thinking in manic, schizophrenic, and borderline patients were viewed as reflective of a generic psychosis factor, not specific to any one diagnostic entity.

Despite this viewpoint, clinicians are routinely asked to help make difficult differential diagnostic decisions. For example, referral sources tell us that this patient is psychotic but ask whether he has schizophrenia or a bipolar disorder. Furthermore, referral sources ask, "Is the patient a decompensated borderline or schizotypal; or does he suffer from schizoaffective psychoses?" Although most would accept that knowing the patient's history and administering a battery of tests are necessary for effective differential diagnosis, the question of qualitative differences in thought disorder among different psychotic and borderline patients remains an important issue for diagnosticians who are interested in answering difficult diagnostic questions.

Is there something unique about the qualitative patterning of thought disorder scores in patients diagnosed with schizophrenia that sets them apart from other patients who manifest disturbances in their thinking? Can the Rorschach assist in the recognition of a phenotypic schizophrenic-like thought disorder? To answer these questions, Rorschach variables associated with schizophrenia are first organized into four overlapping categories: Pathognomic Signs; Indices; Qualitative Differences; and Positive and Negative Symptoms. Each is examined separately along with illustrative clinical examples.

PATHOGNOMIC SIGNS

In chapter 11, I reviewed empirical data that support the claim that a single contamination response is pathognomic of schizophrenia. It seems true that in the contamination response we have a clear diagnostic indicator of schizophrenia. However, once again, the extreme rarity of this score detracts from its general utility as a diagnostic marker.

Koistinen (1995) found that the most severe level of TDI scores (1.0) occurred predominantly among schizophrenic subjects. In addition to the specificity of the contamination response, neologisms and incoherent responses occurred principally in the records of schizophrenic patients. Even when contrasting schizophrenic subjects with those who had a range of schizophrenia-spectrum diagnoses (schizoaffective disorder, schizophreniform disorder, schizotypal disorder, delusional disorder, and psychotic disorder, NOS), these three 1.0 level scores were found to be most specific to schizophrenic Rorschachs. A review of Koistinen's data indicates that none of his schizophrenia-spectrum subjects produced a neologism and only one schizoaffective subject gave a contamination response. Unfortunately, like contamination, the frequency of the other 1.0 level severity scores is similarly rare. For example, of Koistinen's 542 subjects, 1.0 level scores occurred only 13 times (2.4%). Furthermore, although they virtually never occurred in the records of nonschizophrenic subjects, they made up only 18.2% of the thought disorder scores among schizophrenic subjects.

SCHIZOPHRENIA INDICES

Early Indices

Recall how schizophrenia indices flourished in the 1950s when Rorschach researchers attempted to employ a diagnostic sign approach to identify schizophrenia. In chapter 2, we reviewed the Alpha Index (Piotrowski and Lewis, 1950), the Thiessen Patterns (Thiessen, 1952), the Delta Index (Watkins and Stauffacher, 1952), and the Weiner Signs (1961), each of which claimed empirical support for the diagnosis of schizophrenia. The product of flawed methodology and anachronistic diagnostic criteria, virtually none of these indices has survived the test of time.

TDI

Of these early efforts, only the Delta Index survived as a viable diagnostic instrument in the form of its reincarnation, the TDI. As a contemporary measure of disordered thinking, the TDI has stood alone in its comprehensive and detailed analysis of the components of pathological forms of thought as they emerge on the Rorschach. However, as with each of the earlier quantitative measures of schizophrenic thinking, there is little to no diagnostic specificity of the total TDI score. Based solely on total score values, schizophrenic subjects do not achieve significantly higher total scores than acutely manic or schizoaffective patients. For this reason, the TDI shifted from being a scale to assess schizophrenic thinking to becoming a more general measure of disordered thinking.

SCZI

Can the same be said about Exner's (1993) SCZI? Because they chose to call it the "Schizophrenia Index," Exner and his colleagues have implied that the SCZI should be sufficiently sensitive and specific to schizophrenic conditions. Extensive research has gone into refining the SCZI in order to maximize accurate identification of schizophrenic patients and minimize false positive and negative rates (see chapter 6). Exner's studies suggest that a SCZI of 4 should be interpreted with great caution, while a SCZI of 6 indicates a much greater likelihood that schizophrenia is present.

Hilsenroth, Fowler, and Padawer (1998) investigated the reliability, internal consistency, and diagnostic efficiency of the SCZI in classifying schizophrenic and other psychotic subjects in comparison with other groups. Although they demonstrated that the total value of SCZI is significantly positively correlated with the presence of a DSM IV psychotic disorder, Hilsenroth and his team indicated that the SCZI assesses a continuum of disordered thinking, with lower relative values among borderline and Cluster A personality disorders (a mean SCZI of roughly 3.0). They suggested that a value of 4 seems adequate for the purposes of distinguishing psychotic disorders from milder personality disorders, whereas a value of 5 improves diagnostic efficiency with more disturbed borderline and Cluster A personality disorders. More importantly for our purposes, Hilsenroth et al. concluded that the SCZI is probably not diagnostically specific to schizophrenia, as the name of the index would suggest. As a measure of perceptual inaccuracy, impaired reality testing, and fabulized thought processes, they stated that the SCZI would be elevated in bipolar, delusional and, schizoaffective psychoses as well. Thus, they suggested that the SCZI should be employed as a dimensional measure of psychosis and renamed a "Psychosis Index" to assesses the extent of impaired reality testing and thought disorder among a wider variety of patients.

Ego Impairment Index (EII)

Although not formally introduced as an index of schizophrenic thinking, the Ego Impairment Index (EII) was developed to measure the composite of ego functions along a continuum from healthy functioning to schizophrenia (Perry and Viglione, 1991; Perry, Viglione, and Braff, 1992). The EII was originally empirically developed on a sample of melancholic depressives (Perry and Viglione, 1991) and subsequently cross validated on a sample of schizophrenic patients (Perry et al., 1992). The results of the study with a schizophrenic sample led the authors to conclude that the EII is a useful method of assessing thought disorder.

The EII is made up of the following five Rorschach measures, based on variables derived from the Comprehensive System (Exner, 1993): (1) sum of poor form quality responses (FQ–), as a measure of poor reality testing; (2) wSUM 6, measuring strained reasoning and inappropriate perceptual condensation; (3) primitive contents, termed "de-repressed contents" (Perry and Viglione, 1991), which are thought to signal repressive failure (contents reflecting aggressive, sexual, morbid, and dependency themes); (4) human movement and/or content responses that are essentially either distorted (M–, F–), aggressive, or associated with Level 2 special scores, believed to measure both thought disturbance due to primitive aggression and difficulties in self-other differentiation (termed poor human experience); (5) good human experience (essentially Mo responses without special scores).

As expected, the schizophrenic sample demonstrated considerably more impairment on the EII (with a mean EII score of 1.6) than did their original sample of depressed inpatients (mean EII of 0). Furthermore, the authors demonstrated that the EII correlated significantly with the SCZI, the Magical Ideation Scale (Eckblad and Chapman, 1983), and MMPI Scales 6, 8, and 9. Perry and his colleagues concluded that the variables that make up the EII assess failures in reality testing, all thought organization, defensive functioning, and interpersonal relationships, thought to be the hallmarks of schizophrenia. Interestingly, they also demonstrated that the EII differentiated between subtypes of schizophrenic patients. Paranoid and nonparanoid subjects, who scored similarly on the SCZI, scored differently on the EII, with nonparanoid subjects scoring significantly higher than the paranoid subgroup.

Perry and Braff (1994) extended the use of the EII as a measure of disordered thinking among schizophrenic subjects by demonstrating the link between information processing failures and disordered thought. The researchers showed that the poor human experience variable of the EII was significantly correlated with each of their information processing measures. The three information processing measures were entered into a simultaneous regression equation to predict the poor responses of the EII human experience variable. A measure of auditory prepulse inhibition of a startle reflex was determined to be the most significant predictor of the poor human experience variable.

Perry and Braff concluded that poor human responses reflect a tendency for the individual to be overwhelmed by primary process material. However, it is not clear on what basis Perry and Braff chose to focus only on the poor human experience variable of the EII, which they referred to as "a specific, highly sensitive measure of thought disorder" (p. 366). That only responses reflecting poor human experience should be spotlighted as specific and sensitive indicators of disturbed thought processes (apart from the other aspects of the EII that more directly measure disordered thinking) is a rather curious assumption that begs further explanation. Furthermore, it would be useful to know how non-schizophrenic psychotic and borderline subjects perform on the EII.

QUALITATIVE DIFFERENCES

Researchers have concluded that schizophrenic Rorschachs contain more preservations, overly concise and contracted communications, incoherence, interpenetration of one idea by another, contaminations, confusion, absurd responses, fluidity, idiosyncratic language, and neologisms than the records of nonschizophrenic subjects (Holzman et al., 1986; Solovay et al., 1987; Koistinen, 1995). However, before studying these qualitative aspects of Rorschach verbalization associated with schizophrenia, it is useful to discuss some of the more general characteristics of schizophrenic thought organization. An understanding of the nature of schizophrenic thought can provide a conceptual basis for understanding why schizophrenic subjects give certain kinds of responses on the Rorschach.

Information Processing and Attentional Deficits

Many of these characteristic schizophrenic responses can be understood in terms of impairments in information processing and attentional focus. There is an extensive body of literature that looks at the key role of deficits in attention and information processing in schizophrenia (Bleuler, 1911/1950; Cameron, 1939; Shakow, 1950, 1962; Payne, Mattusek, and George, 1959; Venables, 1960; McGhie and Chapman, 1961; Braff and Geyer, 1991; Butler et al., 1991; Braff, Grillon, and Geyer, 1992; Judd et al., 1992). Cameron noted the difficulties that schizophrenic subjects have in focusing on relevant stimuli. Shakow (1950) concluded that schizophrenic individuals have problems maintaining focus or a major cognitive set. McGhie and Chapman underscored the problems that schizophrenic patients have attending to and organizing sensory data in order to reduce the "chaotic flow of information reaching consciousness" (p. 111). They demonstrated that individuals with schizophrenia have difficulty attending to the most relevant aspects of a stimulus field and screening our irrelevant stimuli. Perry and Braff (1994) demonstrated a significant relationship between information processing deficits, cognitive fragmentation, and thought disorder in schizophrenia. Perry and Braff hypothesized that when attentional and information processing functions are disturbed, individuals may be flooded by poorly modulated stimuli, leading to increased distractibility, cognitive fragmentation, and thought disorder.

In his theoretical contribution to understanding the nature of thought pathology in schizophrenia, Meissner (1981) discussed the link between attentional processes and concept formation. Meissner contrasted schizophrenic and paranoid processes in terms of the ability to organize perceptual stimuli into conceptual categories. According to Meissner, the paranoid process is characterized by forming and maintaining rigid conceptual categories that are refractory to the corrective influence of perceptual input. The schizophrenic process, on the other hand, reflects a deficit in conceptual organization, leading to cognitive confusion, fragmentation, and disorganization. Whereas the paranoid, according to Meissner, organizes stimuli in a rigid and "hyperconceptualized" manner, the schizophrenic does so in a loose or "hypoconceptualized" way.

As a consequence of this deficit in the capacity to form conceptual categories, schizophrenic individuals have trouble organizing, regulating, and integrating perceptual material into conceptual categories. Meissner added that if the ability to organize perceptual into conceptual categories is lacking, then attention is left without regulation and is subject to increased variability, instability, and distraction. As a result, stimuli competing for attention are not organized conceptually or hierarchically, leading to fluid attentional focus and an impairment in the ability to screen out irrelevant stimuli.

In reviewing forms of thought disorder in schizophrenia, Weiner (1966) not only spoke about failures in establishing a focus but also about failures in maintaining and shifting one's cognitive focus. Experimental studies have suggested that there are several distinct types of attention, including *selective attention* (the ability to filter relevant information); *sustained attention* (the capacity to maintain vigilance and alertness over time); and *switching attention* (the ability to shift attentional sets from one modality to another). Failures in each of these aspects of focusing may well reflect deficits in information processing.

Adaptive information processing requires the capacity first to establish, then sustain, and ultimately, when appropriate, shift one's attentional focus. Weiner suggested that a failure to maintain or hold an appropriate attentional focus (or cognitive set) allows for the intrusion of irrelevant external or internal stimuli into a previously established attentional set, which may lead to the expression of idiosyncratic associations and verbalizations on the Rorschach. Weiner described two categories of Rorschach verbalizations, "dissociation" and "deviant verbalizations," that may reflect a failure to maintain cognitive focus. Dissociation refers to a disconnection between adjacent ideas. Weiner indicated that dissociation could also be expressed in the form of irrelevant and loosely connected thoughts. In chapter 8, I mentioned that the inappropriate phrase Deviant Response (DR) category in the Comprehensive System (Exner, 1986a, 1993)—for instance, "It looks like a bat; my neighbor shot one in his backyard,"—and vague and looseness scores in the TDI are examples of a loss of cognitive focus, leading to a dissociation between ideas and the intrusion of irrelevant material into the response.

According to Weiner, peculiar and queer verbalizations may result from the "intrusion of idiosyncratic modes of expression and impede verbal communication" (Weiner, 1966, p. 42). DV and DR categories in the Comprehensive System and peculiar, queer, and neologistic responses from the TDI may all reflect a failure to maintain cognitive focus

Weiner also pointed out that adaptive cognitive focusing requires that an individual be able to *shift* focus as perceptual stimuli change from one situation to another. The inability to shift attentional focus from one stimulus (either internal or external stimuli) to another leads one to continue responding to new situations with old representations or cognitive schemas. Bleuler (1911) referred to this process as "perseveration," which he described as a common phenomena in schizophrenia. According to Weiner, the individual with schizophrenia becomes fixed on a train of thought and is unable to take into account the changing stimulus properties of the environment. As a result, the schizophrenic subject maintains an inflexible cognitive set and is unable to modify his schema regardless of changing environmental circumstances. Although common in other conditions, Rorschach perseveration responses are generally understood to reflect inflexibility in holding onto cognitive sets.

Although not studying information processing or the Rorschach per se, Jampala, Taylor, and Abrams (1989) demonstrated that disturbances in focusing are more characteristic of disordered thinking in schizophrenic individuals than in other psychotic subjects. Jampala et al. rated semistructured interviews of manic and schizophrenic subjects according to a narrowly defined definition of formal thought disorder. Although it is problematic to think that the presence of any one type of thought disorder is diagnostic of any particular disorder, they demonstrated that different forms of thought disorder do have some differential diagnostic value. In particular, they found that tangentiality, drivelling speech (defined as "double talk," in which the syntax appears to be intact but the meaning is lost), neologisms, private word usage, or paraphasias (a inappropriate word or phrase that has an approximate meaning, such as saying "head-covering" instead of "hat") were more likely to occur in subjects with schizophrenia than in those with mania.

Approaching thought disorder from the listener's perspective, Hoffman, Stopek, and Andreasen (1986) applied discourse analysis in comparing the speech of schizophrenic and manic subjects. Listeners generally experience multisentence speech as coherent if they can organize the propositions expressed into a hierarchic format. Discourse is experienced as loose or incoherent when the listener cannot organize the speech sample into a "treelike" hierarchical structure (Deese, 1978, 1980). Hoffman et al. demonstrated that schizophrenic subjects tended to generate hierarchies that were subnormally small in size (when compared to normal and manic subjects) and deficient in their elaboration of any discourse structure. In contrast, manic discourse was generally longer and more elaborate.

Research in each of these areas provides a basis for understanding why schizophrenic subjects tend to produce more peculiar verbalizations, fluid and interpenetrating responses that reflect the subject's confusion and perseverative tendencies. Fluidity and interpenetration represent the tendency to ignore categorical boundaries or distinctions between concepts, ideas, or objects (Shenton et al., 1987). In general, schizophrenic Rorschachs tend to convey private meaning, not easily shared by the listener. Examiners may experience a sense of alienation from the subject and be struck by extreme oddness that might leave the listener feeling ill at ease and confused. Records may be constricted and barren, demonstrating a dearth of variability and a tendency to perseverate from one card or response to another. Despite the appeal of this characterization, research has not consistently supported these findings. A recent study by Khadivi, Wetzler, and Wilson (1997) failed to demonstrate a greater amount of idiosyncratic verbalization, confusion, absurd, or fluid thinking in the records of schizophrenic, compared with samples of manic and schizoaffective subjects.

What might we expect *not* to appear with great frequency in the Rorschach records of schizophrenic subjects? Impressive findings emerged comparing the TDI profiles of schizophrenic, schizoaffective, and manic subjects (Shenton et al., 1987; Solovay et al., 1987). As mentioned in chapter 5, a principal component analysis demonstrated that the TDIs of schizophrenic subjects *were not* characterized by combinatory thinking (defined as playful confabulations, incongruous combinations, flippant responses, and fabulized combinations). The infrequency of combinatory thinking in the records of schizophrenics was replicated by Khadivi et al. (1997) in their study that contrasted thought disorder in manic, paranoid schizophrenic, and schizoaffective subjects.

Although Exner has yet to contrast disordered thinking between a group of manic and schizophrenic subjects, data from his psychiatric reference samples (Exner, 1993) do not support this finding. For example, his schizophrenic sample demonstrates a substantial number of inappropriate combinations responses. However, the greater frequency of combinative thinking in the records of schizophrenic subjects is most apparent for the severe Level 2 INCOMs, FABCOMs, and DRs. Unfortunately there are no comparable data for manic subjects in the Comprehensive System.

POSITIVE AND NEGATIVE SIGNS AND SYMPTOMS

In the first chapter, I noted that classifying schizophrenia into negative and positive features has proven to be somewhat controversial, as some researchers now question whether the positive-negative dichotomy is an oversimplification that fails to capture the complexity of forms of schizophrenic (and nonschizophrenic) thought disorder. For example, it is sometimes assumed that negative and positive signs and symptoms bear an inverse relationship to one another. If an individual is floridly psychotic, manifesting a great number of positive symptoms, then it is assumed that the person will not exhibit negative signs, which are generally associated more with chronicity. However, actual ratings of negative and positive features have been found to be uncorrelated with each other (Mortimer, Lund, and McKenna, 1990; Koistinen, 1995), implying that a patient could exhibit the features of either or both together. Patients with negative signs may simultaneously have positive features as well. For example, Frith (1992) noted that patients with a poverty of speech may simply not reveal their incoherence or speak about their delusions.

Despite the overly simplistic nature of this typology, researchers continue to find the negative-positive distinction a useful way to conceptualize cognitive functioning in schizophrenic spectrum disorders. Furthermore, in treatment settings, psychodiagnosticians can help clinicians target specific symptoms and signs for both psychological and pharmacological treatment. To this end, the Rorschach may weigh in as a useful technique for distinguishing between negative and positive symptom complexes.

Positive Symptoms and the Rorschach

Positive symptoms have probably received the most attention from Rorschach researchers who associate bizarre-idiosyncratic thinking and more flagrant impairments in speech and perception with the most severe signs of Rorschach thought disorder. Rapaport's concept of "an increase in distance" from the inkblot certainly implies an idiosyncratic departure from the reality, which may be associated with positive symptomatology.

In Schuldberg and Boster's (1985) factor analytic investigation of Rapaport's "distance" hypothesis, they suggested that high scores on Dimension I (personalized meaning responses, including incoherence, neologisms, self-reference verbalizations, and autistic logic) were associated with autistic personal associations and global amount of thought disorder present. Aronow et al. (1994) noted that personal meaning responses, especially incoherent responses, indicate severe cognitive dysfunction of a floridly psychotic nature.

On the other hand, high scores on Schuldberg and Boster's Dimension II (fluid responses such as absurd responses, fabulized responses, reference ideas, fabulized combinations, confabulations, and neologisms) were associated with flamboyant and fluent behavior. Arnow and his colleagues concluded that schizophrenic patients scoring high on Dimension II (and those who give incoherent responses) "are likely to be characterized by positive symptoms of the disorder, such as hallucinations and delusions" (p. 115).

However, there might not be a one-to-one relationship between individual thought disorder scores and positive symptomatology. As O'Connell et al. (1989) pointed out, the link between individual scores, such as confabulation and contamination, and the presence of clinically detectable psychotic symptoms may be less direct and more complicated than we think. Despite this caveat, O'Connell et al. found that a high total TDI score increased the risk that a psychotic condition was present. Furthermore, other researchers have found more of the scores loading high on Dimension II in the records of recently hospitalized schizophrenic patients than in the records of chronic and deteriorated schizophrenic subjects (Johnston and Holzman, 1979). Thus, it seems reasonable to conclude that most of the scores from severity levels .75 and 1.0 of the TDI, Level 1 formal variables in the PRIPRO, and Level 2 Special Scores in the Comprehensive System can be generally viewed as Rorschach representations of positive symptoms. Additionally, the poor human experience variable on the Ego Impairment Index (Perry et al., 1992) has been shown to be significantly correlated with the Scale for the Assessment of Positive Symptoms (Andreasen, 1984).

Negative Signs

Although Rorschach thought disorder scores are usually associated with positive forms of disordered thinking and flagrantly disturbed reality testing, we have enough information about the nature of negative signs/symptoms to know what to look for on the Rorschach to identify these aspects of the illness. Negative symptoms such as constricted affect, poverty of speech and thought content (alogia), apathy and anhedonia, cognitive rigidity, stereotyped behavior, and social ineptness lend themselves to a Rorschach structural analysis.

In the Comprehensive System (Exner, 1993), affective constriction may be reflected by an absence of color, or the presence of pure color scores (Shapiro, 1960), high Lambda (L) and low Affective Ratio scores (Afr); alogia and apathy by a low number of total responses (R), high Lambda, absence of signs of cognitive complexity (low W, low Zf and Zd, no blends), no human movement responses (M), restricted range of contents (such as high Animal movement percentage); social inadequacy by a low number of human content and no M responses; and cognitive inflexibility by perseveration (PSV) and DW responses (CONFAB). Caution is necessary, however, when making inferences from structural data to clinical syndromes. All of the structural variables and indices mentioned above in relation to negative symptoms could also occur in patients with depression, neurological, or intellectual impairment. In terms of specific thought disorder scores, Schuldberg and Boster indicated that scores that loaded low on Dimensions I and II corresponded to Goldstein's and Scheerer's (1941) concept of schizophrenic concreteness. These included scores such as confusion, reference ideas, position responses, DW responses, relationship verbalizations, and perseverations. Arnow et al. suggested that most of these scores were consistent with negative symptoms.

Loading at the extreme low end of Dimension I (Objective meaning responses) were confusion responses. A loss of distance on the Rorschach may result in confusion as the subject attempts to recognize, instead of interpret, the inkblots. Johnston and Holzman found these responses to be more common among schizophrenic subjects, especially those classified as chronic/deteriorated. Since chronic schizophrenia is associated with more negative symptomatology, we might expect, as Arnow et al. suggested, that confusion responses are more common among individuals with affective, social inadequacy, and other negative symptoms.

One noteworthy example loading on the low end of Dimension II (Rigid responses) was the perseveration response. Perseverations, especially those of the mechanical variety which occur with poor form and in brief records, may reflect both cognitive rigidity and a poverty of thought content. Relationship responses also loaded low on Dimension II, but these generally occur infrequently. Arnow and his colleagues suggested that when relationship responses occur in the context of other objective meaning responses, they be interpreted as manifestations of negative symptoms and a more unfavorable prognosis.

Regarding perseveration responses, it is important to keep in mind that perseveration on the Rorschach is not unique to schizophrenia.

Twenty-two percent of Exner's inpatient depressives, 14% of character disorders, and 11% of general outpatients had perseverations in their records (Exner, 1993). Contrast this to only 11% of inpatient schizophrenic subjects who gave at least one perseveration response. Johnston and Holzman also found a similar frequency of perseveration responses in the records of schizophrenic (26%) and nonpsychotic subjects (24%).

The medication studies with chronic schizophrenics (Spohn et al., 1986) provided further support for the Rorschach distinction between positive and negative symptoms. Spohn et al. found that neuroleptics significantly reduced the positive symptoms or the "vivid, dramatic, gross distortions of reality, delusions, and hallucinations typically associated with an acute episode" (p. 405). In particular they found that on the TDI, the frequency of .75 and 1.0 level scores nearly vanished with neuroleptic treatment. At the same time, medication did not affect the presence of milder levels of thought pathology, those associated with concreteness, vagueness, perseveration, confusion, looseness, and fabulization (reflected by TDI levels .25 and .50). These milder forms of thought disorder were present in both acute episodes and clinical remission, leading Spohn and his team to wonder about the illness-specific nature of these milder "negative" features that appear as residual "thought disorder scars" on the Rorschach.

SPECTRUM DISORDERS

What kinds of Rorschach thought disorder differences exist in the records of patients who fall along the schizophrenia spectrum? Although there are varying opinions about how to classify disorders along the continuum of schizophrenic illness, I make rather broad divisions in keeping with generally accepted diagnostic standards. Beginning with a review of the nature of Rorschach thought disorder among schizotypal personalities, I then discuss the quality of disordered thinking on the Rorschach in paranoid schizophrenic and schizoaffective individuals.

Schizotypal Personality

Disagreement exists as to whether the schizotypal personality is a variant of borderline personality or a distinct entity phenotypically related to schizophrenia. Rorschach studies have also differed in this respect. Edell (1987) found borderline and schizotypal patients indistinguishable on the TDI. However, Exner (1986b) found distinct Rorschach differences between samples of schizotypal and borderline subjects. In Exner's study, schizotypal subjects produced 5.6 critical special scores, which was not significantly different from the mean number produced by schizophrenic subjects at admission and just before discharge (7.3 and 7.17 respectively). By contrast, borderline subjects had a significantly lower mean number of critical special scores (mean = 3.44), suggesting a closer relationship between the schizotypal and schizophrenic groups. When contrasted on the weighted sum of the special scores (WSUM 6), the differences between the borderline and the other two groups were even more dramatic. Although the schizotypal group's mean WSUM 6 was almost twice as high as that of the borderline group, it was also significantly lower than that of the schizophrenic groups (at admission and before discharge). The data suggest that schizotypal individuals give about as many thought disordered responses as do schizophrenic subjects but at a lower level of severity.

This study was also published before Exner began distinguishing between Level 1 and Level 2 special scores, which allow for further refinement in the scoring of pathological Rorschach responses. Nonetheless, as can be seen from Table 13-1, his summary data show differences in the frequency with which each group produced different special scores.

The data in Table 13-1 suggest that, in terms of the kinds of disordered thought processes, schizotypals are more similar to schizophrenics than to borderlines. In particular, they demonstrate significantly more Deviant Verbalizations (DV) than the borderline group and even more than the schizophrenic sample. This finding is supported by another study which used the TDI to assess thought disorder in psychometrically identified schizotypic individuals (Coleman et al., 1996). These subjects were nonpsychiatric undergraduates who scored high on a 35-item Perceptual Aberration Scale (PerAb; Chapman, Chapman, and Raulin, 1978), which measures body image and perceptual distortions associated with schizotypy, a less malignant and more common variant of schizophrenia (Meehl, 1962). High PerAb scores defined the schizotype group (not necessarily diagnosable as schizotypal personalities), which scored significantly higher on the TDI (total mean TDI = 8.83, SD = 15.30) than the low PerAb group (total TDI = 3.65, SD = 4.97). The groups also differed in terms of the number of idiosyncratic verbalizations, with the schizotypic group giving significantly more responses containing peculiar language and odd expressions (peculiar and queer responses). The authors concluded that the schizotypic individuals displayed qualitatively similar thought disorder scores as schizophrenic subjects and their first-degree relatives, adding support to the biogenetic link between the two phenomena.

In terms of reality testing, Exner showed that both the schizotypal and borderline groups had similar good form level percentages (X + %)

Table 13-1 Percentage of Subjects Producing Special Scores

Special Score	Borderline (n = 84)	Schizotypal (n = 76)	Schizophrenic+ (n = 80)
DV	40	76*	67.5
DR	23	13	55
INCOM	56	71	75.6
FABCOM	34	52	75.5
ALOG	13	26	39.8
CONTAM	3.6	0	13.7
PSV	9.5	5.3	15

From Exner (1986).
+ Average percentage for two testings of schizophrenic subjects (admission and discharge).
* Significantly different proportional frequency (p < .05) between schizotypal and borderline group.

of 69%, significantly greater than the admission and discharge schizophrenic groups, whose X + %'s were 54% and 51% respectively. The mean minus form level percentages (X – %) for the groups, in descending order, was 13% (borderlines), 18% (schizotypals), and 31% and 34% for the two schizophrenic groups at admission and discharge. Exner set a cut-off of > 15% for X – % to indicate the presence of reality testing problems severe enough to interfere with effective functioning. In this comparison, the groups differed similarly, with 27% of the borderlines having an X – % > 15, 63% of the schizotypals, and 87% and 90% of the schizophrenic groups.

In sum, Exner's data suggest that schizotypal individuals can be distinguished from both borderline and schizophrenic subjects in terms of level of disturbed thinking and reality testing. In these two areas of functioning, schizotypals seem to occupy a middle range of severity between schizophrenia and borderline personality disorders. In many of the other structural respects, the schizotypal and schizophrenic groups were indistinguishable, supporting the hypothesis that both groups are phenotypically related. Like schizophrenic individuals, schizotypals tended to be introversive, detached, ideationally oriented, and affectively constrained.

Schizoaffective Disorder

In 1933, Kasanin introduced schizoaffective disorder as a diagnostic category to describe a group of patients who exhibited a combination of schizophrenic and manic-depressive symptomatology. Numerous studies indicated that these individuals demonstrated a better outcome than patients with schizophrenia but a poorer outcome than those suffering from bipolar disorder (Hunt and Appel, 1936–1937; Clayton, Rodin, and Winokur, 1968; Croughan, Welner, and Robins, 1974; Tsuang, Dempsey, and Rauscher, 1976; Angst, Felder, and Lohmeyer, 1980; Harrow and Grossman, 1984; Stone, 1990). The diagnostic integrity of schizoaffective disorder has for years been surrounded by controversy regarding its place in diagnostic nomenclature and the very nature of its existence. Researchers in psychopathology have attempted to discover whether schizoaffective disorder is a variant of schizophrenia or affective disorder; a separate diagnostic phenomenon; a midpoint along a continuum between schizophrenia and bipolar illness; or a combination of schizophrenia and affective disorder.

Prior to the 1980s, the Rorschach literature contributed little to this debate. It was not until 1987 that Rorschach researchers investigated schizoaffective psychosis in a rigorous empirical manner. Shenton and her colleagues (1987) contrasted the quality of TDI scores between a carefully selected group of schizoaffective (N = 22) and schizophrenic subjects (N = 43). Because of the variability in the schizoaffective group, subjects were divided into schizoaffective-manic (N = 12) and schizoaffective-depressed (N = 10) subgroups. The researchers also contrasted TDI scores from these groups with those from their manic group (N = 20) (Solovay et al., 1987).

The results of their study showed that schizoaffective-manic subjects resembled both schizophrenic and manic subjects in the quality of their thought disorder patterns on the TDI. The schizoaffective-depressed group resembled the normal control group in most areas. Although the four patient groups overlapped considerably, the total TDI means (and standard deviations) for the schizophrenic, schizoaffective-manic, manic, and schizoaffective-depressed groups were 34.6 (± 38.8), 31.20 (± 25.6), 25.0 (± 16.2), and 13.0 (± 8.6) respectively. Response productivity also showed a similar pattern, with the manic group giving the highest number of responses and the schizoaffective-depressed and schizophrenic groups giving the lowest number.

In the Solovay et al. (1987) post hoc comparisons of manic and schizophrenic subjects, Fluid Thinking (relationship verbalizations, fluidity, and contaminations), Confusion (word-finding difficulty, confusion, absurd responses, incoherence, and neologisms), and Idiosyncratic Verbalizations (peculiar verbalizations) emerged as the factors that best distinguished schizophrenic subjects. In the Shenton et al. (1987) post hoc analyses, the schizoaffective-manics resembled schizophrenic subjects most on the confusion and idiosyncratic verbalization factors. Both schizoaffective-manics and manics gave few responses on the Fluid

Thinking factor, unlike schizophrenic subjects who gave significantly more of these responses.

Schizoaffective-manic subjects resembled manic subjects in more superficial ways compared to their similarities with schizophrenic subjects. Although the schizoaffective-manic subjects demonstrated combinatory activity and some irrelevant intrusions, like the manic subjects, they were most similar to the schizophrenic group in terms of their confusion, idiosyncratic thinking, and disorganization. By contrast, they were more verbal and expansive than the schizophrenic subjects; however, unlike the bipolar manic group, the schizoaffective-manics were less humorous and playful in their combinatory activity, which often struck the listener as peculiar, distant, and overly private.

The schizoaffective-depressed differed generally from each of the clinical groups and resembled the normals in many ways. They produced more contracted records, devoid of more dramatic combinatory activity and idiosyncratic verbalizations. However, they were strikingly similar to the schizophrenic group on an Absurdity factor from the principle components factor analysis. This factor included loadings from response categories such as neologisms and absurd responses. This noteworthy feature led researchers to claim that schizoaffective-depressed patients can be distinguished from constricted normals and patients with primary depressions (Holzman et al., 1986).

Lending further support to their typology of disordered thinking, Shenton conducted additional research that demonstrated that the quality of thought disorder in the groups of first-degree relatives was similar to that of the schizoaffective, schizophrenic, and manic subjects themselves (Shenton et al., 1989). Interestingly the relatives of schizoaffective-manic subjects showed the highest quantity of thought disorder and the highest number of idiosyncratic verbalizations, followed by relatives of the state hospital schizophrenics. As expected, relatives of schizoaffective-depressed subjects showed the lowest amount of thought disorder (next to normals); however, their constricted records revealed isolated examples of disordered thinking.

The same qualitative distinctions on the TDI among schizoaffective and schizophrenic patients have not been found elsewhere. As mentioned above, the recent study by Khadivi et al. (1997) did not support the fine discriminations that the researchers at McLean Hospital found between these different groups of psychotic patients. In particular, Khadivi's group did not find that their schizoaffective subjects demonstrated more combinatory activity, idiosyncratic verbalizations, and confusion. However, it should be noted that their sample size was small and did not distinguish schizoaffective-manic from depressed subjects.

Paranoid vs. Nonparanoid Schizophrenia

Although some feel that attempts to define diagnostic subcategories of schizophrenia (e.g., catatonic, hebephrenic, paranoid, and undifferentiated) have not proven useful or reliable (Frith, 1992), the paranoid-nonparanoid distinction is still commonly used in clinical diagnosis. In general, paranoid schizophrenic individuals are perceived as less overtly disturbed than individuals with nonparanoid or disorganized forms of the disorder. Meissner's (1981) contrast between paranoid and schizophrenic processes provides a framework for understanding this distinction. Viewing the schizophrenic process as a deficit in conceptual organization, Meissner characterized the paranoid process as a tendency to organize stimuli in a rigid and "hyperconceptualized" manner. According to Meissner, the interacting mechanisms of introjection and projection, despite their reality distorting effects, help lend coherence and structure to the individual's sense of self and personality organization. In cases of paranoid schizophrenia, both molar processes (schizophrenic disorganization and paranoid compensation) are at work. Meissner indicated that

> in the face of the ravages of the schizophrenic process, the paranoid process can be brought into play to provide the patient with a semblance of inner coherence and stability. In a sense, then, the paranoid schizophrenic is willing to pay the price of the sacrifice and distortion of his relationship to the outside world in order to gain some degree of inner organization and internal coherence [p. 629].

Given this conceptual distinction, one would expect to find greater structural organization and fewer of the "schizophrenic thought disorder factors" discussed above in the records of individuals with paranoid schizophrenia. The Rorschach literature offers some support for this expectation. Probably the most authoritative work in this area is that of Weiner (1966), who devoted much of this classic volume to identifying subtle psychodiagnostic differences between the various subtypes of schizophrenia. Weiner presented a number of case examples of paranoid schizophrenia, in which the subjects demonstrated greater organization and relatively fewer areas of impaired ego functioning.[1] Weiner's subjects demonstrated more intact reality testing (average F+% = 77.5), an introversive orientation (M > SUM C), an interest in small details (Dd

---

1. It is important to emphasize that Weiner, like all competent psychodiagnosticians, stressed the importance of relying on a convergence of data from a number of tests in order to make inferences. Likewise, his case examples include data from a number of different psychological tests.

and Hd), and fewer formal thought disorder scores (average per record=7). Table 13-2 shows the distribution of formal thought disorder scores in Weiner's two paranoid schizophrenic subjects. Clearly, these subjects demonstrated levels of disturbed thinking that would be considered relatively mild and generally meriting .25 and .50 weighting in the TDI. Weiner also placed great emphasis on content and patient-examiner relationship variables that reflected suspicion, perception of external danger, and need for protection.

Weiner presented five additional cases to demonstrate active schizophrenic conditions not characterized primarily by a paranoid orientation. These cases (which Weiner listed as acute, chronic, and incipient) showed greater structural disorganization manifested by poorer reality testing (average F+% = 62.6) and more severely disturbed thinking (average thought disorder signs per record = 15.8). Table 13-3 shows the distribution of scores for this group.

One can see that thought disorder scores from this group are more frequent and at a higher level of severity. A final observation about Weiner's case examples is worth noting. The low incidence of confabulatory and combinative thinking and the higher incidence of peculiar verbalization, autistic logic, and perseverations in his schizophrenic examples is quite consistent with other findings.

Exner (1991) presented one case example of paranoid schizophrenia that demonstrated some of the organizational features and content variables described above (e.g., R = 16; Zd = +3.5; positive Hypervigilance Index; Introversive EB; FC:CF+C = 4:1; masks, themes of secrecy, evil, revenge, judgment, and hostility). However, Exner's record demonstrates two minus human movement responses (M– = 2), a SCZI of 5, and a weighted total special score sum of 27 (DR1 = 3; FAB1 = 1; INC2 = 1; and ALOG = 2). It is interesting that even though the SCZI is positive at 5, three of the special scores are considered milder in severity, while the remainder would be rated by Exner as "serious" ("serious" was Exner's moderate level, between "mild" and "severe") on his continuum of cognitive dysfunction (see chapter 6). Unfortunately, there are no cases of nonparanoid subjects with which to compare these data. It would be interesting to see if more disorganized, nonparanoid schizophrenic individuals would demonstrate a greater number of Level 2 scores (at the serious and severe level) relative to those at Level 1.

Perry et al. (1992) used the Ego Impairment Index with an outpatient and inpatient schizophrenic sample. In addition to demonstrating the usefulness of the EII in identifying disordered thinking, the authors found a significant difference between the EII scores between a paranoid and nonparanoid (undifferentiated and disorganized) group. As

Table 13-2 Distribution of Thought Disorder Scores Among
Weiner's Paranoid Schizophrenic Case Examples

Thought Disorder Score	Frequency	Mean
Fabulized Responses	4	2.0
Peculiar Responses	5	2.5
Queer Responses	1	0.5
Incongruous Combinations	1	0.5
Incongruous Combinations-tend	1	0.5
Fabulized Combinations	1	0.5
Contamination-tendency	1	0.5
Autistic Logic	0	0.0

From Weiner (1966).

expected, the paranoid group had a lower mean EII (less impairment) than the nonparanoid group. This difference was all the more impressive in that the two groups were not differentiated on the basis of their SCZI scores.

Using a total TDI score of 25.00 to separate high from low scoring subjects, Koistinen (1995) determined that his paranoid schizophrenic subjects demonstrated both low levels of positive thought disorder and low levels of negative symptomatology as well. Given the relative lack of definite TDI signs associated with paranoid schizophrenia, Koistinen concluded that making diagnostic use of the TDI may be especially problematic when attempting to assess individuals with the paranoid subtype of the disorder.

Finally, as noted above, the recent study by Khadivi et al. (1997) did not find distinctive TDI profiles in their samples of schizophrenic and schizoaffective subjects. However, it is interesting to observe that their schizophrenic subjects met the Research Diagnostic Criteria (RDC; Spitzer, Endicott, and Robins, 1978) for Schizophrenia, paranoid type. If these individuals truly suffered from paranoid schizophrenia, then the relative absence of idiosyncratic verbalization, fluid and autistic thinking, and confusion may be explained, in part, by the generally lower levels of thought disorder and ego impairment demonstrated by this group. Notice that the mean TDI score for their paranoid schizophrenic sample was 12.4, almost one-third the size of the general schizophrenia mean of 34.56 in the Solovay et al. (1987) study. Furthermore, the crude comparison between Weiner's paranoid and other schizophrenic cases showed that the "other" (not primarily paranoid) schizophrenic subjects had more than twice the average frequency of TDI scores as did the paranoid subjects (15.8 vs. 7). Thus, it may not be entirely unexpected that Khadivi's schizophrenic group did not

Table 13-3 Distribution of Thought Disorder Scores Among
Weiner's "Nonparanoid Schizophrenic" Case Examples

Thought Disorder Score	Frequency	Mean
Fabulized Responses	24	4.8
Peculiar Responses	13	2.2
Queer Responses	3	0.6
Incongruous Combinations	4	0.8
Perseverations	9	1.8
Fabulized Combinations	5	1.0
Confabulation	2	0.4
Fluid	4	0.8
Autistic Logic/Position	10	2.0
Contamination	1	0.2

From Weiner (1966).

demonstrate the expected schizophrenic TDI profile. Given the information reviewed here, the Rorschach thought disorder profiles of paranoid schizophrenic subjects *may not* be representative of general thought disorder patterns in schizophrenia.

CONCLUSIONS

Available evidence seems to support the conclusion that the contamination response is pathognomic of schizophrenia. Unfortunately, as we have seen, the extreme rarity of this response, even among schizophrenic individuals, limits its overall diagnostic utility. "Schizophrenia indices" are certainly sensitive to schizophrenia, but their specificity is considerably lower. As Hilsenroth et al. (1998) pointed out, the SCZI seems misnamed. To continue to call this the "Schizophrenia Index" may be misleading. The "schizophrenia factors" derived from the factor analytic studies of TDI researchers may offer the most help to clinicians in making difficult differential diagnostic decisions. Available information supports the contention that disordered thinking in schizophrenia manifests itself in terms of idiosyncratic and bizarre verbalizations (peculiar, queer, or DV responses), and confused, fluid, or perseverative responses, that strike the listener as odd and devoid of consensual meaning. Confabulatory and combinatory responses may occur, but they are not the hallmark of a schizophrenic Rorschach. Schizophrenic subjects, and especially schizoaffective-manic individuals, may give combinatory responses, but these lack the dramatic, coherent, and playful flair that we expect to see in the records of manic patients.

CHAPTER

14

AFFECTIVE DISORDERS

Few psychiatric conditions occur as frequently as affective disorders. Not only are they relatively common disturbances, but depression and mania are also associated with a range of syndromes of varying types and intensities. The presence of psychotic symptoms in some patients suffering from manic or depressive disorders, or both, has long been observed; however, it was not until the last 35 years that researchers have begun to study the nature of thought processes in these patients.

In the 1960s and 1970s researchers interested in both depressive and manic conditions began to question the diagnostic specificity of thought disorder and to investigate its occurrence and nature in affective disorders (Beck, 1963, 1964, 1967, 1971; Braff and Beck, 1974; Andreasen, 1976, 1979a,b; Harrow and Quinlan, 1977; Pope and Lipinski, 1978). Findings from many of these studies challenged the dichotomous view of thought disorder as either "present or absent" and led to more sophisticated, multidimensional approaches to conceptualizing and diagnosing disturbances in thinking. However, with new research findings came disagreements about whether disordered thought in depressed and manic patients could be reliably distinguished from the thought disturbances observed in individuals with schizophrenia.

To understand the Rorschach contributions to the differential diagnosis of disordered thinking in patients suffering from depression, or mania, or both, it is useful to begin by reviewing broader diagnostic and conceptual issues related to the presence of thought pathology associated with affective disorders. Beginning with a brief review of the diagnostic taxonomy of affective disorders, I then examine non-Rorschach research that has looked at the occurrence and nature of disordered thinking in individuals with affective disorders. Turning then to the Rorschach literature, I review empirical findings that have identified Rorschach thought disorder variables associated with manic and depressive conditions and hypothesize about further connections between varieties of Rorschach thought disorder scores and affective disorders.

CLASSIFICATION OF AFFECTIVE DISORDERS

Affective disorders seem traditionally to have been separated into two categories. Kraepelin (1921) initially proposed two categories: involutional melancholia (to describe an anxious depressive condition occurring later in life) and manic-depressive insanity. Responding to scientific inquiry about whether it was justified to separate these two disturbances, Kraepelin later collapsed involutional melancholia into his manic-depressive category. Decades later, researchers agreed that there was substantial evidence for classifying two broad categories of affective disorders.

Perris (1966) is credited with coining the distinction between "bipolar" versus "unipolar" depression to reflect the differences between these two categories of affective disturbance. This distinction has led to over 30 years of research showing different courses, familial patterns, and treatment responses for patients suffering from each type of illness. It has also gained ascendancy in the modern DSM systems that currently adopt these two major diagnostic subdivisions under the category of affective disorders.

Two additional popular diagnostic dichotomies were proposed for classifying depression. Distinguishing "neurotic" from "psychotic" forms of depression seemed a logical outgrowth of psychoanalytic theory of neurotic conflicts. However, over the years there has been debate about whether these were two distinct syndromes or simply endpoints on a single continuum. "Endogenous" versus "reactive" depression is another distinction that has appeared in diagnostic circles for decades, as researchers and clinicians puzzled over the relative contributions from biology and the environment to the onset of a depressive illness.

Introducing the terms "primary" and "secondary" to the diagnostic lexicon of affective disorders, Winokur (1973) proposed another binary classification schema that encompassed some of the other approaches to diagnosis. According to Winokur, primary affective disorders are depressions or manic conditions that occur in the absence of other types of psychiatric or medical illnesses. Thus, primary affective disorders would include bipolar and unipolar depressions that could occur either with or without accompanying psychotic features. Secondary affective disorders would include depression or mania that occurred as a reaction to a more central medical or psychiatric illness or environmental condition. Table 14-1 depicts a contemporary revision of Winokur's (1991) classification schema.

This chapter focuses only on disorders of thinking that have been found in bipolar and unipolar affective disorders (with and without manifest psychotic features). Disordered thinking in mania (or bipolar manic disorder) is considered first, followed by a review of the literature on thought disorder in depression (both unipolar and bipolar types). A review of the research into the quality of thought disturbances associated with both of these syndromes (mania and depression) provides a conceptual framework for examining the utility of the Rorschach as an aid in differential diagnosis.

Manic Thought Organization

Formal Thought Disorder in Mania

"Manic-depressive insanity" was part of Kraepelin's (1921) early diagnostic schema. Clinicians have always considered psychosis as one possible manifestation of mania; however, historically, it seems that most of the diagnostic emphasis was placed on the striking affective and behavioral characteristics of manic individuals. With the exception of the concepts of "pressured speech" and "flight of ideas," the quality of thought in mania received comparatively little attention from early psychiatric experts. Until more recently, diagnosticians accepted the possibility of delusions and hallucinations in manic psychosis, but reserved special qualities of disordered thought for schizophrenia alone. For example, Bleuler (1911) indicated that the speech of manic individuals is "flighty" but that, unlike schizophrenia, there are no specific signs of affective psychosis. Proposing a list of "first rank systems" that he believed were pathognomic of schizophrenia, Schneider (1959) stated that he was unable to find any first rank symptoms in mania.

However, a strikingly different picture began to emerge in the 1970s. Lipkin, Dyrud, and Meyer (1970) found that the cognitive phenomenology of mania overlapped considerably with that of schizophrenia. Carpenter, Strauss, and Muleh (1973) looked specifically at the quality of thought processes and reported a high frequency of first-rank Schneiderian symptoms of schizophrenia in manic individuals. Andreasen and her colleagues conducted a number of studies comparing thought processes in manics and schizophrenics (Andreasen and Powers, 1974, 1975; Andreasen, Tsuang, and Canter, 1974; Andreasen, 1979a,b; Andreasen and Akiskal, 1983). The collective conclusions of Andreasen's

Table 14-1 Winokur's (1991) Classification of Affective Disorders
AFFECTIVE DISORDERS

Organic Affective Syndrome	Bipolar Disorders	Unipolar Disorders	Schizoaffective Disorder
-structural -physiological -withdrawal	Bipolar I Bipolar II		
Reactive Depression	Endogenous Psychotic Depression		Neurotic
Bereavement Depression secondary to medical illness	Familial Pure Depressive Disease (FPDD) Sporadic Depressive Disease (SDD)		Depressive Spectrum Disease (DSD) Depression secondary to neurosis, personality disorders, & substance abuse

From Winokur (1991).

studies were that (1) manic subjects had high levels of thought disorder characterized by overinclusive and bizarre conceptual thinking, whereas schizophrenic subjects were more underinclusive and bizarre in their concept formation; (2) based on responses to a proverbs test, clinicians diagnosed thought disorder more frequently in manic subjects than in those with schizophrenia; and (3) Bleulerian and Schneiderian symptoms are not specific to schizophrenia but occur in many manic subjects as well.[1] Taken together, these and other influential studies at the end of the

---

1. It is worth noting that some research has indicated that Schneiderian symptoms do have differential diagnostic value. Akiskal and Puzantian (1979) found that only 10% of subjects with "pure" affective psychoses had clear evidence of first rank symptoms and that those who did usually had concurrent psychiatric or medical conditions. Andreasen concluded that Schneiderian symptoms carry diagnostic weight when they are "massively" present and when known organic conditions are ruled out.

decade contributed significantly to greater diagnostic precision and reliability for both schizophrenia and manic-depressive illness. The studies conducted by Morrison and Flanagan (1978) and Pope and Lipinski (1978) influenced the evolution of the modern DSM systems by concluding that many patients with bipolar (manic) illnesses were commonly misdiagnosed as schizophrenic on the basis of their having disturbances in formal thought processes.

Descriptive Characteristics

In addition to being characterized as distractible, self-referential, and grandiose, mental activity in mania is most commonly described as expansive, rapid, pressured, circumstantial, and tangential (Belmaker and van Praag, 1980). In her study of affective disorders and creativity, Jamison (1993) found that both creative and hypomanic thinking is characterized by fluency, rapidity, and flexibility. A greater speed of thinking leads to a greater quantity of thoughts and associations that may produce some unique ideas and associations. However, whereas healthy creative individuals may demonstrate a richness in their unusual associations, manic subjects may have difficulty maintaining a focus and filtering out distractions that give their associations a bizarre quality (Andreasen and Powers, 1975).

Jamison mentioned another key aspect of manic thought which is the ability to combine ideas or categories of thought in order to form new and original connections (combinative thinking). Using object sorting tests, researchers have showed that manic subjects demonstrate overinclusiveness in their conceptual thinking in that they tend to combine test objects into categories in a way that broaden, shift, and blur conceptual boundaries (Andreasen and Powers, 1974, 1975). Harrow et al. (1982) also demonstrated that manic subjects tend to be more active and behaviorally overinclusive than schizophrenic individuals.

However, manic thought may not simply be overinclusive; it may be bizarre and idiosyncratic as well (Harrow et al., 1982). Harrow and his colleagues also used a proverb and object sorting test to assess bizarre and idiosyncratic thinking in manic, schizophrenic, and nonpsychotic patients. Harrow and his team found that 94% of their manic subjects, compared to 79% of their schizophrenics, demonstrated moderate to severe "bizarre-idiosyncratic thought" (their name for diverse types of speech and behavior associated with positive thought disorder or florid psychosis).

Despite the possible presence of bizarreness, overinclusiveness, and first-rank symptoms, manic speech has also been described as more reality based and logical enough to invite involvement by others (Janowsky,

Leff, and Epstein, 1970). Harrow and his group also noted how manic subjects attempted to interact with others, albeit in bizarre and inappropriate ways, whereas schizophrenic individuals tended to be more private, autistic, and inwardly directed. Perhaps it is this interactivity that, according to Janowsky et al., makes people dismiss the schizophrenic individual as "crazy" and accept the manic patient's pseudologic more easily. Echoing this idea, Lipkin, Dyrud, and Meyer (1970) reported that "The ideation of the patient with a manic episode, although at times delusional, shows reasonably good form; and the associations, although often occurring as a flight of ideas or even clang associations, have a different quality than the puzzling symbolic looseness of associations demonstrated in schizophrenia (p. 266).

As mentioned in the last chapter, Hoffman et al. (1986) conducted a discourse analysis to contrast the different processing requirements that manic and schizophrenic speech impose on the listener. Their linguistic analysis of speech samples of manic, schizophrenic, and normal subjects provided some support for the claim that manic thought/speech disorder is, in some way, less incoherent or alienating than that which is found in schizophrenia. Hoffman and his team based their investigation on the psycholinguistic studies of Deese (1978, 1980), which proposed that an extended, multisentence text will be experienced as coherent if the listener can organize the propositions expressed by the text into a hierarchical discourse plan or structure. If a speech segment can be organized by the listener into a propositional hierarchy, with some of the propositions dependently linked to others, then all of the propositions expressed by the speaker can be logically related to each other.

Hoffman et al. determined that, unlike schizophrenic subjects, manic speakers could construct complex, well-organized discourse plans that sound incoherent only when the speaker abruptly shifts from one plan to another. As a result of this finding, they concluded that the disorganized, but more comprehensible, speech of the manic would be characterized by a "structural shift" from one well-formed message or discourse plan to another, whereas the disorganization of the schizophrenic speaker was characterized more by a "structural deficiency" in generating any clear plan whatsoever.

These reports suggest that illogical and incoherent speech in mania may somehow be less alienating and difficult for the listener to understand (or simply tolerate) than the speech and logic of schizophrenic individuals. It may be that the interpersonal orientation of the manic also helps make it easier for the listener to attend than the more distant demeanor of the subject with schizophrenia. The delusions of manic patients often reflect themes of ecstasy and communion as opposed to the more ominous and fearful delusions of the schizophrenic patients that seemed oriented more toward seclusiveness and segregation. Perhaps it is also the infectious mood of the manic subject that is more amusing and less frightening than the affective flatness or incongruity of the schizophrenic which increases the listener's tolerance for deviance. Andreasen and Pfohl (1976) conducted a linguistic analysis of manic speech and found it to be colorful and filled with adjectives and action verbs; however, curiously, it reflected more interest in things than in people.

Rorschach Indices of Manic Thought Disorder

In describing the general structural characteristics of "manic mood disorders," Rorschach (1921) stated that (1) the total number of responses (R) would be greater than average, (2) reaction times would be low, (3) form level (F+%) would be between 60–70%, (4) the sequence of responses loose, (5) whole responses (W) between 8–10, (6) great variability in responses, (7) percentage of original responses would be high but associated with poor form, and (8) experience balance (EB = Sum Color : Sum Human Movement responses) would reflect a greater number of color than movement responses. In discussing thought disordered scores in particular, Rorschach stated that "in manics there are confabulatory responses which are vague and of indifferent quality, W responses confabulated from various parts, and poor forms" (p. 170).

For decades, subsequent research did not add much to Rorschach's findings. A smattering of studies in the next three decades generally confirmed Rorschach's data. For example, Levey and Beck (1934) compared Rorschach responses during depressed and manic phases and found a greater number of confabulations, more W–s (minus level Whole responses), and a tendency to combine details into unrealistic wholes. Looking primarily at structural variables, Wittenhorn and Holzberg (1951) found that manic subjects differed from paranoid schizophrenics, depressives, and involutional melancholics in terms of having a higher number of CF (Color-dominated form responses). Schmidt and Fonda (1954) contrasted 42 manic-depressive and schizophrenic subjects with Beck's (Beck et al., 1950) normative data on nonpsychiatric individuals. They found that, compared to normals, manic subjects responded more rapidly and demonstrated (1) greater emotional dilation (as measured by Beck's lambda), (2) greater organizational energy (Beck's Z score), (3) higher W%, (4) F+% around 62, (5) greater Sum of color responses (Sum C), and (6) fewer vista responses, suggesting less self-criticism. Compared to schizophrenic subjects, manics demonstrated greater use of color (higher Sum C), more organizational capacity (greater Z score), and more human movement and content scores, suggesting greater involvement with the outside world and people.

Klopfer and Spiegelmen (1956) contrasted manic and schizoaffective subjects and found that both gave an abundance of color and human movement (M) responses. They suggested that the difference lay in the quality of Ms, with the schizoaffective group giving M-s with bizarre quality and content and the manic subjects giving M-s, without bizarre quality, that resulted more from carelessness.

Unlike Rorschach, Bohm (1958) expected manics to have lower form levels (50–70%), fewer originals, and an increase in both human movement and color responses, resulting in a dilated EB ratio. However, like Rorschach, Bohm mentioned that a greater number of DWs, successive combinatory wholes, and "confabulatory-combinatory" responses would characterize the manic Rorschach.

Weiner (1966) also contrasted manic and schizoaffective Rorschach and agreed with most of the findings regarding structural data, in terms of lower reaction times, higher R, and higher Sum C. Regarding the quality of ideation in both groups, Weiner stated, "They [manics] employ both movement and color freely, extend their interpretations far beyond conventional animal and popular percepts, and obvious D locations, and embellish their responses with numerous fanciful specifications, combinations, and peripheral associations" (Weiner, 1966, p. 433).

Perhaps the most detailed and rigorous Rorschach analysis of disordered thinking in mania was conducted by Holzman's TDI research group (Solovay et al., 1987), which has been discussed a number of times thus far. The mean TDI score for their 20 manic subjects was 25.02 (± 16.15) compared to a mean of 35.58 (± 38.77) for the group of 43 schizophrenic subjects. Although the schizophrenic group was rated as significantly more disorganized (in terms of GAS ratings) and with more chronicity than the manic group, there was not a significant difference between total TDI scores. This was apparently due to the greater variation within the schizophrenic sample. In a principal components factor analysis, one factor correctly identified 73.3% of the manic group. Termed "Combinatory Thinking," this factor was comprised of the following individual TDI scores (and their respective loadings): playful confabulation (0.83); incongruous combination (.60); flippant response (.58); and fabulized combination (.53). An additional factor that distinguished the manic from the schizophrenic group was called "Irrelevant Intrusions" (made up of flippant and looseness responses). In terms of severity levels, the schizophrenic group showed thought disorder at all four levels of severity on the TDI. In contrast, none of the manic subjects demonstrated thought disorder scores at the most severe level of 1.0. Both groups had equivalent amounts of thought disorder at the .25 and .75 levels, while the manic group produced more thought disorder scores at the .50 level than the schizophrenic group. It is the .50 level scores that include such factors scores as playful confabulations and fabulized combinations.

Based on their data, Solovay et al. (1987) concluded that "manic thought disorder manifests itself as ideas loosely strung together and extravagantly combined and elaborated. . . . One prominent outcome of such an arbitrary integrative process is the appearance of irrelevant intrusions into social discourse that at times may appear inappropriately flippant and playful" (p. 19).

Khadivi et al. (1997) cross-validated some of these key findings as they pertained to manic subjects. Contrasting six overarching thought disorder categories (Combinatory Thinking, Idiosyncratic Verbalization, Autistic Thinking, Fluid Thinking, Absurdity, and Confusion), among paranoid schizophrenic, manic, and schizoaffective subjects, Khadivi et al. found that the manic group had significantly more combinatory thinking than the other two groups. They concluded that combinatory thinking reflects a tendency to connect things normally kept apart. Here, the subject's effort to integrate disparate elements outstrips adherence to reason, reality, and intellectual capacity. Khadivi and his colleagues associated this combinatory process with distractibility or problems in maintaining one's focus. They noted that since manic individuals are driven to respond to unrelated stimuli, they become overinclusive and are unable to screen out irrelevant stimuli. The authors also conjectured that this combinatory quality may be related to the concept of "flight of ideas."

Despite my earlier criticisms of the Deviant Response category (DR) in the Comprehensive System, I believe that DR scores capture these inappropriate intrusions that disrupt the flow of thought or disturb the subject's focus of attention. In fact, although he did not present any data on manic subjects, Exner (1986a) indicated that DR scores are most common among subjects with affective problems. Later, Exner (1993) added that DR2 scores represent problems in "ideational impulse control" and occur commonly in "hypomanic subjects whose affective disorganization impairs their ability to stay 'on target'" (p. 480). In his interpretative guide to the Comprehensive System, Wilson (1994) indicated that bipolar patients are characterized by high Zf scores, many blends, DR2s, and ALOGs.

Unfortunately, there are no separate Comprehensive System norms for manic or hypomanic subjects. In his major text, Exner (1993) included norms for 315 inpatient depressives. However, since he did not provide a differential diagnostic breakdown for this psychiatric reference group, there is no way of knowing whether this group contained bipolar as well as unipolar depressives. Singer and Brabender (1993) used the Comprehensive System to examine differences and similarities between bipolar manic, depressed, and unipolar depressed subjects. They found that the bipolar manics had significantly higher SUM 6 Special Scores and WSUM 6 Special Scores, more scores at Level 2, higher SCZI, and a higher X-% than the other two groups. Seventy seven percent of the manic group had at least one DR1; 56% had one or more DR2s; 50% had INCOMs; 56% FABCOMs; and 22% ALOGs. Interestingly, none of the manics had level 2 Deviant Verbalizations (DV2), which would include neologisms or extremely odd word usage. This is quite consistent with TDI studies that have shown that idiosyncratic verbalizations are less reflective of manic thinking.

DISORDERED THINKING AND DEPRESSION

Investigations of the relationship between thought pathology and depression have revealed conflicting findings due, in part, to the different ways that researchers have operationally defined the variables of depression and thought disorder. For example, regarding the variable "thought disorder," it matters whether one is referring descriptively to a traditional psychiatric taxonomy of thought disorder types, as one would find, for example, in Andreasen's (1986) TLC scoring system,[2] or trying to deconstruct the concept of thought disorder by dissecting it into its cognitive components such as impairments in concept formation, reasoning, focusing, attention, and so on. On the other hand, some researchers have defined "thought disorder" in terms of cognitive distortions and unrealistic views of oneself and the future (Beck, 1964).

Regarding the variable of "depression," it matters whether one is referring to depression diagnostically or phenomenologically. In other words, some studies classify subjects on the basis of depressive diagnosis, whereas others do so on the basis of self-reporting of depression (e.g., scores on a depression inventory) in diagnostically heterogeneous subjects. Furthermore, given that illness acuity may contribute to the

---

2. Recall, from chapter 1, that Andreasen (1986) devised a scoring system that consists of 18 different forms of thought disorder including familiar categories such as Poverty of Speech, Poverty of Content of Speech, Pressure of Speech, Distractible Speech, Tangentiality, Derailment, Incoherence, Illogicality, Clanging, Neologisms, Word Approximations, Circumstantiality, Loss of Goal, Perseveration, Echolalia, Blocking, Self-Reference, and Paraphasias.

quality of thought (dis)organization, it matters whether depressed subjects are inpatients or outpatients. It matters also whether one is studying thought disorder in psychotic depressives, in particular, or all depressives, regardless of the presence or absence of psychotic features. Finally, it matters greatly whether we are studying thought disorder in unipolar versus bipolar depressives.

Thus, conceptual differences in how key variables have been defined has led to a schism in the literature between those researchers who argue for the existence of a form of thought disorder in depression and those who believe that thought disorder does not exist in any meaningful way in this population. What follows is a brief summary of positive and negative findings regarding the presence of certain types of disordered thinking in depression.

Positive Findings

COGNITIVE DISTORTION AND DEPRESSION. Beck (1963, 1964, 1967, 1971; Braff and Beck, 1974) first wrote that thought disorder may be an underlying causal mechanism of depression as opposed to an artifact of changes in mood. Of course Beck's definition of thought disorder was a broader, more generic one than that used in traditional psychiatric circles. Beck was interested in cognitive distortions that produced low self-esteem and other symptoms of depression. He reasoned that self-criticism and pessimism about the future cause distortions, misperceptions, and eventually lead to a depressed mood. Andreasen (1976) raised questions about using such an atypical definition of "thought disorder" that lacks precision and deviates from psychiatric norms.

DISTURBANCES IN FORM AND CONTENT. Other researchers studied the relationship between disturbances in thinking and both bipolar and unipolar depression. Using structured mental status examinations and cognitive tests, Winokur, Clayton, and Reich (1969) identified thought content and process disturbances in a heterogeneous group of depressive subjects. Roughly 20% of the total depressive sample of 89 subjects were found to have moderate to severe formal thought disorder (including such thought disorder manifestations as paralogical or unrelated responses, tangentiality, flight of ideas, neologisms, echolalia, perseveration, clanging, and word salad). Of their 47 confirmed unipolar subjects, a surprisingly high 40% had moderate to severe formal thought disorder.

Ianizito, Cadoret, and Pugh (1974) studied disorders of thought content and form in unipolar depressives and found that 78% of unipolar patients who demonstrated moderate to severe disturbances in the formal structure of their thinking had poor outcomes as measured by longer lengths of stay and referral for ECT. Thus, the authors concluded that formal thought disorder at the time of admission may predict a severe episode of depression that might be more refractory to treatment.

IMPAIRED ABSTRACTING ABILITY. Other researchers have studied specific cognitive functions, such as abstracting ability, that have traditionally been associated with thought disorder. Braff and Beck (1974) looked at the relationship between abstracting ability and diagnosis, in this case, schizophrenia, depression, and normal controls. Not surprisingly, the schizophrenic group showed more idiosyncratic and concrete answers on the Abstraction portion of the Shipley Hartford; but the depressed group demonstrated poorer abstracting ability than the normal controls. However, Braff and Beck did not find that the diagnosis of depression was associated with impaired abstraction, only the subjects' rating of their own depressive symptomatology on the BDI. Braff and Beck concluded that the presence of an abstracting deficit may or may not be consistent with a primary diagnosis of depression.

Sprock et al. (1983) looked at cognitive functioning in subjects complaining of depression. Specifically, they investigated the presence of thought disorder in chronic pain patients who complained of depressive symptoms. They were subjects who were not considered to be suffering from primary affective illness but were instead classified as "depressed" on the basis of rating themselves extremely depressed on the Beck Depression Inventory. The researchers found three significant areas of deficit on a tachistoscopic procedure designed to test information processing speed: (1) abstracting ability, (2) associative intrusions, and (3) speed of processing. Impairment in each area was significantly correlated with ratings of depression.

The Category Test has also been used to study abstraction ability in both unipolar and bipolar depressives (Donnelly et al., 1980; Savard, Rey, and Post, 1980). In these studies, investigators discovered a significant degree of abstraction impairment in hospitalized depressives (of both types) as compared with nondepressed controls.

FOCUSING AND PERSEVERATION. Silberman, Weingartner, and Post (1983) looked for evidence of illogical reasoning and inefficient use of feedback by the depressed sample on an impersonal, abstract, problem-solving task. Using a procedure in which subjects must generate, test, and ultimately narrow down a problem-solving hypothesis based on feedback from the examiner, Silberman et al. found that a combined sample of unipolar and bipolar depressives demonstrated significantly impaired performances. Specifically, the depressed group had more trouble focusing and tended to make more perseverative errors than a nondepressed control group. Perseveration was said to occur when subjects stuck to incorrect solutions despite being given negative feedback. Interestingly, the researchers found that their depressed subjects performed qualitatively similar to subjects with right and left temporal lobectomies. They concluded that some organic dementias with perseverative tendencies might be useful as models for aspects of the dementia associated with depression.

Negative Findings

Contrary to the findings of others, Andreasen (1976) did not find impairments in abstracting abilities or associational deficits leading to a poverty of thoughts in her subjects. Later, Andreasen used her TLC Scale and found that 53% of her depressive subjects had global TLC ratings of 1 or greater, suggesting the presence of some type of thought disorder in over half of these patients (1979a,b). However, Andreasen noted that only the mildest forms of thought disorder occurred in these subjects and that the occurrence of each individual subtype was relatively uncommon. Table 14-2 depicts the frequency of different forms of disordered thought, language, and communication in her depressed subjects.

Andreasen maintained that the more severe signs of disordered thinking do not occur in depression. For example, derailment, which occurred in only 14% of the depressives, was found in 56% of the manics and schizophrenic patients. The milder forms that do seem to occur in depression are, according to Andreasen, products of primary affective symptoms.

Carter (1986) conducted a study to assess the presence of formal thought disorder in psychotically depressed individuals. In particular, she was interested in contrasting the nature of disordered thinking in psychotic depression and chronic paranoid schizophrenia. Carter found that the psychotic depressive subjects demonstrated as much idiosyncratic thinking (including such qualities as looseness, incoherence, and illogicality) as subjects classified as paranoid schizophrenic.

Carter focused on the similarities between the two groups but noted some subtle differences as well. For example, although both groups were overly concrete on the Proverbs Test, only the schizophrenic group showed this pattern on the Object Sorting Test. Since a higher level of conceptual ability may be assessed on the Proverbs Test, Carter reasoned that the psychotic depressives only became concrete as the task became more demanding and required more complex abstracting skills.

Carter concluded that the presence of psychosis equalizes thought disorder among different diagnostic groups. Like Harrow et al. (1982), she believed that the kinds of positive thought disorder found in her subjects were products of psychotic disorganization, and that distinctions between different diagnostic groups were less significant. In

Table 14-2 Frequency of TLC Disorders in Andreasen's (1979) Depressive Group

Type of Disorder	% of Patients
Circumstantiality	31%
Tangentiality	25%
Poverty of Speech	22%
Poverty of Content	17%
Loss of Goal	17%
Derailment	14%
Self Reference	11%
Pressured Speech	6%
Perseveration	6%
Blocking	6%
Stilted Speech	3%
Incoherence	0%
Neologisms	0%
Illogicality	0%

From Andreasen, 1979b.

essence, Carter was saying that, among psychotic depressive subjects, the presence of thought disorder was a product, not of depression, but of the associated psychotic disorganization. She suggested that a general psychoticism profile would include idiosyncratic thinking, restricted abstraction ability, linguistic errors, content deficiencies, intermixing, and loss of goal-directedness.

Kay (1986) took issue with Carter's conclusions that thought disorder is not qualitatively associated with diagnosis but is primarily a product of psychotic disorganization. Among other things, Kay criticized Carter's decision to contrast psychotic depressives with paranoid schizophrenics who have demonstrated less severe cognitive impairment than other subtypes of schizophrenia. As seen in the last chapter, paranoid schizophrenia yields relatively fewer signs of positive thought disorder (on interview ratings and testing) than nonparanoid subtypes. Thus, as Kay argued, it should not be surprising that a schizophrenic subgroup known for its lesser degree of thought impairment would fail to demonstrate more positive thought disorder than another actively psychotic group.

Kay also noted that two noteworthy differences between the groups were deemphasized by Carter. Kay drew attention to Carter's finding that psychotic depressives demonstrated more "intermixing" (either the mixing or blending into the response of extraneous personal material from the subject's past or current experience, or the extensive elaboration of a theme or idea, which does not fit into the structure of the response [Marengo et al., 1986]) and less conceptual overinclusion than the paranoid schizophrenic subjects. Kay wondered whether these findings actually supported the existence of distinct qualitative differences between the thought disorder profiles of the two groups, quite apart from the general disorganizing effects of their psychoses.

Although empirical support for a general "thought disorder profile" for depression remains ambiguous, there are some useful Rorschach findings that may prove helpful in making differential diagnostic decisions between such clinical syndromes as bipolar versus unipolar depression and psychotic depression versus other psychotic disorders.

Rorschach Indices of Unipolar vs. Bipolar Depression

Singer and Brabender (1993) pointed out that the issue of distinguishing bipolar from unipolar depressives has been largely neglected in the Rorschach literature. They found that bipolar depressives had a significantly greater mean SUM 6 and WSUM6 than their unipolar counterparts. Regarding the presence of Special Scores, the bipolar group demonstrated significantly more Level 1 DR and INCOM responses than the unipolar depressives. In fact, the bipolar depressives did not differ significantly from the bipolar manics on these two measures. It was particularly noteworthy that 60% of the bipolar depressives gave DRs, compared to 77% of the manics and only 14% of the unipolars. Qualitatively, Singer and Brabender found that the responses of the bipolar depressives were "less fantastic, less playful, and less sanguinely toned than the bipolar manic subjects" (p. 342).

As mentioned earlier in this chapter, the manic subjects scored significantly higher on WSUM 6 (with a greater number of Level 2 Special Scores) and SCZI than either the bipolar or unipolar depressives. The bipolar and unipolar groups did not differ on frequency of Level 2 scores. The researchers concluded that Level 2 Special Scores are the realm of the manic bipolar subjects (72% of the manics had more than one Level 2 score, compared to 33% of the bipolar depressives and 18% of the unipolars).[3]

In addition to having more Level 1 INCOMs and DRs than the unipolars, the bipolar depressed group obtained a higher percentage of

---

3. Although the two depressive groups did not differ significantly on frequency of Level 2 Special Scores, there was a trend for the bipolar depressives to give more of these responses (33%) than the unipolars (18%). Although not statistically significant, the bipolar depressives also showed a trend toward giving more ALOGs (20%) and CONTAMs (6%) compared to the unipolars (ALOGs, 7%; CONTAMs, 0%).

minus form level responses than the unipolars (X–% = 21 vs 14 for unipolars), leading the authors to conclude that when depression "is manifest (either from the Rorschach or from other modes of observation) and a relatively high number of special scores is present, particularly in combination with a deficit in reality testing, the hypothesis of the presence of a bipolar disorder should be raised" (p. 343).

Looking more closely at Singer and Brabender's data on unipolar depressives, one can see that they demonstrated a relatively low frequency of disordered thinking. In every category, they showed fewer Special Scores than bipolar subjects. In most categories, their frequency of Special Scores is similar to that of nonpatient adults (Exner, 1993).

Psychotic Depression and Rorschach Thought Disorder

Using the TDI, Makowski et al. (1997) examined disordered thinking in adolescent onset schizophrenia and psychotic depression. Like Carter (1986), the researchers noted that the thought disorder patterns of both groups were characterized by idiosyncratic word usage, illogical reasoning, perceptual confusion, loss of realistic attunement to the task, and loosely related ideas. Likewise, they found no significant difference in mean TDI scores for each group (schizophrenics = 20.81 ± 26.4; psychotic depressives = 14.13 ±12.63).[4] However, unlike Carter, who found little difference in the nature of disordered thinking between paranoid schizophrenics and psychotic depressives, Makowski et al. found qualitative distinctions in thought disturbance patterns between schizophrenic and psychotic depressive subjects.

Following the methodology of earlier differential diagnostic TDI studies (Shenton et al., 1987; Solovay et al., 1987), Makowski and his colleagues factor analyzed their data and identified seven empiric factors, shown in Table 14-3.

Both groups scored high on the Psychotic Disorganization factor (incoherence, neologisms, and peculiar verbalizations). Although the schizophrenic group showed elevations on all seven factors, Psychotic Reasoning (queer verbalization, looseness, autistic logic), Loss of Set (inappropriate distance and flippancy), and Confusion (confusion and autistic logic) seemed to define the main schizophrenic factors. On the other hand, Associative Looseness (idiosyncratic symbolism and

---

4. The authors noted that the nonsignificant difference in mean TDI scores may have been an artifact resulting from the high number of schizophrenic subjects, compared to psychotic depressives, who were medicated at the time of testing, thus most likely reducing the elevations of their TDIs. One might infer that if they had been nonmedicated, the schizophrenics would probably have scored higher than the psychotic depressives.

Table 14-3 Principal Components Analysis of TDI Scores

Factor	TDI Scores
Psychotic Reasoning	Queer Verbalization, Loose, Alog, Clang
Psychotic Disorganization	Incoherence, Neologisms, Peculiar Verbalizations
Loss of Set	Inappropriate Distance, Flippant
Associative Looseness	Idiosyncratic Symbolism, Confabulation
Psychotic Looseness	Incongruous Combination, Contamination
Confusion	Confusion, Alog
Playful Looseness	Relationship Verbalization, Playful Confabulation

From Makowski et al., 1997.

confabulation) and Psychotic Looseness (incongruous combination and contamination) characterized the affective psychosis factors. Makowski et al. concluded that the scores making up these affective psychosis factors reflect a style of thinking in which responses are arbitrarily embellished by personal meaning to the extent that reality testing is compromised.

Conclusions

There is convincing evidence of a "manic Rorschach thought disorder profile" characterized primarily by combinatory thinking, playful confabulations, and flippant remarks. Qualitative features such as pressured, rapid speech, use of active verbs, affective language, and ambitious integrative efforts may bolster the characteristic thought disorder signs to strengthen diagnostic inferences. There is also evidence that bipolar depressives can be identified (and distinguished from unipolar depressives) on the basis of combinatory activity, poorer form level, and constriction.

Psychotic unipolar depression seems to manifest a great deal of thought disorder that overlaps with schizophrenia and other psychotic conditions (bipolar mania). However, as Carter pointed out, the presence of psychosis may bring with it a general disorganizing effect that tends to mask the qualitative distinctions between different subtypes of depression. For example, distinguishing whether a patient is suffering from a psychotic unipolar or psychotic bipolar depression may be particularly difficult on the basis of the Rorschach alone. Although both disorders could possibly be distinguished from schizophrenia and manic psychosis, it may be difficult to make a finer discrimination between the two subtypes of psychotic depression.

CHAPTER

15

BORDERLINE SYNDROMES

In a comparatively brief period of time, the borderline concept developed into one of the most captivating and controversial diagnostic phenomena in the history of psychopathology. Although it has been with us in one form or another since the beginning of the century, its "rise to fame" in the world of psychiatric diagnoses has occurred within the last few decades. Aptly captured by the title of a book about borderline personality disorder called "Imbroglio" (Cauwels, 1992), the borderline concept has eluded and confounded us as much as it has intrigued us. Yet despite the decades of confusion and controversy and the countless volumes written to sharpen and tidy up the concept, there still does not exist unanimous agreement of just what the borderline concept "borders" on or between.

Traditionally seen as occupying the border of its older and more well established cousin schizophrenia, borderline disorders have also been conceptualized as the "borderland" between neuroses and psychoses. Viewed this way, borderline becomes a superordinate realm for a heterogeneous group of personality disorders that have certain structural features in common. Others have argued that borderline is better understood as a specific type of personality disorder, not as a broader category of personality functioning. Not content with any of these explanations, some have proposed that the borderline syndrome lies along the border of primary affective disorders, which are thought to give rise to the myriad cognitive, affective, interpersonal, and adaptive problems that are observed in borderline patients. More recently, researchers have wondered whether borderline disorders border on being characterological adaptations to chronic complex post traumatic stress. Finally, there are those among us who would probably state that the borderline concept should be relegated to the border of the diagnostic wastebasket!

Following a brief overview of the development of the borderline concept, I turn to the linkage between the phenomena of thought disorder, psychosis, and borderline disorders. The majority of the chapter addresses the interface between the Rorschach and borderline-level thought pathology.

DEVELOPMENT OF THE BORDERLINE CONCEPT

One can understand the development of the borderline concept from three different vantage points, which have focused on four different conceptual domains of borderline phenomena. The vantage points consist of three different epistemological traditions, each of which has studied the borderline concept from its own theoretical and methodological orientation. These traditions included (1) psychoanalytic ego psychology and object relations theory that focused on the concepts of borderline schizophrenia and borderline personality organization or BPO (Stern, 1938; Zilboorg, 1941; Deutsch, 1942; Hoch and Polatin, 1949; Knight, 1953; Kernberg, 1967); (2) empirically based descriptive psychiatry, which gave rise to the DSM diagnosis of Borderline Personality Disorder or BPD (Grinker, Werble, and Drye, 1968; Gunderson, 1977, 1984; Gunderson and Singer, 1975; Gunderson and Kolb, 1978; Gunderson, Kolb, and Austin, 1981); (3) biopharmacological psychiatry, which studied both borderline schizophrenia and the relationship between borderline and subclinical affective disorders (Kety et al., 1968; Rosenthal et al., 1968; Wender, Rosenthal, and Kety, 1968; Klein, 1975, 1977; Stone, 1977, 1978; Wender, 1977; Akiskal, 1981; Kroll et al., 1981; Soloff and Ulrich, 1981; Pope et al., 1983; Akiskal et al., 1985; Gunderson and Phillips, 1991).

PSYCHOSIS, THOUGHT DISORDER, AND THE BORDERLINE SYNDROME

Regardless of which tradition one favors, all definitions of borderline disorders include some mention of the propensity for psychotic, or primary process, thinking. Knight (1953) was interested in what he termed "ego weaknesses" in normal-appearing patients undergoing transient psychotic episodes. In particular, he noted that psychotic manifestations would become evident to experienced interviewers. In describing the "microscopic" and "macroscopic" signs of schizophrenic illness, Knight suggested that the borderline patient could demonstrate a spectrum of thought pathology, ranging from subtle peculiarities of expression to fully autistic thought content. Knight wrote, "Occasional blocking, peculiarities of word usage, obliviousness to obvious implications, contaminations of idioms, arbitrary inferences, inappropriate affect, and suspicion-laden behavior and questions are a few possible examples of such unwitting betrayals of ego impairment of psychotic degree" (p. 103).

A colleague of Rapaport, Gill, and Schafer at the Menninger Clinic in the 1940s, Knight learned that the Rorschach was a sensitive instrument for assessing autistic thinking in borderline patients. Kernberg also believed that psychotic-like thinking would appear in unstructured situations, such as projective testing.[1] According to Kernberg, primary process thinking would appear in the form of primitive fantasies, problems adapting to the demands of the test materials, and peculiar verbalizations.

Kernberg included the "tendency toward primary process thinking" and "weakening of reality testing" among his diagnostic criteria for BPO. He downplayed the presence of a formal thought disorder in these patients and stated that reality testing is usually intact in the borderline individual. However, he emphasized that it may be temporarily lost under the press of heightened emotionality, alcohol or drugs, or in the throes of a psychotic transference. Both borderline and psychotic patients are vulnerable to psychotic transferences; but, according to Kernberg, lapses in reality testing for the borderline individual tend to be circumscribed to the treatment setting and do not generally affect the patient's functioning outside of treatment. Kernberg also indicated that different levels of boundary disturbances distinguish the borderline from the psychotic-level transference psychosis. Psychotic patients may manifest fusionlike experiences in which they feel a common identity with the therapist. In contrast, the borderline's psychotic transference is not predicated on a merger experience, in which the distinction between self and other is lost, but on the fantasy that the separate patient and therapist are exchanging aspects of their personalities. Instead of feeling like one is becoming the therapist, the borderline patient may regressively assert that the therapist either hates or loves him based on a projected fantasy that the patient is trying to disown.

---

1. Again, it is no accident that Kernberg considered projective testing an important diagnostic tool since he developed his seminal theory of borderline personality organization while at Menninger, a decade after Knight introduced the concept and two decades after Rapaport, Gill, and Schafer had introduced the concept of the diagnostic testing battery.

Gunderson has been a major proponent of the school that views a tendency toward psychotic thinking as a chief characteristic of border-line personality disorder. He stressed that the psychotic symptoms in borderline patients were typically ego dystonic and mild, characterized by paranoid ideation, psychotic-like reactions to drugs, depersonalization, or derealization. Citing a series of empirical investigations that found the presence of mild psychotic experiences to be diagnostically useful (Gunderson, 1977; Gunderson and Kolb, 1978; Perry and Klerman, 1980), Gunderson lobbied to make the proneness to brief psychotic regression one of the diagnostic criteria for the DSM definition of borderline personality disorder. However, this criterion was excluded from both DSM III and III-R primary diagnostic criteria and mentioned only as an ancillary feature of the disorder. It was finally added as a ninth criterion for borderline personality disorder in DSM IV (American Psychiatric Association, 1994) in the form of "transient stress related paranoid ideation or dissociative symptoms."

Although a believer in the presence of psychotic-like symptoms in borderline patients, Gunderson indicated that these phenomena should not be expected to occur in every borderline patient. However, he believed that when they occurred, they had considerable differential diagnostic value. In other words, Gunderson agreed that what the presence of mild ego-dystonic psychotic experiences lacked in sensitivity, they made up for in specificity.

Gunderson (1984) attempted to characterize the phenomenology of psychotic reactions in borderline patients by describing five qualities of experience: (1) affective phenomena, (2) disturbances in the sense of reality, (3) audio-visual perceptual distortions, (4) paranoid beliefs, (5) self-boundary confusion. Affective phenomena involve unrealistic pre-occupations with inner badness, worthlessness, or sinfulness reaching delusional proportions. Disturbances in one's sense of reality include signs and symptoms of derealization and depersonalization, character-ized by out-of-body experiences and perceptual changes in the size and shape of one's body. Auditory and visual pseudoperceptions may or may not involve actual hallucinatory experience. Usually the patient experiences transitory perceptual distortions that are brief and unelaborated. Examples might include hearing sound or one's name called. Borderline-level paranoid beliefs include ideas of reference, around which some reality testing is maintained. For example, the patient may believe that he is being talked about but then reminds himself that this is probably his imagination. Finally, self-boundary confusion essentially involves a type of boundary impairment associated with a certain level of reality testing difficulty, in particular, the failure to distinguish "inner from outer." While maintaining a sense of separateness from the other and an accurate perception of the external world, the borderline patient may confuse his thoughts with those belonging to the other.

Several studies have supported the presence of a range of these mild psychotic experiences in borderline patients (Perry and Klerman, 1980; Koenigsberg, 1982; Chopra and Beatson, 1986). Episodic depersonalization and derealization, psychotic transference reactions, distorted perceptions of others, and brief paranoid experience were the most common experiences in inpatient and outpatient borderlines. For example, Chopra and Beatson found that all of their inpatient borderline subjects had some type of brief psychotic experience. At least 77% of their borderline patients had brief paranoid or other psychotic experiences and/or symptoms of depersonalization and derealization. On the other hand, only 53% reported transient auditory or visual hallucinations.

Stone (1980) described "soft signs" of disordered thinking characteristic of borderline patients. Whereas the psychotic patient may have delusions, the borderline may have "overvalued ideas" and magical thinking. Stone included among these soft signs phenomena such as heightened superstitiousness, vague or murky speech, attention to irrelevancies, rigid attitudes, tangentiality, and circumstantiality.

In addition to proposing that borderline individuals are especially prone to develop brief psychotic reaction under the influence of mind altering substances (Gunderson and Singer, 1975; Gunderson, 1977, 1984), Gunderson also discussed other conditions under which borderline patients would be most vulnerable to brief psychotic decompensation. These are characterized chiefly by threats to important primary object ties. According to Gunderson,

> When this object tie is threatened by frustration or the possibility of loss, the relationship to reality becomes shaky, but the reality testing capacity remains intact. When there is a felt absence of a primary object, the reality testing function itself becomes shaky or—as in the dissociative reaction—the feeling of reality is clearly disrupted. In other words, the reality testing function is regressively and defensively sacrificed in response to the perception that there is no single enduring and basically caring person available [Gunderson, 1984, p. 120].

Gunderson went on to state that the regressive shift in thought organization is accompanied by the emergence of primary process thinking, overelaborate affects, and a breakdown in reality testing (in this case, the ability to discriminate one's inner world from outer influences). Gunderson pointed out how each of these psychotic-like phenomena has an object-restitutive function in that each is a means of attempting to restore the lost object. If dissociative episodes remove the borderline individual from the immediacy of internal or interpersonal pain, self-mutilative behavior functions to counteract nihilistic terror and reconnect the patient to his or her body and the interpersonal world.

Despite the array of empirical findings and clinical experience supporting the presence of brief psychotic vulnerability and regressive thinking in borderline individuals, there have been a chorus of voices who have questioned the association between borderline personality, and disordered thinking, or psychosis proneness (Grinker et al., 1968; Spitzer, Endicott, and Gibbons, 1979; Loranger et al., 1982; Pope et al., 1983; Frances et al., 1984; Jonas and Pope, 1984; Pope et al., 1985). Grinker et al. originally concluded that, in contrast to schizophrenia, borderline patients do not present formal disturbances in thinking such as autistic reasoning, delusions, or hallucinations.[2] Spitzer et al. also questioned the presence of true psychotic features in borderline patients. Frances et al. (1984) looked at outpatient borderlines and found that psychotic episodes occurred infrequently among their sample.

Pope et al. (1985) criticized the methodology of previous studies that had found a relationship between borderline personality and psychotic vulnerability. One of their criticisms was that some of these studies employed diagnostic criteria for assigning subjects to borderline groups that were inconsistent with DSM III criteria. For example, in Gunderson and Singer's (1975) study, many of the so-called borderline subjects would be classified today as schizotypal. Another criticism of these studies, is that many did not control for the factitious elements or the presence of major affective disorders. This latter criticism is particularly important given that a number of researchers have pointed out the high comorbidity of affective disorders with borderline personality disorder (Akiskal, 1981; Carroll, 1981; Stone et al., 1981; Pope et al., 1983).

Pope et al. (1985) reviewed case histories of 33 DSM III borderlines and found that only eight (24%) met the "narrow" DSM III definitions of psychosis.

In all of these subjects, the psychotic symptomatology was attributed to another Axis I condition such as substance abuse or major affective disorder. On the other hand, the majority of the borderline subjects displayed "broadly" defined psychotic symptoms, which the authors attributed to autohypnotic phenomena. In other words, while agreeing that most borderlines experience such broadly defined psychotic symptoms as dissociative episodes, impaired reality testing, and periods of regression during therapy, the authors considered such symptoms at best

---

2. Gunderson (1984) pointed out that Grinker (1979) later indicated that the presence of brief psychotic experiences is a useful diagnostic sign for discriminating borderline from schizophrenic patients.

"factitious" (under voluntary control) and at worst due to "hysterical psychosis." In any event, like Spitzer et al., they did not consider these quasi or "soft" signs of regressive thinking bonafide indications of psychotic symptoms. In essence, Pope and colleagues shared similar observations as Gunderson and his colleagues, but the two groups are using different definitions of what they consider "psychotic" or "psychotic-like" experience.

At this juncture, it is important to point out that those who argue against the presence of psychotic symptoms in borderline patients may be missing the essential point of Gunderson and Kernberg's positions on this matter. It is not the *presence* of "hard core" signs of thought disorder or psychotic symptoms that is at question but the *vulnerability* toward regressive, primary process thinking that is most relevant. Gunderson has always emphasized that borderline patients may experience *mild* psychotic phenomena (which he defines), not the more severe symptoms characteristic of psychosis. Similarly, Kernberg stated clearly that the presence of overt psychotic symptoms would likely rule out the diagnosis of borderline. Specifically Kernberg argued that BPO is characterized by "a shift toward primary process thinking," while also stating that the presence of hallucinations or delusions is indicative of psychosis, not BPO. Those arguing against the presence of "transient," "mild," or "micro" psychotic phenomena in borderline patients seem to view psychotic experience in a dichotomous fashion—one is either comletely psychotic, or one is not. Such a position harkens back to the earlier viewpoint that disordered thinking is a discrete, instead of continuous, variable. As we have seen, most contemporary researchers studying disordered thinking with the Rorschach have concluded that it exists along a continuum of severity.

RORSCHACH THOUGHT DISORDER AND THE BORDERLINE CONCEPT

Early Rorschach References to Borderline Phenomena

The Rorschach Test and the borderline concept are by no means strangers to one another. Beginning with Rorschach, the inkblots have been used to study individuals who appear "normal" on the surface but give schizophhrenic-like responses to the Rorschach cards. Although he never used the term "borderline," Rorschach (1921) presented a case of a 45-year-old woman, referred to as "Nervous Exhaustion," whose abnormal responses to the inkblots came as quite a surprise. The patient had held a responsible job for years and consulted a physician because of "nervous" complaints. Rorschach noted that her protocol was characterized by a surprising number of "responses involving self-reference, the repeated indication of belief in the reality of the pictures interpreted, and the emotional coloring in the answers" (p. 157). He also indicated that the variability in the quality of her responses, many of which reflected absurd and abstract verbalizations, would normally suggest a diagnosis of schizophrenia. However, he stated that this was not the case, and that the test may confuse individuals, such as this patient, with patients suffering from active schizophrenic illnesses. He ended his discussion of this case example with the somewhat cryptic statement that "A comparison of this protocol with the examples of schizophrenic records below will show that the results in many cases of manifest schizophrenia approach the normal result more closely than is the case in latent schizophrenia" (p. 158). Rorschach's conclusion led a generation of Rorschach clinicians to assume that borderline individuals (borderline or "latent" schizophrenics) could look quite normal in more familiar and predictable settings but that their Rorschach records would demonstrate greater deviance than would be observed even in the records of overtly schizophrenic individuals.

Rapaport et al. (1968) did not use the term borderline, either, to describe their group of 33 "preschizophrenic" patients, who in some ways presaged the contemporary bifurcation of the borderline concept into two separate groups (i.e., borderline and schizotypal personalities). Referring to their sample of "preschizophrenics", Rapaport et al. identified one subtype as an "overideational" group and the other as a "coarctated" one. The overideational preschizophrenics demonstrated an "enormous wealth of fantasy, obsessive ideation, and preoccupation with themselves and their bodies" (p. 436). Their responses were frequently characterized by a tendency to embellish their ideas with vivid affective elaboration, to combine their associations, and to use odd language. The "coarctated" preschizophrenics, on the other hand, tended to respond to the inkblots in a more constricted manner, giving odd responses that reflected a sense of alienation. The responses were delivered in a flat, dull manner, often revealing form level that was characteristically poor.

Rapaport and his colleagues also observed that these individuals performed relatively well on the Wechsler-Bellevue Scales in contrast to their idiosyncratic performances on less structured tasks like the Sorting Test and especially the Rorschach. With this observation, Rapaport et al. introduced what was to become a popular inter-test psychodiagnostic sign, namely that the borderline's performance would be expected to be quite intact on the Wechsler and impaired on the Rorschach.

Schafer (1948) dropped the term "preschizophrenic" and divided this quasi-borderline group into three subgroups, consisting of incipient schizophrenics, schizoid characters, and schizophrenic characters. Each group differed slightly but all were stable "pre-psychotic" personalities that did not present with either hallucianations or delusions.

According to Schafer, the Rorschachs of his incipient schizophrenics tended to contain several human movement responses (M) with poor form level (M−) and arbitrary Form-Color responses (essentially incongruous combinations based on inappropriate integration of color into a response). One to two confabulations were present "which are very likely to involve sexual or aggressive content" (p. 89), along with several fabulized combinations, and some near contaminations. Schizoid characters also produced records characterized by arbitrary Form-Color responses, fabulized combinations, and peculiar verbalizations. Finally, the schizophrenic characters gave long records with as many as 40 responses. Many overt signs of disordered thought were present in these records; however, they were also characterized by marked variability.

Weiner (1966) defined borderline and pseudoneurotic schizophrenia as stable conditions in which there is an underlying schizophrenic disturbance with overt manifestations of neurotic or characterological adaptation. He also included the criterion that these individuals would be expected to reveal their vulnerability in unstructured settings. As for their Rorschach performances, these individuals tended to produce a range of thought disorder verbalizations including fabulized responses, fabulized and incongruous combinations, autistic logic, peculiar and queer responses, and even contaminations.

This brief introduction to the early writings about the Rorschach and borderline phenomena is by no means an exhaustive review of the research during the 1940s–60s on Rorschach performances of borderline-level patients. Interested readers will find more thorough reviews by Singer (1977), Widiger (1982), and Gartner, Hurt, and Gartner (1989).

The best way to organize the rest of the discussion of the Rorschach assessment of borderline-level thought disturbances is to divide the subject into three areas. The first has to do with the diagnostic utility of inter-test comparisons between the Wechsler and Rorschach, the so-called "good WAIS/bad Rorschach" hypothesis. The second area concerns empirical findings regarding formal Rorschach variables associated with borderline-level thought disorder (in particular form level and specific thought disorder scores). Finally, the third has to do with the content or thematic aspects of responses that reflect thought pathology in borderline patients. Certain kinds of response content not only reflect the intrusion of primary process material but also, I believe, help distinguish certain formal scores (e.g., combinatory and confabulatory responses) in borderlines from those that occur in other types of disorders.

Wechsler-Rorschach Comparisons

Rapaport was the first to observe that "preschizophrenics" presented little to no thought disturbance on a structured test such as the Wechsler, while demonstrating strikingly deviant responses on the Rorschach. A number of studies in the 1950s and 1960s offered support for this hypothesis (Forer, 1950; Mercer and Wright, 1950; Zucker, 1952; Schafer, 1954; Shapiro, 1954; Fisher, 1955; Stone and Dellis, 1960; McCully, 1962; Weiner, 1966). Confident in these findings and the results of her own studies, Singer (1977) asserted that an adequate performance on the WAIS together with a Rorschach characterized by "highly elaborated, idiosyncratic associative content and peculiar reasoning . . . is almost axiomatic that a borderline diagnosis should follow" (p. 194). Echoing Rorschach's (1921) own statement about the relative bizarreness of borderline versus schizophrenic Rorschach, Singer also claimed that the Rorschach of the borderline patient is often more pathological looking than that of the schizophrenic person.

Despite the widespread support for the WAIS-Rorschach hypothesis, Stone (1980) questioned the specificity of this pattern among borderline patients, noting that intellectually gifted patients with a psychotic structure may also exhibit this same kind of qualitative WAIS-Rorschach split. In his thorough review of the literature on psychological testing and borderline diagnosis, Widiger (1982) questioned the empirical support for the "good WAIS/bad Rorschach" hypothesis. Widiger criticized aspects of the methodology in many of the studies that offered support for this hypothesis. In particular, he found no evidence to support Singer's (1977) claim that the Rorschachs of borderline patients are more bizarre and unusual than those generally found among schizophrenic individuals. Widiger also noted that the empirical evidence in support of the WAIS-Rorschach hypothesis is flimsy. He cited only one study by Carr et al. (1979) that he believed provided some suggestive support for the hypothesis. However, Widiger raised questions about the use of Kernberg's BPO, vs. the narrower DSM BPD definition, to identify the borderline subjects in this study. While acknowledging that Carr et al. found that the Rorschachs of the borderline and psychotic patients were indistinguishable and that the WAISs of the borderline group were less disturbed than those of the psychotic group, Widiger highlighted the fact that the study never demonstrated that the WAISs of the borderlines were normal and free from signs of pathology.

In their more contemporary review of the literature on the use of psychological testing to diagnose borderline personality disorder, Gartner et al. (1989) again addressed the empirical evidence supporting the good WAIS/bad Rorschach hypotheses. They concluded that research done since Widiger's critique has substantiated three findings related to the hypothesis. The first is that psychotic WAISs can be differentiated from those of borderline subjects on the basis of degree of thought disorder present on the WAIS, while both groups produce equal amounts of thought disorder on the Rorschach (Carr et al., 1979; Hymowitz et al., 1983). The second is that adolescents with thought disordered Rorschachs and WAISs manifested a significantly higher percentage of psychotic symptoms, whereas those with thought disordered Rorschachs and intact WAISs demonstrated symptoms more consistent with severe characterological problems (Armstrong, Silberg, and Parente, 1986). Third, Edell (1987) found that borderline, schizotypals, and schizophrenic subjects demonstrated equal amounts of thought disturbance on the Rorschach, but that the borderline and schizotypal groups performed much better on a structured test of cognitive slippage than did the schizophrenic group. Edell also noted that the borderline, schizotypal, mixed personality disordered, and normal groups all performed at an equivalent level on this test.

Despite differences in literature, some general conservative conclusions seem warranted. First, it is safe to say that borderline-level individuals will probably struggle more with the ambiguity of the Rorschach than with the familiarity and conventionality of the WAIS (WAIS-R, WISC III, or WAIS III). As such, their Rorschachs will reveal more overt signs of disordered thinking than will their WAISs. However, the assumption that their WAISs should be "intact" and free of signs of disturbed thinking is more questionable. As Berg (1984) observed, the WAISs of borderline patients may be "speckled with lapses in logical thinking" (p. 123), especially on tasks that require more extensive use of language and verbal reasoning such as on the Comprehension and Similarities subtests. Finally, the assertion that the Rorschachs of borderlines are more disturbed than those of schizophrenic or other psychotic patients not only seems overly simplistic, but it has not been supported by contemporary findings (Lerner et al., 1985; Wilson, 1985; Exner, 1986b). Most important, what this simplistic hypothesis overlooks are the intriguing qualitative differences in the nature of thought disorder profiles between psychotic and borderline patients. These formal or qualitative Rorschach features of borderline patients are discussed next.

Formal Rorschach Variables

If there has been an "axiomatic" conclusion about the qualitative nature of borderline-level Rorschach thought disorder scores, it is that borderlines manifest moderate levels of disturbed thinking. Beginning with Rapaport, most researchers have found fabulized combinations and confabulations to be the most typical of these moderate-level scores. Singer

(1977) emphasized the borderline's tendency to embellish ideas with affect or overly specific attribution and to combine images based on proximal contiguity. However, there has been some disagreement regarding whether combinatory or confabulatory thinking is most characteristic of thought disorder on the borderline Rorschach.

COMBINATORY THINKING (FABULIZED COMBINATIONS). Some studies have emphasized that fabulized combinations are the hallmark of the borderline Rorschach (Larson, 1974; Gunderson and Singer, 1975; Singer, 1977; Singer and Larson, 1981; Patrick and Wolfe, 1983). Although not identifying the specificity of the fabulized combination response per se, Rapaport et al. indicated that their "overideational preschizophrenic" group had a greater number of fabulized responses and fabulized combinations than confabulations. In Singer and Larson's study, the presence of two or more fabulized combinations characterized the records of almost two-thirds of the borderline group. However, Singer and Larson's sample was comprised primarily of subjects who would have probably met the DSM III criteria for schizotypal personality.

From a theoretically reasoned, developmental object relations vantage point, Smith (1980) distinguished Rorschach thought disorder features of patients who fell at the lowest versus the highest ends of the borderline continuum (Smith was using Kernberg's superordinate BPO, versus the DSM III BPD, definition, which holds that borderline disorders occur across a range of functioning). Although he presented no empirical data, Smith suggested that the presence of several fabulized combinations and FCarbs distinguished borderline from neurotic patients. According to Smith, the fabulized combinations would be expected to be milder in nature as opposed to more bizarre or malignant. Higher level borderline fabulized combinations are expected to be of good form and devoid of bizarre content. Smith went on to state that it would be even more unlikely for bizarre or malignant fabulized combinations to occur within the borderline range. According to Smith, fabulized combinations such as Card IX, "Two witches with machine guns for arms" (p. 66), strongly suggest a psychotic process.[3] In his efforts to distinguish the borderline from the psychotic structure, Smith suggested that one would not expect to find contaminations, malignant fabulized combinations, or primitive symbolic imagery in the Rorschachs of borderline individuals.

---

3. Smith, like Blatt and his followers, believed that malignant combinatory responses were closer to contaminations and therefore more indicative of a psychotic organization. As indicated earlier, however, this hypothesis has not received empirical support.

Patrick and Wolfe (1983) tested a sample of subjects diagnosed as borderline according to DSM III and confirmed Singer and Larson's finding that fabulized combinations occurred frequently in the Rorschachs of borderline individuals. Similar to Singer and Larson's findings, two-thirds of their subjects produced one fabulized combination, while 57.14% gave at least two fabulized combinations. On the other hand, 33.33% gave one confabulation and only 19.05% gave two or more.

Another interesting study looked at the Rorschachs of a group of depressed DSM III borderline subjects (Steiner et al., 1984). Unlike Singer and Larson's sample, which were predominantly schizotypal, Steiner et al.'s borderlines were rated as chiefly affective on the basis of both the SADS and a Rorschach subtyping technique (Carsky and Bloomgarden, 1981). Despite this difference in sample makeup, Steiner et al. found fabulized combinations percentages strikingly similar to those found in Singer and Larson's schizotypal/borderlines. In Singer and Larson's study, two or more fabulized combinations occurred in 64% of their sample and in Steiner et al.'s study, the frequency was 61% (and 57.14% in Patrick and Wolfe's study). Form level percentages (F+%) were also remarkably similar in both groups (71% for Singer and Larson's subjects and 67% for those of Steiner et al.). Such similar findings in structural features between differently defined groups of "borderline" subjects lend support to the concept of a borderline level of ego functioning that runs across character types or clinical syndromes (Wallace and Martin, 1988).

Exner (1986b) contrasted the Rorschachs of borderline, schizotypal, and schizophrenic subjects and found that from one-third to over one-half of his borderline group gave at least one combinatory response (34% gave a FABCOM, while 56% had at least one INCOM). Combinatory thinking occurred in schizotypal records at a frequency of 52% FABCOM and 71% INCOM. In contrast, only 23% of the borderlines had at least one DR score (the closest score in the Comprehensive System to confabulation). If the schizotypal group were combined with the borderline one (as in Singer and Larson's study), the frequency of combinatory responses increased to 63% for INCOMs and 43% for FABCOMs. The combined frequency for DRs in the two groups would have been 18%. Thus, although Exner's data would suggest some degree of combinatory thinking (INCOM) in over half of his borderline subjects, he would by no means agree that FABCOM (or INCOM for that matter) is the hallmark of borderline record. This is even more the case if one compares these scores among the borderline (and schizotypal) subjects to those of his schizophrenic group. Whereas Singer and Larson's combined group of borderline and schizotypal subjects produced more fabulized combinations than their schizophrenic group, Exner found the opposite. In his sample of 80 schizophrenic subjects, tested at admission and then again before discharge, between 74 and 78% gave at least one INCOM and 73 to 78% at least one FABCOM.[4]

CONFABULATORY THINKING. As mentioned above, Rapaport was quite specific in attributing fabulized and fabulized combination responses to his overideational preschizophrenic subjects. He offered less regarding the specific diagnostic implications of confabulation responses except to say:

> When fabulized combinations and confabulations begin to enter the picture, the ideation is taking a pathologically autistic turn, and the suspicion of at least a preschizophrenic condition is raised. When the confabulations begin to predominate, with or without a sizable incidence of the other responses, we are most likely dealing with a full schizophrenia, and more likely with a chronic than an acute one [p. 436].

Thus, although Rapaport allowed for the presence of some confabulatory thinking in his quasi-borderline group (the overideational preschizophrenics), his emphasis seemed to be on fabulized and fabulized combinations.

Kim Smith (1980) also discussed the role of confabulation in borderline records. Dividing borderlines into upper and lower ranges, Smith suggested that confabulations are expected among lower level borderlines and occasionally among borderlines who function at the upper end of the continuum. Smith indicated that lower level borderline confabulations have a story telling quality that flouts reality. He gave the following Card X example of a confabulation response given by a patient functioning at the lower end of the borderline range.

> Two blue crabs . . . almost looks like they have human faces . . . and you know how a scorpion has a long claw, it's like a mixture of parts of a monster . . . the green thing looks like it's alive . . . some little animal that they're using to fight with . . . the little green guys have a

---

4. Not only do these findings not support the specificity of Singer and Larson's findings regarding a greater number of fabulized combinations among borderline/schizotypal patients, but they also show how little reduction occurred in these thought disorder scores between admission and discharge. This is even more surprising given that one would guess that these schizophrenic patients had been treated with medication during their hospitalizations, which would have been expected to reduce the severity of their thought disorder as it appears on the Rorschach.

horn coming out of their lip, that's how they fight, they're all angry . . . and the brown part looks like two animated monsters, they're also angry and fighting, they are competing with the crabs over who's gonna get the red part (p. 66).

Smith said that upper level borderlines tend to give confabulations that have a more detached, pictorial quality that is based more in reality. His example of a higher level borderline confabulation is as follows: "It looks like looking through a glass-bottom boat with mermaids in the red, blue crabs . . . then shells, different fish . . . the crab looks like it caught something . . . and two people . . . in suits of armor . . . what are they doing? maybe dancing . . . I don't know what they're doing down there" (p. 66).

Wilson (1985) and Lerner et al. (1985) found that their borderline samples were distinguished by varying degrees of confabulatory thinking. To be more specific, Wilson (1985) demonstrated that his borderline subjects (DSM III BPD and Schizotypals) had higher confabulation tendency scores (as well as higher Fabulized Combination Benign scores) than his neurotic and psychotic groups. At the same time, Lerner et al. (1985) found that inpatient borderlines (DSM III BPD and Schizotypal personality disorders) gave more confabulations than neurotics, outpatient borderlines (not operationally defined), or schizophrenic subjects. If we assume that many inpatient borderlines may occupy the lower end of the borderline continuum, then Lerner's findings are consistent with Smith's observations that confabulations are seen frequently in lower level borderlines.

Based on their research, Lerner et al. and Sugarman (1986) theorized that confabulation scores reflect a borderline-level structural impairment in the formation of the "inner-outer" boundary. Furthermore, Lerner and Sugarman reasoned that borderline individuals do not fully recognize the inkblots as having an existence separate from themselves. Sugarman suggested that borderlines tend to shape external reality according to their inner needs and relational paradigms. Thus, both Lerner and Sugarman viewed borderline-level ego disturbances as indicative of a developmental arrest at the level of transitional objects, and that patients giving confabulations are treating the inkblots as transitional phenomena, investing them with attributes coming from themselves.

As seen in chapter 9, Exner's (1986b) DSM III borderlines did not have a greater frequency of DRs than subjects in the schizophrenic sample. As mentioned above, even if the schizotypal and borderline samples were collapsed into one larger group, the frequency of DRs among this expanded "borderline group" was still only 18%. As I concluded in chapter 9, the discrepancy between Exner's findings and those of Wilson and the Lerner group support my contention that DR and traditional confabulation scores are not equivalent.

The "embellished DR" (Kleiger and Peebles-Kleiger, 1993) is a term given for DR responses that reflect a confabulation-like infusion of affect, specific details, or fantasy elements into the response (narrower than the general DR category in the Comprehensive System). Distinguishing a "tendency" toward embellishment from extreme embellishment and poor form level from unusual and good form level could help differentiate borderline DRs from those given by other diagnostic groups. For example, some of the literature reviewed thus far demonstrates that if borderline persons give confabulations, they will most likely be less severe in nature, or confabulation-tendencies. In keeping with Smith's observations, these confabulations would be more attuned toward reality (unless, as Smith suggested, the patient is organized at the lower end of the borderline range).

In writing about the phenomenology of borderline experience, Cauwels (1992) quoted a borderline patient who spoke about her tendency to *perceive* accurately but *misinterpret* what she perceives.

People say I distort a lot, and one of my major problems is hypersensitivity. But I know that a lot of what I pick up on is true. My interpretation of it and reaction to it may be off, but my initial perception is accurate. . . . Now what I might do is think that someone's anger, for instance, is caused by me. My perception of the anger is true, but my interpretation of it is a distortion [Cauwels, 1992, p. 78].

This combination of reasonably accurate perception together with misinterpretation, or overly subjective or inferential judgment, seems to capture the borderline tendency to combine accurate (or unusual) form with moderate degrees of confabulatory thinking.

FORM LEVEL. Briefly, several of the studies that looked into the nature of the borderline Rorschach included information about the mean form level of their samples compared to those of schizophrenic and other samples. Most of the sources cited in this chapter suggest that borderline patients will typically achieve a moderate degree of disturbance in reality testing as measured by form level percentages somewhere between 60 and 70%. Singer and Larson's (1981) borderline/schizotypal group had a mean form level percentage of 67%; Exner's (1986b) separate borderline and schizotypal groups both had form level percentages of 69%; and Steiner et al.'s (1984) borderlines had a mean of 71%. Based on their review of the literature, Gartner et al. (1989) concluded that BPD patients typically achieve F+ and X+%'s between 65 and 70%, roughly 10 to 15% higher than schizophrenics and 10 to 15% lower than normals.

Thematic Aspects of Borderline Responses

Affect-laden fantasies reflecting themes of malevolence, aggression, loss, reunion, or merger may characterize some of the responses of borderline patients. These themes cluster into two primary content categories relevant to the dynamics of borderline functioning—malevolence/aggression and symbiosis/separation. Whether these themes are reflected in the content of an ordinary or fabulized response, a fabulized combination, or a confabulation, borderline patients have an uncanny way of focusing their attention on primitive affect-laden psychological issues. Most often responses containing themes of destructive aggression and malevolence or primitive dependency will merit one of Holt's primary process content scores. Research concerning both of these content categories is presented below.

MALEVOLENT, DESTRUCTIVE, AND AGGRESSIVE THEMATIC CONTENT. Several investigators have found greater malevolence in the test imagery of borderline subjects compared to other groups of patients (Lerner and St. Peter, 1984; Stuart et al., 1990; Westen et al., 1990; Nigg et al., 1992). Lerner and St. Peter found that borderlines produced more malevolent human representations than did schizophrenic subjects. Stuart et al. reported similar findings in their group of borderline subjects who produced more malevolent figures than did subjects with major depression and normal controls. According to their findings, borderlines also perceive human action as more highly motivated than do either depressives or normal subjects.

Singer (1977) reported an unpublished study by De Sluttitel and Sorribas (1972) that found that borderlines gave fabulized combination responses with "unpleasant content," unlike artists who gave creative combinatory responses with more positive content. Stuart and her colleagues (1990) gave the following examples of highly motivated malevolent activity that occur within the context of either a combinatory or confabulatory response. "These are two people that are half male and half female, and they're mixing a potion in a large bowl. Looks like it might be some kind of evil ritual. Their hearts are exposed" (p. 313); and "These two pieces here [look like] you know, like in Casper the Ghost? These look like the bad guys that are trying to get [Casper] to do mean things" (pp. 313–314). Another typical fabulized response (and incongruous combination) of borderline-level severity can be seen in a common response to Card X: "Angry insects, yelling at each other."

Researchers have found similar phenomena in other tests with borderline subjects. For example, Westen et al. used the TAT to demonstrate that borderlines construct more malevolently-toned relational paradigms than do major depressives. Nigg et al. used the Early Memories test to show that borderline patients represent early caregiving figures more malevolently, sadistically, and as having been less helpful.

Nigg and his colleagues speculated that the origins of these malevolent relational schemata lie in the individual's difficulty in self-soothing. Whether as a result of abusive, neglectful, or misattuned parenting or because of constitutional or neurological factors, the borderline youngster is unable to learn to regulate internal tension states and ends up attributing the source of internal discomfort to others in his environment. Nigg et al. reasoned that such a child is likely to "respond with increased aggression, which leads to an escalating cycle of malevolent attributions, aggressive reactions, and angry or vengeful counterreactions" (p. 66).

SYMBIOSIS AND SEPARATION THEMATIC CONTENT. Kwawer (1980) developed a Rorschach scale to assess borderline interpersonal relations and found that borderline subjects gave at least one response that symbolized symbiotic relatedness and difficulties in separating and differentiating from a primary object. Included among his scoring categories were responses reflecting themes of engulfment; symbiotic merging; violent symbiosis, separation, and reunion; malignant internal processes, including primitive incorporation; birth and rebirth; metamorphosis and transformation; narcissistic mirroring; separation-division; boundary disturbance; and womb imagery.

Using her developmental object relations scale, Coonerty (1986) found that borderline subjects produced significantly more responses indicative of separation-individuation concerns than did a sample of schizophrenic subjects, whose concerns reflected preseparation issues. Consistent with Mahler's theory, Coonerty found that her borderline subjects were rated higher on both the practicing (narcissism) and rapprochement scales of her instrument than were the schizophrenic subjects.

Coonerty constructed three scales thought to reflect the subphases of separation-individuation, including Early Differentiation, Practicing, and Rapproachment. The Early Differentiation subphase was characterized by hatching, engulfment, and merging responses, such as "These are two girls, maybe not, they seem to be together with the same head" (p. 510). The Practicing subphase was characterized by responses that reflected narcissistic mirroring, pairing, and omnipotence or insignificance. Finally, the Rapprochement scale reflected themes of figures who were enmeshed, stuck, and unable to separate. Figures could be depicted as having unstable form or affect and were seen as struggling to either come together or separate, with resulting damage to one or both. The following are examples of both combinatory and confabulatory responses from her Rapprochement scale that may be characteristic of borderline-level pathology. Note the degree of malevolence contained in the second response as well. "I don't know, this seems like some people doing something but they seem stuck together somehow, all struggling in every direction but whatever is doing it, they can't get free" (p. 510). "They're touching hands but it's as if one of them is trying to save the other from electrical shock and they both get fried" (p. 510).

DIFFERENTIAL DIAGNOSIS

If we return to the beginning of this chapter, we are reminded that the borderline concept has been regarded as a fickle one, viewed and defined differently by different experts. As with efforts to categorize other complex phenomena, the borderline concept has lent itself to "lumping" and "splitting" approaches. We have seen how some have strived to construct broad categories that lump together seemingly heterogeneous disorders into a borderline realm of functioning, while others have sought to split up this heterogeneity and limit the construct only to a narrow range of individuals. Regardless of whether one prefers to be a borderline "lumper" or "splitter," these conceptual difficulties become especially apparent when one is using the Rorschach to assess so-called borderline phenomena.

One of the persistent difficulties has to do with the relationship between borderline disorders and related diagnostic syndromes. Regardless of whether one employs the narrow or broad definition of "borderline," the issue of co-morbidity makes differential diagnosis especially challenging. In his novel *When Nietzsche Wept*, Irvin Yalom (1992) told a tale about an imaginary conversation between Joseph Breuer and Sigmund Freud in which Breuer shared with the young Freud his "trade secret" about differential diagnosis:

> "Sig," said Breuer, rising and speaking in a confidential tone, "I'm going to give you a trade secret. One day it'll be your bread and butter as a consultant. I learned it from Oppolzer, who once said to me: 'Dogs can have fleas and lice, too.'"
>
> "Meaning that the patient can—"
>
> "Yes," Breuer said, putting his arm around Freud's shoulders. The two men began to walk down the long hallway. "The patient can have *two* diseases. In fact, those patients who reach a consultant generally do" [p. 45].

Like dogs, sometimes people have *two* illnesses; and borderline patients, in particular, are notorious for presenting with a complex interplay of problems. Borderline patients frequently have concurrent affective disorders and trauma histories. Likewise, they often meet diagnostic criteria for schizotypal and narcissistic personality disorders as well.

On the other hand, dogs may have only fleas and not lice, or vice-versa, making the issue of differential diagnosis all the more relevant. Co-morbidity aside, differential diagnosis is harder when each illness produces similar signs or symptoms. For example, are the lesions from a flea infestation distinguishable from those of a lice infestation? In terms of Rorschach indices of disordered thinking, how can we be sure if the patient's combinatory, confabulatory, affectively charged, or symbiotic responses reflect a primary borderline personality disturbance and not an affective disorder, the residual of chronic trauma, or the psychic imprint of a schizotypal or narcissistic personality disorder?

The final section of this chapter is devoted to a review of the question of differential diagnostic signs. Most studies reviewed thus far have contrasted borderlines to schizophrenic, depressed, and normal subjects and found a characteristic borderline thought disorder profile. Are there ways to distinguish borderline-level thought pathology from that of a bipolar type I or II patient, or a patient with a trauma history, a narcissistic, or a schizotypal personality disorder? Can we combine the collective findings reviewed in this chapter and compile a differential borderline thought disorder profile? In proposing such a profile, one must, however, be mindful of the existence of co-morbidity with the other diagnoses mentioned here, which may make efforts to distinguish borderline personality from these other entities at times controversial and fraught with conceptual problems.

Borderline and Affective Disorders

Gunderson and Phillips (1991) acknowledged that depression and borderline personality may coexist, but they concluded that the two disorders are related in only weak and nonspecific ways.[5] Given the prevalence of affectively charged Rorschach content associated with both syndromes and the literature concerning the presence of cognitive disorders in unipolar depression (see chapter 14), how can we distinguish disturbances in thought organization of these two diagnostic entities?

Several studies reviewed here have used depressed subjects as control groups and found significantly fewer confabulatory, combinatory, and either malevolently-tinged or symbiotic content or both in unipolar

---

5. The exception, according to these authors, seems to be patients suffering from nonmelancholic unipolar depression, who have an especially high prevalence of borderline personality disorder, thus, making differential diagnosis largely irrelevant.

depressives compared to borderlines. Form level percentages in both groups may be similar, with the depressives having a slightly lower F+ and X+% than the borderline groups.

Bipolar thought disorder may also be confused with that of the borderline patient. Both groups give thought disordered responses characterized by affectively charged combinatory and confabulatory thinking. Assuming the absence of both conditions in the same patient, how do we distinguish Rorschach thought disturbances in borderlines from thought disturbances in patients with bipolar (manic or depressive) depressions? Sticking just with indices of disordered thinking (and artificially ignoring the rest of the testing protocols), the clues to differential diagnosis perhaps lie in the nature of the fabulized and combinatory content. While all of these patients will produce affective content, Khadivi et al. (1997) demonstrated that manic patients' content revealed more playfulness (e.g., animals playing pattycake), energy (e.g., a rocket ship blasting off), excitement (e.g., two happy clowns at a circus), and celebration (e.g., animals dancing at a party). The content may also reveal depressive themes, as well as images of instability, and fairy tales scenarios. Additionally, manic patients may produce larger numbers of responses, a lower F+ and X+%, use movement and color liberally, and intersperse a personal commentary along the way. Flippant side comments, some of which may amuse the examiner, may also be expected. In contrast, we have seen how the affectively charged content in fabulized, confabulatory, and combinatory responses in the borderline patient is often characterized by malevolence and destructive aggression or by themes of conflicted symbiosis and separation.

Finally, are the psychological processes that lie behind the abundance of combinatory thinking in manic and borderline patients different? Although this is speculative, one might conceive of combinative responses in borderline individuals as a loss of distance, in which the reality of the blot is taken too literally. This is similar to Bruce Smith's (1990) notion of a collapse of potential space that occurs in the borderline Rorschach record and in the treatment setting with these individuals. By contrast, the combinative activity of the manic patient may reflect ideational expansiveness, typically referred to as a "flight of ideas," in which the subject's energy-driven integrative efforts outstrip the available cognitive resources. One might add that this rapid linkage of disparate ideas comes close to the kind of divergent thinking that is observed in creative individuals.

Borderline and Schizotypal Personality Disorder

As we have seen, some consider schizotypal personality disorder to be subsumed under the rubric of the broader borderline personality organization concept (the "lumpers"), while others view it as a distinct type of personality disorder, different from borderline personality (the "splitters"). A number of studies lumped borderline and schizotypal subjects together into a "borderline" group and found that this group produced either high numbers of fabulized combination or confabulation responses (Singer and Larson, 1981; Steiner et al., 1984; Lerner et al., 1985; Wilson, 1985). Most interesting were the observations of Wallace and Martin (1988) that pointed out that Singer and Larson's predominantly schizotypal sample yielded equivalent structural data as did Steiner et al.'s sample of predominantly BPD subjects. Both of these studies showed that two or more fabulized combinations were produced by 61 to 64% of the subjects in each sample.

Exner's (1986b) data showed some similarities and differences between DSM III BPD and schizotypal personality disordered subjects, relative to indices of reality testing and thought disorder. To begin with, the schizotypal group had a significantly higher weighted SUM 6, suggesting an overall greater number of thought-disordered responses than the borderline group. Both groups had mean X+%'s of 69, but the schizotypals tended to give a greater number of distorted responses (higher X-%) than the borderline subjects.

Regarding qualitative differences in thought disorder scores, the borderline group achieved a greater frequency of DRs (23% vs. 13%), while the schizotypals had a greater frequency of FABCOMs (52% vs. 34%) and INCOMs (71% vs. 56%). However, these differences did not reach the .05 level of significance. The only statistically significant difference was in the proportional frequency of DV responses, with 76% of the schizotypal group giving at least one DV response as compared to 40% of the borderline group. Furthermore, the mean number of DVs among the schizotypals was 2.37 (SD = 2.56) compared to a mean of 1.01 (SD = 1.87) in the borderline group. There were no significant differences in content scores between the two groups; however, 52% of the borderlines gave aggressive movement scores (AG) compared to only 39% of the schizotypals. Morbid content occurred with equivalent frequency in both groups, in roughly 58 to 60% of the subjects from each group.

In general, Exner's data revealed that the thought organization of the schizotypal subjects was characterized by more "strangeness and slippage" (p. 466) than that of the borderline group, but less than that of the schizophrenic subjects. The greater frequency of DV responses in the schizotypals seems to capture this difference. Exner's study highlighted other important structural differences between the two disorders that are important to note. The borderline protocols were characterized by greater affective arousal and instability than the records of both the schizophrenic and schizotypal subjects. The schizotypal subjects, like the schizophrenics, tended to be more ideational and introversive. Although the schizotypals demonstrated less emotional reactivity and greater affect and impulse control than the borderlines, they were more vulnerable to distorting reality and taking flight in fantasy

Carsky and Bloomgarden (1981) rated Rorschach content in order to distinguish between subtypes of BPO patients. They distinguished between unstable affective (BPD) and schizotypal subgroups on the basis of whether the content reflected primarily affect-laden themes (depicting oral deprivation or aggression and the presence of "good/strong" vs. "bad/weak" figures) or themes reflecting autistic thinking or paranoid attention to eyes, bizarre detail, or fluid boundaries and changeable identities. The first type of patient gave the following response to Card I: "See also two Santa Clauses, even though they're black, tugging at one of the witches from Shakespeare; in the center—two witches with hoods over their heads. (Tugging?) . . . The impression of trying to pull apart the witches" (p. 110). Contrast the aggressive, confabulated, combinatory quality of this response to the more distant and peculiarly worded one given to Card II by a more schizotypal subject. "Again, it's highly symmetrical. Hands raised in prayer. (Why looked like hands?) I really can't say . . . maybe the effect of the contrasting red. (How so?) I guess the way that formation was surrounded by the red shape that looked like hands, the elongated shape with the thin line made it look like hands. The red around it made it look more together" (p. 112).

Borderline and Narcissistic Disorders

As with the schizotypal-borderline comparisons, the boundaries between the borderline and narcissistic diagnostic categories are sometimes unclear. However, fewer studies comparing Rorschach variables in narcissistic and borderline patients have appeared in the literature. Farris (1988) compared DSM III BPDs and narcissistic personality disorders (NPDs) on a number of Rorschach scales. One of these was Friedman's Developmental Level scoring system (1952). Recall that lower scores on Friedman's scale reflect the presence of poorly structured and amorphous responses, including those manifesting evidence of fabulized combinations and contaminations. Farris showed that BPDs had lower scores on Friedman's scale than NPDs, suggesting the greater likelihood of finding combinatory and poorly structured responses in the records of BPD patients. Farris pointed out that this finding is also consistent with Smith's (1980) observation that narcissistic personalities produce fewer merged or fused responses.

Lerner (1988) also discussed the Rorschach structure of the narcissistic personality. Although he did not produce empirical data to support his claims, Lerner suggested that narcissistic patients may exhibit subtle boundary disruptions on the Rorschach, manifested by the appearance of benign, and some severe, fabulized combinations (boundary laxness) and confabulations (disruptions in the inner/outer boundary). He also suggested that the narcissistic patients are often egocentric and self-referential on the Rorschach, giving many elaborated personalizations. As far as combinatory and confabulatory responses, Lerner suggested that the content of these responses may reflect condensed representations of the real self, grandiose self, and idealized other. One of his narcissistic patients gave the following combinatory response to Card IX that Lerner thought condensed an image of narcissistic grandiosity with oral aggressive content. "A weird-looking guy on the back of an eagle sniffing coke. The bird is part lion and part bird" (p. 271). Another of Lerner's narcissistic patients gave a circumstantial DR response to Card VI that reflects both grandiosity in content and an exhibitionistic process of verbalization. "Looks like a sword in a rock or crown, it looks like the crown of Hungry. Franz Josef was the Emperor of Austria and also the King of Hungry. The double sword of the Hungarian crown" (p. 271).

Paul Lerner (1991) suggested that narcissistic patients tend to give a higher number of mirror, reflection, and pair responses, suggesting a tendency to relate to others on a narcissistic basis. Furthermore, Lerner believed that the concept of "false self," a prominent feature of pathological narcissism, may be captured by the color arbitrary score (FCarb). In chapter 8, I reviewed Lerner's rationale for linking the false self with the FCarb score, which is essentially a variant of an incongruous combination response.

Finally, narcissistic individuals may produce thought disordered responses that reflect their tendencies to indulge themselves in a capricious, egocentric view of the task and reality in general. For example, it is not unusual for these patients to add or comment on things that are not in the blot or to project color into achromatic cards. Furthermore, as mentioned in chapter 8, they may embellish human movement (M) responses with affects related to their own situations. According to Mayman (1977), "The perceived action [in these M's] is largely fabulized rather than inherent in the percept itself. . . . The response is reported with intense absorption . . . he infuses himself into the figure he is describing, vicariously sharing in the other's experiences" (p. 246). A good example of this kind of self-absorbed confabulation is the highly embellished response of "two matrons having a talk over coffee" presented in chapters 8 and 9.

Trauma and Borderline Disorders

There may currently be no other area where the issues of co-morbidity and causality are more relevant than in the interface between trauma and borderline personality. A number of studies that have looked at the relationship between history of trauma (in particular, sexual, physical, and emotional abuse and neglect) and borderline personality disorder have found an extremely high incidence of physical or sexual abuse in the backgrounds of borderline patients (Stone et al., 1981; Herman et al., 1986; Goodwin, Cheeves, and Connell, 1990; Westen et al., 1990). Frequencies of abuse in the backgrounds of borderlines have reportedly ranged from 30 to 80% (Cauwels, 1992), with frequencies of incest ranging from 19 to 41% (Stone, 1990). The strikingly high incidence of childhood trauma in borderline patients has led some researchers to view borderline personality as a trauma-related disorder or a "complex post-traumatic stress disorder" (Arnold and Saunders, 1989; Herman, 1992).

Several studies have looked at the constellations of Rorschach features in borderline subjects with trauma histories (Cerney, 1990; Saunders, 1991). Saunders demonstrated that borderline patients with histories of sexual abuse tend to produce more flamboyant and graphically violent responses than borderlines with other kinds of trauma histories. Cerney confirmed this finding by mentioning that one of her subjects, who was later found to have had a history of sexual abuse, gave "some of the most vicious and brutal responses in the entire sample: 'a giant monster nailed onto a post in the middle with two animals crawling into his arms' area, eating away at him'; 'two angels trying to pull a person apart and she is screaming and yelling so much that a lot of dust is rising. She's bleeding all over'" (p. 785).

In summary, it may not be possible to disentangle Rorschach manifestations of a borderline personality disorder per se from the psychological imprint of complex trauma. In most cases, the two conditions occur together and, according to some, they may be one in the same. As we see in the next chapter, psychological trauma, whether co-morbid or synonymous with borderline personality disorder or not, may be expressed on the Rorschach in a florid pattern of disturbed thinking, lapses in reality testing, and graphically violent imagery.

Table 15-1 presents a comparison of Rorschach variables related to thought organization in borderline and other diagnoses. The data in this table are based on findings from a number of the studies reviewed in this chapter and can be used as a rough guide in making differential diagnosis. In using this table, several caveats are worth mentioning and repeating. First, I have artificially limited the focus to Rorschach indices of disordered thinking, while ignoring other critical aspects of the Rorschach and other tests that one would typically use in clinical assessments. Diagnostic accuracy is obviously increased significantly when one makes inferences based on convergence from multiple data points. Finally, it bears repeating that the boundaries between many of the diagnostic concepts discussed here remain at best controversial and at worst clear as mud.

Table 15-1 Differentiating Rorschach Indices of Disordered Thinking in Borderline and Related Syndromes

Rorschach Variable	Clinical Syndrome				
	Borderline	Bipolar (Manic)	Unipolar	Schizotypal	Narcissistic
Form Level	69a	54b	61b	69a	?
Total TDI Score	12–13c	25d	?	16–17c	?
Qualitative Features	Combinatory (FABCOM, INCOM) Confab-tend DR	Combinatory (FABCOM, INCOM) Playful Confab Flippant	Few, if any	DV Combinatory (INCOM, FABCOM)	FCarb
Combinatory Rationale	Loss of distance Loss of "as if" Collapse of space	Expansive Flight of Ideas			
Thematic Content	Aggressive Malevolence Symbiosis-Separation	Playful Excitement Festive Sad	Damaged Morbid	Distant Bizarre Autistic	Grandiose Insignificant

a. From Exner (1986).
b. From Singer and Brabender (1993).
c. From Edell (1987).
d. From Holzman, Shenton, and Solovay (1986).

CHAPTER
16

DISORDERED THINKING
ASSOCIATED WITH OTHER
CONDITIONS

No clinical syndrome can claim exclusive rights over the domain of disordered thinking. In addition to finding pathological thought organization in patients with schizophrenia, affective psychoses, and borderline conditions, disturbances in the process and content of thinking can be found in a range of other conditions as well. How useful is the Rorschach in identifying and conceptualizing thought disturbances in other psychiatric conditions? The clinical syndromes reviewed in this chapter include (1) Posttraumatic Stress and Dissociative Disorders, (2) Obsessive-Compulsive Disorder, (3) Delusional Disorder, and (4) Organic Brain Impairment.

TRAUMATIC AND DISSOCIATIVE DISORDERS

Posttraumatic Stress Disorders

As suggested in the last chapter, psychological trauma has a profound effect on the structure and content of the survivor's internal world, leading in some cases to chronic deformations in character development, ego functioning, self-experience, and object relational paradigms. An array of studies on heterogeneous survivors of childhood and adult trauma has amassed a constellation of Rorschach variables that operationally define the signs and symptoms of PTSD (Carr, 1984; van der Kolk and Ducey, 1984, 1989; Armstrong and Lowenstein, 1990; Cerney, 1990; Hartman et al., 1990; Armstrong, 1991; Kaser-Boyd, 1993; Levin, 1993; Briere, 1997). Included in this Rorschach trauma profile are elevations in inanimate movement (m) and diffuse shading (Y), both indicating anxiety and helplessness related to unintegrated experiences; unmodulated affectivity (CF + C > FC); the presence of violent and morbid imagery, often having to do with anatomical or sexual content; and elevated indices of disordered thinking and impaired reality testing, reflected by the presence of either combinatory or confabulatory thinking and minus form level responses (X–). Comprehensive formulations of the relationship between each of these features and the phenomenology of trauma can be found in the works of van der Kolk and Ducey (1989), Levin (1993), and Briere (1997). Our focus here is principally on those indices having to do with thought organization.

CONFABULATION IN TRAUMA RECORDS. Armstrong (1994b) introduced the term "traumatic thought disorder" (TTD) to describe the unique sort of confabulatory responses produced by traumatized patients. She defined TTD as a dynamic, state-dependent phenomenon, triggered by the traumatic stimulus. Most characteristic of this process is its affectively driven loss of distance or flooding, as the subject becomes immersed in the blot characteristics and the response that follows. According to Armstrong, the response itself can be disorganized and perseverative and can have the quality of an encapsulated traumatic reaction. There is typically a striking loss of reality testing as the intensity of the imagery that is triggered by the inkblot overshadows the subject's critical capacity to perceive reality accurately. Graphic and primitive imagery, tinged with aggression, sadism, and sexual-anatomical violence, reminiscent of Holt's Level 1 Aggression scales, may color the patient's confabulatory immersion in the blot.

The following examples from the records of a sexual abuse survivor and a combat veteran, respectively, express such a degree of unmodulated aggression:

Card II: "The first thing I see is my art which tends to be black and covered in blood!" (Inquiry) "That's what I did before; I cut myself and had a black marker which I wrote with. I cut myself and covered the black with blood."

Card IV: "Looks like a long dark road where there's been an explosion. Something's gotten killed, blown to bits. Blood and bodies all over, people yelling for help, crying, and screaming to get 'em."

Trauma researchers reject the traditional explanation that the primitive imagery and extreme loss of distance represented in these responses reflects the "breakthrough of primary process" material or signals the presence of a borderline-level thought disorder or worse, an incipient psychotic regression. Instead, researchers like Armstrong, Levin, Briere, and van der Kolk view such responses as unmetabolized reexperiencing of the traumatic event. According to Carlson and Armstrong (1995), the Rorschach ceases to be a projective test and instead becomes a trigger for reliving the trauma. Van der Kolk has argued that trauma survivors lose the capacity to represent traumatic experiences symbolically and instead express graphic images of trauma concretely on the Rorschach.[1] Thus, according to Armstrong (1994b), TTD, with its trauma-laden confabulatory quality, which contains self-reference and graphically primitive imagery, is almost seen as a Rorschach equivalent of a flashback experience.

COMBINATORY THINKING IN THE TRAUMA RECORD. In her study of a heterogeneous group of adult trauma survivors, Levin (1993) found an increased number of FABCOM2 responses among her samples. In her effort to explain this finding, Levin and Reis (1996) suggested that combinatory responses may be a metaphor for the incongruity of the survivor's traumatic experiences. For example, the response "a foot sticking out of the ground" is combinatory but, according to the traumatologist's argument, may represent an implausibility of the survivor's experience captured by an actual witnessing of a scene of violence and death. On a more symbolic level, the combinatory response such as "looks like a weasel climbing on a butterfly" is probably less reflective of a literal trauma experience and more indicative of a sadomasochistic relational paradigm, perhaps itself the product of some sort of interpersonal trauma bonding (see chapter 8).

Levin and Reis also compared the frequency of FABCOMs among groups of "pure trauma" adults, combat veterans, and patients suffering from dissociative disorders. The descriptive statistics showed little

---

1. Although this is a compelling viewpoint, one should not overlook the roles of fantasy and conflict in these responses. Kowitt (1985) pointed out how Rorschach responses can be seen as creations that "borrow" images from the traumatic event and incorporate these with symbolic expressions of underlying internal conflicts. I believe that to ignore completely the role of fantasy and conflict in trauma responses runs the risk of too literal a translation of response content, just as interpreting manifest dream content or recovered memories of abuse, without taking into account unconscious motivation and fantasy, misses the complexity and layering of intrapsychic experience.

difference in mean number of FABCOMs, with the dissociative group giving an average of .40 compared with the two trauma groups, which averaged between .52 and .56. Although substantially greater than the adult nonpatient mean of .17, the FABCOM means of these trauma-related groups are smaller than those of Exner's (1986b) BPD (.62) and schizotypal (.79) groups and roughly equivalent to the mean of his depressed inpatients (.52).

Levin also noted the increased number of perseveration responses (PSV) among her adult trauma survivors. Together with a positive hypervigilance index (HVI) (Exner, 1993) and graphic depiction of traumatic content, Levin understood elevations in perseveration scores as a composite of variables that depict the survivor's psychological guardedness and preoccupation with repetitive traumatic themes.

Dissociative Disorders

Closely related to trauma, dissociative disorders have also received special attention in the Rorschach literature (Wagner and Heise, 1974; Lovitt and Lefkof, 1985; Armstrong and Loewenstein, 1990; Armstrong, 1991, 1993, 1994a; Scroppo et al., 1997). Most thoroughly represented by the work of Armstrong, dissociative patients (DD/MPD) have been shown to have distinctive Rorschach profiles similar to but also different from those of other trauma groups. According to Armstrong (1991), DD/MPD subjects gave at least one developmentally advanced human movement response (M+). Although their overall good form level percentage (X+%) was not significantly different from that found in schizophrenic samples, the DD/MPD group produced more unusual (Xu) responses than severely distorted ones (X–). Furthermore, they gave extremely high numbers of responses with aggressive, anatomical, blood, morbid, or sexual content. Finally DD/MPD subjects often gave playful and artistic responses and FABCOMs that reflected the experience of dividedness or multiplicity. Scroppo et al. (1997) confirmed these findings in their sample of dissociative identity disordered (DID) subjects who gave significantly more FABCOMs, lower X+%'s, and more responses containing morbid, bloody, or anatomical contents than a control group.

In terms of the thematic nature of the combinatory activity, Armstrong (1991) gave the following example of a combinatory response that depicts the theme of multiplicity: "Card VII. These are two girls and they're the same person, but there are two of them and they're always checking each other. And this is another part of the female anatomy that they share. This is where the vagina is, why the two of them know they're the same person. And it's why you know they're girls" (p. 543).

The bizarre combinatory quality of this response is quite apparent but so is the confabulatory-tendency ("they're always checking each other") and the strained logic ("This is where the vagina is . . . it's why you know they're girls). This significantly thought-disordered response is also consistent with Armstrong's finding of an elevated SCZI and WSUM 6 in these patients.

Compared to military and nonmilitary survivors of trauma, and to Exner's borderline and schizotypal samples, Armstrong's DD/MPD subjects had the highest WSUM 6 mean (WSUM 6 = 19.73). Reminiscent of Levin's explanation of the greater presence of FABCOMs in her adult trauma survivors, Armstrong (1991) concluded that elevated thought disorder indices in DD/MPD patients not only reflect the disorganizing impact of traumatic reexperience, but also the fact that "Multiplicity is, at one level, a nonlogical self-construction that affirms the primacy of fantasy over logical, external restrictions. The Rorschach, as a measure of phenomenologic experience, captures the efforts of MPD patients to bend the constraints of linear logic and language to express their internal reality" (p. 543).

Putman (1997) has labeled this phenomenon "dissociative thought disorder" to describe the kind of "trance logic" that is typical of dissociative patients who have the ability to tolerate mutually contradictory propositions without seeming awareness of their logical discordance.

DELUSIONAL AND OBSESSIVE-COMPULSIVE DISORDERS

At first glance, delusional and obsessive-compulsive disorders (OCD) may seem to be strange bedfellows, one traditionally understood as a psychotic syndrome and the other a classically neurotic or anxiety-related one. However, a number of pre-Freudian writers observed the close connection between obsessive-compulsive phenomena and delusional states (Hunter and MacAlpine, 1963). Even Freud (1908) noted that obsessive-compulsive symptoms may not always occur in the context of a neurosis but, in some cases, may be a form of psychosis. The association between obsessive-compulsive disorders and schizophrenia also has a long lineage of scientific inquiry (Bumke, 1906; Mignard, 1913; Stern, 1930; Stengel, 1931; Schneider, 1939; Claude, Vidart, and Longeut, 1941; Sullivan, 1956; Sadoun, 1957; Eggers, 1969). More recently, Insel and Akiskal (1986) argued that OCD represents a spectrum of disorders ranging in severity from anxiety disorders to psychoses. In particular, they discussed the shift from overvalued ideas or obsessions to delusions in some OCD patients.

Putting aside traditional psychopathological taxonomies, one can easily see that paranoid or delusional and obsessive-compulsive disorders share a number of structural similarities. Pathology in both forms of disorder is based on aberrant beliefs that are usually unaltered by discomfirmations from external reality. Both disorders may be hidden and can occur in individuals who have adaptive and conflict-free spheres of functioning that are not contaminated by their pathological beliefs. Likewise, both disorders usually occur in the absence of disorganized thinking or signs of formal thought disorder. Both paranoid and obsessive-compulsive disorders have less severe characterological variants that may or may not predispose the individual to the more severe syndromes. Finally, the characterological variants share a number of similar ego or cognitive/perceptual features that can be studied with tests like the Rorschach. For example, both syndromes are characterized by a keen attention to details, an overvaluation of thinking or "ideational richness," as Rapaport termed it (Rapaport et al., 1968), emotional guardedness and constriction.

Aside from these stylistic features, are there specific underlying anomalies in the form or content of the thought processes of these patients that are captured by Rorschach indices of disordered thinking? The question actually becomes two questions: First, do both of these disorders have characteristic cognitive vulnerabilities or defects in logical reasoning and inference making that predispose sufferers to develop their respective symptoms; and if so, is the Rorschach sufficiently sensitive to such underlying vulnerabilities? Both questions will be addressed in the following sections.

Delusional Disorders

Delusional disorders (formerly referred to as "Paranoia" or "Paranoid Disorders") need to be distinguished from delusional beliefs that can occur in other psychiatric or medical conditions. In fact, delusions have been observed to occur in over 75 different clinical conditions (Maher and Ross, 1984; Manschreck, 1979, 1997). What we are talking about here is a discrete psychotic syndrome characterized by a stable and well-defined delusional system that occurs within a relatively normal-functioning personality. Although the individual may eventually become overwhelmed and dominated by the delusional beliefs, they may exist in "encapsulated" form for much of the time.

It is also important to distinguish the dimension of delusional thinking from a more general dimension of paranoid mentation (or paranoid cognitive style). Not all delusional disorders need be based on a paranoid style of thinking. The recognition that encapsulated delusions did not have to be paranoid in nature eventually led framers of the DSM to change the name of the syndrome from "Paranoid" to "Delusional" Disorder.

Cognitive-psychological characteristics, and Rorschach indices, of this paranoid stylistic dimension and the vulnerability to forming delusional beliefs are both examined in the following sections. A central question concerns whether there exists an inherent cognitive defect that predisposes an individual to delusional thinking, and if so, can it be identified by the Rorschach.

RORSCHACH INDICATORS OF A PARANOID STYLE. Rapaport et al. (1968) delineated a number of Rorschach structural features indicative of a paranoid style. They found that the emotional constriction and guardedness of the paranoid to be reflected in (1) a low total number of responses (R), (2) a propensity to reject cards (refusal to see anything in the inkblot), (3) fewer color responses, and a greater number of form-dominated and general form responses versus those that were dominated by color, suggesting heightened concern over emotional control. Rapaport also indicated that a high number of space responses (S) would be characteristic of paranoid conditions, reflecting the individual's oppositionality and underlying hostility. One would expect these space responses, and most other responses, to be accurately perceived (higher F+%) because of the paranoid person's rigidity and sharp attunement to external reality.

Regarding overtly disordered thinking, Rapaport and his associates indicated that "these patients are very sparing in their use of any of these pathological verbalizations" (p. 435). According to Rapaport's group, confabulations are unlikely to occur in paranoid states; however, some queer and relationship verbalizations may be seen. In terms of relationship verbalizations, Rapaport was talking about the paranoid subject's tendency to try to discover the purpose of the test or search for hidden meaning in the Rorschach cards.

Schafer (1948) presented a case of a patient who suffered from an enduring, encapsulated delusion which did not lead to widespread disorganization or deterioration. In attempting to generalize about Rorschach indices, he suggested that these patients may give a few strained symbolic responses in a rather constricted record. He elaborated on these indices in his later work (1954) and added a number of features he thought diagnostic of paranoia. Schafer agreed that paranoid patients will demonstrate their emotional constriction and restraint by achieving high F%s, a low number color responses, more FC than CF + C responses, and a tendency to reject cards. He added that their tendency to ferret out hidden details would be demonstrated by using a greater number of unusual details of the inkblot to form their images.

Unlike Rapaport, who did not feel that the paranoid state was conducive to the production of many Ms, Schafer believed that these patients could give a number of Ms, some of which may be distorted in form. Schafer also suggested that there may be a tendency to ascribe human movement to tiny details of the inkblot. An example of this response was given by a constricted and guarded patient who studied the tiny details on top of what is usually perceived as a human head or face (D9) on Card VII and responded, "This is a town full of people. They are carrying on their business. These people are looking at these others over here." Even with a high-powered microscope, one would not be able to detect any convincing rationale for humans engaging in activity. This response would not only be scored M–, but there is also a distinct confabulatory quality.

Unlike Rapaport, Schafer believed that confabulations could occur in paranoid conditions. Predicated on the tendency to blur reality with fantasy, Schafer reasoned that confabulatory elaboration is a prominent aspect of pathological projection. He stated that confabulatory embellishment requires setting up arbitrary connections between details of the blot. Schafer added that confabulations, in an overcautious and guarded setting, may be especially indicative of paranoia. Overcautiousness could be expressed through the patient's efforts to retain control, by limiting the number of responses, by rejecting cards, or by being overly vague and noncommittal about what one sees in the inkblots.

One of Schafer's (1954) unique contributions was to describe the importance of thematic content as a source for making inference about structural and dynamic issues. Regarding paranoia, Schafer indicated that content reflecting themes of self-protection and external threat could signal the potential to employ projective defenses. Imagery indicative of self-protection could reflect themes of flight, hiding, or exertion of superior power. Content such as shields, armor, shells, and grandiose images of powerful figures could all reflect self-protective concerns. Imagery suggesting external threat may reflect aggressive, accusatory, or erotic themes, including such contents as sinister, evil, or threatening figures; leering faces, eyes, pointing fingers, policemen, detectives, judges, and so on.

Schachtel (1966) and Rapaport et al. (1968) described a particular type of shading response in which the subject would use shading to delineate form or shape. Both sources indicate that the F(c) response was indicative of perceptual sensitivity. Rapaport stressed the watchful and cautious quality of the response, while Schachtel emphasized the "stretching out of feelers in order to explore nuances" (p. 251). As such, the F(c) response has come to be associated with a watchful, hypervigilant stance, possibly suggestive of a paranoid style.

Putting this all together, we can see how the paranoid style (apart from the concurrence of delusional thinking) manifests itself in responses in which the subject looks cautiously for unusual details, including white space; often uses shading to carve out internal shapes in the blot; may perceive human movement that has a distorted and confabulatory quality; and may elaborate themes that suggest external danger or a need for protection. The following response given by an angry paranoid man indicates this constellation of features in one response: Card VIII. "If you look in here (inside of D5) you can see a guy with a hood. Looks like an executioner with hate in his eyes. Ready for the kill. Also looks kinda like a KKK guy with a sheet over his head."

Finally, Exner (1993) developed a special index of structural features to assess paranoid watchfulness. His decision to call this the Hypervigilance Index instead of the "Paranoid Index" was appropriate because "hypervigilance" is a more general, less pejorative, and more conceptually descriptive term. The index hinges on the presence or absence of texture responses (FT + TF + T). If no texture is present in the record, then the examiner looks for any of the following features: (1) Zf > 12, (2) Zd > +3.5, (3) S > 3, (4) H + (H) + Hd + (Hd) > 6, (5) (H) + (A) + (Hd) + (Ad) > 3, H + A : Hd + Ad < 4 : 1, (6) Cg > 3. The index is positive if there is no texture and at least four of the other features are present. Conceptually, the index picks up a subject's wariness about trust and attachment (T = 0); a cautious and detail-oriented approach to scanning the external environment (Zf > 12 and Zd > +3.5); veiled anger (S > 3); and a preoccupation with details about people (H + (H) + Hd + (Hd) > 6). In discussing the empirical underpinnings of the index, Exner (1993) reported that the Hypervigilance Index was found to be positive in 88% of paranoid schizophrenics subjects and 90% of subjects with paranoid personalities.

DELUSIONAL THINKING. Since the DSM IV defines "delusion" as "a false belief based on incorrect inference about external reality" (American Psychiatric Association, 1994, p. 765), we might expect disturbances in formal deductive or syllogistic reasoning to lie at the base of delusion formation. As discussed in chapter 12, faulty reasoning can be conceptualized as predicate thinking, which is best captured by the autistic logic (ALOG) response. Like delusions, ALOG responses reflect the subject's sense of certainty about his or her idiosyncratic interpretation of reality which is usually based on only limited information, while overlooking more obvious and relevant cues.

However, like Rapaport, Exner stated that ALOG responses are most common among schizophrenic patients. Neither presented data suggesting that this score should be expected in a delusional process, absent concurrent schizophrenic disorganization. In other words, ALOG is generally associated more with severe psychosis, and schizophrenia in particular, than with delusional thinking per se.

The death knell for the hypothesis that predicate thinking underlies the formation of delusions actually came in the form of a number of studies that failed to demonstrate that delusional subjects reason any differently than do nondeluded ones (Nims, 1959; Williams, 1964). Thus, psychiatric researchers have concluded that the formation of delusions is not due to some defect in formal reasoning that is absent in nondeluded subjects. Although I know of no Rorschach studies that have attempted to link ALOG responses with nonschizophrenic delusional disorders, it is probably safe to conclude that, based on the available evidence, we should not expect patients with delusional disorders to give more ALOG's than nondeluded subjects.[2]

Absent any evidence of specific impairment of reasoning ability in delusional patients, Maher (1974, 1988; Maher and Ross, 1984) proposed that delusions are rational and systematic explanations of anomalous experiences that are arrived at by the same process that scientists use to account for their observations. Maher argued that delusional theories arise when the subject is presented with a puzzle or discontinuity that requires some form of explanation. The puzzle activates a "search mode" that impels the subject to find an explanation. When an explanation has been developed, it is accompanied by significant feelings of relief and reduction of tension. Data that are discrepant with this explanation evoke cognitive dissonance and are not welcome.

Chapman and Chapman (1988) agreed that Maher's model may hold promise for describing the underlying process of delusion formation in nonschizophrenic delusional subjects, but they also adduced evidence that subjects scoring high on scales measuring distortions in perception and magical thinking demonstrated an upsurge of cognitive slippage when discussing psychotic or psychotic-like experiences, like delusions or aberrant beliefs. These same subjects did not show cognitive slippage when discussing other experiences, including even nonpathological anxiety-arousing ones. When asked about their deviant experiences, these subjects tended to express themselves vaguely, demonstrate word-finding difficulty, and become tangential. The Chapmans, together with Edell (Chapman, Edell, and Chapman, 1980) found that subjects who had more delusional and aberrant beliefs than control subjects also showed

---

2. However, there may be other Rorschach indicators of delusional thinking. Exner (1993) has stated that the presence of more than two passive M-responses "increases the probability that characteristics are present from which delusional operations evolve" (p. 482). Exner has not, however, presented any data to support this hypothesis.

more cognitive slippage. However, the mild cognitive deviancy appeared primarily when the subjects were discussing their anomalous experiences.

What this suggests is that the Rorschach will not likely be sensitive to underlying delusional mechanisms unless the subject's delusional ideas are somehow aroused by the inkblot stimuli. In other words, the non-schizophrenic deluded subject may not reveal any formal disturbance in thought organization on the Rorschach. This may be especially true if the subject is responding to the inkblots in a cautious and constricted manner. This prediction seems consistent with the suggestions of Rapaport and Schafer who both indicated that that delusional patients may be difficult to detect on testing. According to Rapaport, "Patients with paranoid conditions may or may not be coarctated because their ideational productivity takes the form of delusions, they remain exceedingly coherent, and great segments of their intellectual functioning are unimpaired by the delusion formation" (Rapaport et al., 1968, p. 391). Schafer added, "These cases are among the most difficult to diagnose on the basis of test results. Many of them are indistinguishable from normals" (1948, p. 91).

This finding was illustrated by the case of a 35-year-old female patient who had the delusion that she had infected her 5-year-old daughter with the HIV virus years earlier. Despite both mother's and child's repeatedly testing HIV negative, the patient maintained that during an earlier bout of promiscuity, she had gotten semen on her leg, that later got onto a shower cap, and eventually touched her infant daughter's leg. The patient had worked responsibly and did not have a history or other symptoms of schizophrenia.

The patient's Rorschach was striking for its absence of any signs of disordered thought processes or content. Furthermore, there were none of the structural, content, or behavioral manifestations of a paranoid style. She produced several conventional Ms; her X+% was good; and she did not have any special scores. Somehow, the stimulus demands of the Rorschach bypassed her encapsulated delusionality, enabling her to appear "exceedingly coherent" and "indistinguishable from normals." However, her delusional beliefs were abundantly captured by the TAT, on which she produced a number of stories revealing themes of pathological guilt and punishment. Each card revealed the characters' hypertrophied guilt and the perseverative concern that they had done something "terribly wrong" and must be punished.

Obsessive-Compulsive Disorder

There are two interesting and controversial conceptual issues surrounding the diagnosis of OCD. The first has to do with the relationship between between OCD as a clinical syndrome, the older concept obsessive-compulsive neurosis (OCN), and obsessive-compulsive personality style or character (OCC). The second issue pertains to the relationship between OCD and psychotic disorders. Although I do not think that anyone is ready to reclassify OCD as a primary psychotic disorder, the boundary between OCD and schizophrenia or OCD and delusional disorder can, in some cases, become blurred.[3] Both of these issues have implications for our efforts to describe the underlying Rorschach-specific thought organization associated with obsessive-compulsive syndromes.

OCD, OCN, AND OCC. OCD is a newer term for what used to be called obsessive-compulsive neurosis. Is OCD essentially an old package with new wrapping? The answer seems to be yes and no. According to Yaryura-Tobias and Neziroglu (1997), who have written extensively about the syndrome, OCD symptoms have remained essentially unchanged over time. OCD *is* OCN with a new name. Both terms refer to "a strong desire to control the outer environment; to engage in forceful, unwanted, repetitive thoughts; and to perform irresistible mental and motor activities, all within a substratum of doubting" (Yaryura-Tobias and Neziroglu, 1997, p. xiii). However, what has changed dramatically is the understanding of the disorder. No longer viewed as a discrete neurotic condition, OCD is now conceptualized as a neurobiological process that exists along a spectrum of related disorders including hypochondriasis, eating disorders, body dysmorphic disorder, and Tourette's Syndrome.

Unfortunately, there is a great deal of debate about whether OCC is part of the OCD spectrum. Some regard OCD as an extension of OCC, while others reject this view, opting instead for the medicalized viewpoint that separates premorbid character from symptoms and illness (Reed, 1985). Thus, there is no consensus on whether the characteristics of the OCC cognitive-perceptual style also apply to the OCD. The lack of consensus makes the assumption of continuity tenuous. This is unfortunate for our purposes because, as I mentioned above, there is a great deal of information available about the Rorschach characteristics of subjects with obsessive character styles, which may not be applicable to the study of thought organization in OCD.

---

3. A recent study by Fear and Healy (1997) demonstrated that in terms of probabilistic reasoning, patients with OCD are more severely impaired than those suffering from delusional disorders. They noted that when delusional patients are not discussing their delusions, they appear normal. Furthermore, delusional patients typically do not act on their delusions, whereas OCD patients act on their obsessions.

Nonetheless, in what follows, I review some of the Rorschach literature that addresses the qualities of thought organization and disorder in
OCC and OCN. My assumption is that the findings pertaining to OCN
apply equally well to the concept of OCD, while those pertaining to
OCC may or may not.

Rapaport et al. (1968) and Schafer (1948, 1954) commented extensively about the Rorschach indices of OCN. However, in their writings,
it is not always clear whether they are referring to OCN or OCC.
Nevertheless, Rapaport listed the following variables as indicative of
OCN and "obsessive-compulsive cases": (1) high number of unusual
location details (Drs); (2) high number of Ms; (3) M > SumC; (4) FC >
CF + C; (5) great variety of content; (6) high number of original
responses; (7) high number of combination responses; (8) no confabulations and possibly a few fabulized combinations; and (9) high number
of fabulized responses. Schafer (1948) added the following: (1) total R
> 35; (2) F% > 80; (3) F + % > 80; (4) populars > 30%; (5) animal con-
tent > 50%; (6) criticism of accuracy of one's responses; (7) detailed
description of the inkblots; attention to symmetry; and (8) anal content.

Schafer also commented on the presence of a high number of combination responses along with a few fabulized combinations. He explained
that the obsessional patient is striving to make integrative efforts but
that this striving leads to an overly literal interpretation of a situation.
Schafer also cautioned that if the fabulized combinations are too common or contain gory detail, then the diagnosis might be one of incipient
schizophrenia.

Regarding the characteristics of OCC, Reed (1985) compiled a comprehensive list of cognitive features. Although his was not a Rorschach
study, one can easily see the conceptual linkage between his features and
a number of empirically validated Rorschach variables. Reed listed the
following categories of traits: (1) doubt and inconclusiveness; (2) accuracy, concentration, detail, precision, thoroughness; (3) aspiration, con-
scientiousness, perfectionism, persistence; (4) categorization, symmetry,
tidiness; (5) propriety, punctuality; (6) control, discipline, orderliness;
and (7) obstinacy, rigidity. Reed concluded that the central feature in the
obsessional character is the inability to tolerate the absence of order and
structure which undermines spontaneity and leads to an over-structur-
ing of experience. Although describing OCC, and not OCD per se,
Reed's categories fit well with the list of Rorschach features generated
by Rapaport and Schafer to describe patients with OCN.

Unfortunately, there is a dearth of contemporary Rorschach literature
on OCD. I found one study that looked specifically at the structural
organization of patients with OCD (Coursey, 1984). In a sample of 15
DSM-III OCD patients, carefully diagnosed to rule out schizophrenia,

Coursey found an unexpectedly high number of explicitly aggressive responses in 60% of the subjects. If mildly or symbolically aggressive content was considered, then 80% of the subjects gave responses of this quality. Coursey was struck by the contrast between the degree of hostile and aggressive content, on the one hand, and the subjects' timid, inhibited, and fearful demeanor. He also reported that 66% gave mouth or food responses; 33% touching and holding responses; and another 33% responses that had to do with unusual genital or anal content.

Coursey's findings become less impressive if compared to Exner's adult nonpatient norms. For example, 67% of this normative sample had AG scores (aggressive movement) on their protocols, compared to the 66 to 80% that Coursey reported in his sample. Although Coursey included examples of some of the more explicit aggressive responses of his OCD subjects, it is not clear to me that these responses were necessarily qualitatively different from many of the more extreme AG responses found in the normative sample. It does appear that Coursey's sample gave more responses reflecting oral dependent and sexual content than Exner's normative group. Roughly 66% of Coursey's subjects gave food and mouth responses compared to about 19% of the normative sample (Fd) responses. The difference was especially noteworthy when comparing the frequency of sexual responses. Thirty-three percent of the OCD patients gave genital and anal content, whereas only 4% of the normative subjects did.

Regarding formal thought disorder, Coursey reported that 20% of his OCD subjects gave responses with scorable thought disorder. Although he did not provide data indicating what kinds of scores were most characteristic of this group, he did include some examples, probably of the more flagrantly disordered responses. One example is the following response to Card VIII:

> Top part looks like it could resemble some type of face—imaginary or sinister. Looks like he's rather omnipotent, omniscient. . . . It destroys the usual theory that something good is over all. Or at least disputes the theory that the supreme being is a good caliber type of person. Possibly it's the devil. Or if you don't want to look at religious viewpoint, hardship and evil override pleasure. Looks like the sea is cracking; land has a fault in it. It is destroying itself [p. 110].

This highly confabulated response clearly reflects idiosyncratic embellishment of deviant proportions. It is undoubtedly an overly intellectualized DR2 response that is so highly subjective that it is almost autistic. Nonetheless, how representative is this single example of thought organization among the OCD subjects in his study or of OCD patients in general? How many of Coursey's subjects gave such severely disordered responses? Roughly 80% of Exner's normative adult subjects had some type of special score in their records. However, the frequency drops to 3% when one looks at the sum of Level 2 special scores. By comparison, Coursey indicated that among his OCD subjects, "20% had some formal thinking impairments of a variety of types" (p. 110). Since he did not distinguish level of severity, it is impossible to make an adequate comparison of his findings to normative data.[4]

Coursey also noted the defensive styles of his OCD subjects, who typically responded to the eruption of aggression into consciousness with expressions of guilt, embarrassment, apology, or further responses indicative of efforts to undo or deny the impact of their aggressive content. Using Holt's scoring system, Coursey described a number of other defensive maneuvers that these subjects utilized to contain or neutralize the overt primary process material in their responses. He concluded that OCD was marked by the extent to which primitive material has invaded the subjects' consciousness and overwhelmed the neutralizing strategies used to control them. In this, they are like other neurotics in whom primitive material does not enter consciousness, except in symbolic or symptomatic forms, or psychotics in whom primary process material is conscious and defenses have failed. Coursey proposed that OCD patients represent a third group, in which primitive material is conscious but where defenses, other than repression, remain intact.

The Obsessive Style Index (OBS) was added to the Comprehensive System in 1990. Made up of seven variables, the OBS was developed on two samples of obsessional subjects, 32 outpatients diagnosed with OCD and 114 outpatients who had been designated as compulsive personality disorders. Two of the conditions (FQ+ > 3 and X+% > 89) are weighted more heavily than the other five. The final calculation of the OBS includes any four combinations of the following variables that are found to be positive: (1) Dd > 3; (2) Zf > 12; (3) Zd > +3.5; (4) populars > 7; (5) FQ+ > 1. The OBS is positive if one or more is true: (1) conditions 1 to 5 are all true; (2) two or more of 1 to 4 are true *and* FQ+ > 3; (3) three or more of 1 to 5 are true *and* X+% > 89; and (4) FQ+ > 3 *and* X+% > 89 (Exner, 1993, p. 189).

The OBS has similarities to the Hypervigilance Index (HVI), which makes sense given the structural features that obsessional and para-

---

4. Although Coursey reported that the subjects were screened for schizophrenia, it is misleading to think that this screening effort left him with a pure culture sample of OCD subjects. The possibility that his subjects were comorbid for other, nonschizophrenic affective or characterological conditions was not addressed. Although his subjects came from an NIMH OCD project, it would be important to know if conditions other than schizophrenia were also ruled out.

noid/hypervigilant styles have in common. One may also note distinct similarities to the lists of variables proposed by both Rapaport and Schafer and the OCC categories suggested by Reed.

In developing the OBS, Exner did not separate OCC from OCD, but instead combined subjects from both groups into a larger "obsessional" sample. A positive OBS simply indicates that the subject is likely to be perfectionistic, indecisive, preoccupied with details, careful scanners of the environment, and somewhat emotionally constricted. It says nothing about the likely presence of OCD, only that an obsessional style is present. In fact Exner only reported that 101 of the 146 subjects (69%) were correctly identified by the index. He does not indicate how discriminating the OBS was for OCC versus OCD patients. It is conceivable, then, that most of the 101 correctly identified subjects could have come from the OCC group (N = 114), with a lower percentage coming from the OCD group (N = 32).

Curiously, Exner found that OBS is not highly correlated with an introversive, ideationally-oriented, style but can be found among a variety of other kinds of personality constellations. Finally, unlike Rapaport and Schafer, Exner's index includes no mention of the presence of combinatory thinking among obsessional subjects; however, it does not rule out the possibility of INCOMs or FABCOMs either.

OCD AND PSYCHOSIS. As mentioned at the beginning of this section, the search for links between OCD and psychosis has a long history. Early interests in this area concerned either the comorbidity of obsessive-compulsive syndrome with schizophrenia,[5] the occurrence of obsessional symptoms in schizophrenia (Pious, 1950; Rosen, 1957; Huber and Gross, 1989), or the progression of OCD to schizophrenia (Gordon, 1926; Stengel, 1945; Muller, 1953; Rudin, 1953; Kringlen, 1965; Ackhova, 1976; Birnie and Littmann, 1978). Among the implications of these studies was that OCD and schizophrenia were intimately related and that shifts from one condition to the other were relatively common.

Weiss and a team of investigators (Weiss, Robinson, and Winnik, 1969, 1975; Robinson, Winnik, and Weiss, 1976) described the longitudinal course of 36 OCD patients whose obsessional symptoms reached delusional proportions. What was particularly interesting about these individuals was that they did not have premorbid compulsive traits. Furthermore, their delusional obsessions were ego syntonic and aggressive in nature. Weiss et al. proposed the diagnostic category of "obsessive psychosis" to distinguish these patients from those suffering from schizophrenia.

---

5. Comorbidity estimates have ranged between 10% and 15% (Fenton and McGlashan, 1986).

Insel and Akiskal (1986) reviewed the literature on psychotic symptoms and OCD and concluded that OCD and schizophrenia are separate syndromes and that schizophrenia deterioration in well-established OCD is extremely rare. However, they agreed that some form of psychotic decompensation among OCD patients is not that unusual. They reviewed follow-up studies with OCD patients who eventually became psychotic and discovered that as many as 20% may indeed develop psychotic symptoms. Insel and Akiskal concluded that the kind of psychosis that could become superimposed on OCD was related to either a paranoid state or a mood disorder. According to these researchers, the shift from an obsessional idea to a delusional belief occurs when resistance against an obsessional idea or urge is given up and

> may take either (1) an affective form, when the fear of contamination is replaced by the delusional guilt that one has contaminated others, or (2) a paranoid form, when doubts about having committed some reprehensible act are replaced by the delusion that one is being subjected to persecution as if one had actually committed such acts [p. 1529].

Although Insel and Akiskal observed that the distinction between delusional OCD patients and those suffering from primary delusional disorders may be difficult, they suggested that the OCD patient may be more likely to fear hurting others, while the paranoid (delusional) patient is more afraid of being harmed by someone else. Furthermore, OCD patients will have had periods in the past in which they recognized the senselessness of their obsessional delusions.

Nineteen eighty-six seemed to be a popular year for studying atypical forms of psychosis in OCD. Insel and Akiskal recommended that the use of the qualifying phrase "with psychotic features" be incorporated into the DSM system. Two additional teams of researchers proposed diagnostic categories for patients whose obsessional symptoms reached delusional severity. Rasmussen and Tsuang (1986) identified a group of near-delusional OCD patients whom they called "chronic deteriorative OCD" and Jenike, Baer, and Carey (1986) used the term "schizo-obsessive" to describe patients with OCD who simultaneously met diagnostic criteria for schizotypal personality disorder.[6] In general this group was characterized by social isolation, odd speech, paranoia, and deperson-

---

6. More recently, Hwang and Hollander (1993) have used this term more generically to describe delusional symptoms in OCD and obsessive symptoms in schizophrenia.

alization. Furthermore, as a group, they were younger than the typical nonpsychotic OCD patients. In terms of treatment response, Jenike's schizo-obsessive patients were more refractory to pharmacological and behavioral treatments. The patients described by Jenike et al. seem to fall closer to the schizophrenia spectrum, whereas the obsessive psychotics described by Weiss et al. and Insel and Akiskal appear to be more similar to patients with encapsulated delusional disorders.

Regarding the Rorschachs of these obsessive psychotic or schizo-obsessive patients, we are again handicapped by a dearth of available studies of this special subgroup of OCD patients. Nonetheless, assuming that we have a conceptual understanding of these disorders, can we speculate about the Rorschach indices of disordered thinking that we might expect to find in these conditions?

The term obsessive psychosis or OCD with psychotic features implies that the obsessional symptoms have reached delusional proportions. However, as with patients suffering from encapsulated delusional disorders, the Rorschach may not always be sensitive to their circumscribed delusionality. Thus, we may have a Rorschach without signs of disordered thinking, as was the case with the patient described above, who suffered from an OCD that had reached delusional severity. Furthermore, as Weiss et al. found, obsessive psychotic patients may not show any evidence of compulsive personality patterns. Thus, these patients may not demonstrate any of the characteristic Rorschach patterns associated with OCC, as was also the case with our patient. In the absence of demonstrable Rorschach signs of obsessional delusions or an obsessional style, we are left to the use of careful interview and historical data (not to mention the convergence of signs from other tests) to make the differential diagnosis.

An exception to this rather bleak differential diagnostic picture may be the schizo-obsessive patients that Jenike described. Patients whose schizo-obsessive disorders are a product of a comorbid schizotypal personality or schizophrenia and OCD might be expected to show more pervasive signs of thought pathology. For example, we might expect to find peculiar ideas and language, vagueness, confusion, and fluidity in thought organization in the records of these patients, along with possible evidence of an obsessional style. However, some research has suggested that when both disorders are present together, the schizophreniform elements dominate. Abraham et al. (1993) gave the Rorschach (according to the Comprehensive System) to five adolescent patients, comorbid for both schizophrenia and OCD and found that all five were positive on the Schizophrenia Index (SCZI) but that none had a positive OBS Index.

NEUROLOGICAL CONDITIONS

There are at least three problems with using the Rorschach to assess disordered thinking in organic conditions. First, it is not considered a sufficiently sensitive and valid instrument for this purpose, at least not in the United States. The science and practice of neuropsychology has exploded in the last several decades, leading to a sophisticated armamentarium of empirically validated means for assessing brain-behavior relationships. The Rorschach is simply not among these conventional neuropsychological assessment techniques.

Second, the term "organicity" is passé and reflects a conceptual naivete that assumed that "brain damage" was a unitary construct that could be identified by a set of test signs. Unfortunately, much of the pre-neuropsychology research with the Rorschach viewed brain damage in this simplistic way and employed an "empirical sign approach," with all its methological shortcomings (Weiner, 1977). Reitan (1962) rejected the erroneous assumption of the unitary nature of brain damage by demonstrating the differential effects of different types of neurological syndromes and lesions on psychological functioning and behavior.

Third, much of the early neuropsychological research with the Rorschach was predicated on the distinction between "functional" and "organic" disorders. However, this dichotomy is, for the most part, anachronistic, as contemporary psychiatry looks more toward an integration between biopsychosocial factors. Nowhere is this more evident than in the understanding of schizophrenia. Previously considered the archtypal "functional" illness, schizophrenia was a common comparison group in studies testing the validity of Rorschach indices of "organicity." Nowadays, however, schizophrenia itself is increasingly understood as a neurobiologically based spectrum of illnesses that reflects varying degrees of cognitive deficits requiring as much, if not more, neuropsychological rehabilitation as psychotherapy.

Interestingly, there are signs of renewed interest in using the Rorschach as a neuropsychological instrument in this country (Perry et al., 1996; Zilmer and Perry, 1996; Perry and Potterat, 1997), along with evidence that it continues to be used overseas to assess different types of cerebral disorders (Christensen, 1985; Regard, 1985). Nonetheless, most clinical and neuropsychologists would agree that the Rorschach should have a comparatively limited role in the assessment of cognitive deficits among neurologically impaired patients.

So, why drag the Rorschach into this area at all? It would be fine to leave the issue of the differential diagnosis of cortical impairment to trained neuropsychologists, except for the fact that psychodiagnosticians using the Rorschach have always encounted, and probably always will encounter, patients in consultation who suffer from neurological syndromes. Patients with either known or heretofore undiagnosed neuropsychological deficits will continue to be referred for testing to aid in differential diagnosis and treatment planning. Because of this practical reality, it is important for clinical psychologists using the Rorschach to be familiar with patterns of cognitive disturbance that may merit referral for neuropsychological assessment.

The following review of Rorschach indices of neurological impairment is not intended to be exhaustive or to resurrect the Rorschach as a primary instrument in neuropsychology. Instead, I would like to broaden the construct of disordered thinking by applying it to neurological conditions and hence, alert practitioners to those forms of thought pathology that they may encounter in patients with cortical impairment. I begin with a brief historical overview of the use of the Rorschach as a tool to diagnose brain damage and then look more specifically at patterns of disturbed thinking that may be associated with different kinds of neurological conditions.

Organic Signs on the Rorschach

Goldfried et al. (1971) critiqued a number of sets of "organic signs" that appeared in the Rorschach literature between the decades of 1940 and 1970 (Piotrowski, 1937; Ross and Ross, 1944; Aita, Reitan, and Ruth, 1947; Dorken and Kral, 1952; Hertz and Loehrke, 1954; Evans and Marmorston, 1963). In general, they found many of the assumptions and methodology of these studies to be erroneous and lacking and recommended caution in using the Rorschach to diagnose brain damage. Nevertheless, Goldfried et al. and others (DeCato, 1993; Lezak, 1976) praised the Piotrowski Signs as the most successful of all the Rorschach sign approaches. Despite its flaws, a number of studies have supported the clinical utility of some of the signs.

PIOTROWSKI'S SIGNS. With Goldstein as a teacher, Piotrowski set out to investigate the effects of brain damage on Rorschach responses. Out of his efforts emerged a 10-point scale made up of qualitative signs for identifying the presence of brain damage. These signs included: (1) R. Total number of responses is less that 15; (2) T. Average time per response is more than one minute; (3) M. The number of human movement responses is less than or equal to one; (4) *Color denomination, Cn.* Also called color naming, a response is scored Cn if the subject simply names or describes the colors in the blot; (5) $F\%$. Good form percentage is below 70%; (6) $P\%$. The percentage of populars is below 25%; (7) *Repetition, Rpt* (Perseveration). Perseveration is scored when the subject gives the same response to several inkblots; (8) *Impotence, Imp.*

The subject gives a response despite the recognition that it is inadequate. Imp occurs in the presence of perseveration; (9) *Perplexity, Plx*. Here the subject shows mistrust about his or her ability and seeks reassurance; (10) *Automatic phrases, AP*. The subject uses the same phrase repeatedly in an indiscriminant manner.

Piotrowski regarded the presence of at least five signs as a diagnostic indication of personality change that is a result of cortical pathology. He was quite clear, however, in stating that fewer than five signs did not rule out the possibility of brain damage.

In their review of the validity of the Piotrowski Signs, Goldfried et al. reported that the most discriminating of the ten signs was Impotence, and the least M, P%, and Cn. Impotence significantly discriminated brain-damaged subjects in 10 out of 16 studies, while Perseveration, the next most successful sign, was a significant discriminator in 50% of the studies. Perplexity and Automatic phrases were also said to be among the most effective test signs. Lezak (1976) indicated that, except when compared against samples of chronic schizophrenic subjects, Piotrowski's signs correctly identified the correct diagnostic category of no less than 51% and as many as 97% of patients across 11 different studies.

GENERAL SIGNS CONSISTENT WITH BRAIN DAMAGE. Recall how Aronow et al. (1994) used Schuldberg and Boster's (1985) two-dimensional schema to categorize Rorschach deviant verbalizations. Dimension I included the superordinant categories of *Fluid responses* contrasted with their polar opposite, *Rigid responses*. Dimension II consisted of *Personal Meaning*, on one end of the continuum, and *Objective Meaning responses*, on the other. Aranow et al. indicated that scores from the categories of Rigid and Objective Meaning responses could be found in the Rorschachs of organically impaired subjects. Schuldberg and Boster also believed that both Rigid and Object Meaning Responses were consistent with Goldstein's concept of a loss of abstract attitude.

Rigid responses would chiefly include examples of perseveration (scored at the .25 level in the TDI). Several studies have found these responses in the records of brain-impaired subjects (Neiger, Slemon, and Quirk, 1962; Evans and Marmorston, 1964). However, as we saw in chapter 13, perseveration responses are also common in chronic deteriorated schizophrenic patients (Johnston and Holzman, 1979) and associated with negative symptomatology. Object meaning responses include vagueness and confusion scores (scored at the .25 and .50 level in TDI, respectively). Both of these scores reflect the subject's struggle with a loss of distance in which the blots are interpreted in a literal manner, leaving the subject perplexed as to what they really are. Thus, two of Piotrowski's signs are clearly reflected in these response categories.

A more general, but not Rorschach-specific, listing of projective test response tendencies characteristic of brain-damaged individuals was given by Lezak (1976). The reader will spot a number of themes similar to those found in Piotrowski's signs. Lezak's general response tendencies (with Rorschach examples) included: (1) *Constriction.* Responses tend to become reduced in size (e.g., Rorschach low R; high F% or Lambda); (2) *Stimulus-boundedness.* Responses interpret the test stimuli in literal and concrete ways (e.g., "It looks like an ink blotch to me."); (3) *Structure-seeking.* Difficulty making sense or order out of one's experiences without guidance from external sources (e.g., "Now what am I supposed to do here?"; "It's a bug; is that OK?"); (4) *Response rigidity.* Problems shifting sets or flexibly adapting to different conditions (e.g., perseveration responses); (5) *Fragmentation.* Difficulty integrating parts into a whole (e.g., fragmentation responses such as "This is a body . . . I see wings, a stomach"); (6) *Simplification.* Poorly differentiated responses lacking in detail (e.g., global whole responses with little or no detail provided); (7) *Conceptual confusion and spatial disorientation.* Subjects may appear confused by the spatial orientation of the stimulus (e.g., confusion responses such as "A tree but how can it have this thing in the middle?"); (8) *Confabulation.* Lezak indicated that brain-damaged patients tend to produce responses in which unrelated percepts or ideas become irrationally linked because of spatial or temporal contiguity. Lezak seemed to be describing combinative responses which have a stimulus-bound quality. Taking things too literally, brain-damaged patients are more likely to combine or embellish details based on concrete spatial relationships than on conceptual associations; (9) *Hesitancy and doubt.* Patients exhibit ongoing doubt and uncertainty about their perceptions and responses (related to perplexity and impotence).

Not only are these response tendencies characteristic of subjects with brain damage, but they may also be found in mentally retarded subjects (Peebles, 1986). Actually, when the Rorschach is considered as a complex problem-solving test, it is not surprising to find that subjects with low intelligence typically demonstrate many of these features too.

Neuropsychological Functions, Disordered Language, and Thought

Aside from those early studies using the empirical sign approach, there have been only a limited number of studies that actually attempted to correlate patterns of Rorschach thought disorder with deficits in different functional systems of the brain or with certain types of neurological syndromes (Hall, Hall, and Lavoie, 1968; Christensen, 1985; Kestenbaum-Daniels et al., 1988; Perry and Potterat, 1997). There is, however, abundant information about specific kinds of cognitive impairment associated with disturbances of these basic functional systems or the syndromes in which they appear. This information enables us to extrapolate a set of Rorschach variables that we might expect to find in patients manifesting different types of neuropsychological impairment. Both sources of information pave the way for a review of probable Rorschach indices of disordered thinking associated with different types of cortical dysfunction.

The broad categories of neuropsychological impairment selected are admittedly crude, overlapping, and incomplete but give a sampling of how impairment in different functional systems or locations in the brain may give rise to more or less specific patterns of deviant thought or language on the Rorschach. The categories include deficits in (1) verbal, (2) visuoperceptual, (3) executive, and (4) emotional reactions to neurological impairment.

IMPAIRMENTS IN VERBAL FUNCTIONS. Lesions in the dominant anterior and posterior temporal areas create marked disturbances in language and communication. Aphasia is a category of language disorders characterized by errors of grammatical structure, word-finding difficulties, and the presence of word substitutions (paraphasias). Depending on the nature and site of the lesion, aphasic language can vary in fluency, articulation, paraphasic distortion, repetition competence, and comprehension.

Language fluency depends on whether words flow easily with abundant associative connections linking ideas together or are sparse, halting, and effortful. Fluent language is usually delivered at least at a normal rate, but may be devoid of meaningful content and contain abnormal words and syllables, whereas nonfluent language output contains primarily nouns (substantive words), is agrammatic, and reflects word-finding difficulties.

Three primary types of paraphasia have been described by Goodglass and Kaplan (1983). Literal or phonemic paraphasia occurs when the individual produces syllables that are in the wrong order or adds unintended sounds to words. An example is the subject who looks at Card I and says "This looks like a cap . . . uh, a back, no a bat." Verbal or semantic paraphasia consists of unintended words that are inadvertently used in place of another. The substituted words usually are connotatively related to the intended word. For example, a more subtle variation of the Card I response could have been "This looks like a bird, I mean a bat." Extended paraphasia or paragrammatism refers to punning speech that is logically incoherent because either the phrases do not make sense or are due to the intrusion of misused words and neologisms. The traditional psychiatric concept of "word salad" may, in some cases, reflect a severe aphasiac disorder. Two other forms of paraphasic distortion may occur. Remote paraphasias include word substitutions that are arbitrary and seemingly unrelated to the intended word, while perseverative paraphasias are based on words that have just been said in another context. Perry et al. (1996) developed a scale for assessing paraphasic errors, word-finding difficulties, awkward and stilted speech, and executive perseverative errors from the Rorschach. They applied their scoring criteria to a sample of 22 subjects suffering from Dementia of the Alzheimer Type (DAT) and, as one would expect, found significant differences between this group and a group of nondemented subjects in the frequency of these kinds of responses.

The major classes of aphasia typically present with different patterns of disordered language that may yield predictable signs of pathology on the Rorschach. Qualitative Rorschach linguistic patterns that may be associated with two major categories are reviewed below.

(1) BROCA'S APHASIA. Involving damage to the anterior temporal-frontal operculum (areas 44 and 46), Broca's aphasia is characterized by non-fluent language output and a lack of grammatical complexity. Articulation is poor and speech may be halting. Output may range from short phrases, containing only substantive words, to meaningless utterances that are almost unrecognizable (Alexander, 1997). Rorschach responses may be expected to be fragmentary, one- or two-word responses, delivered in a halting and truncated manner. Additionally, the subject may struggle to find the right words to express his or her ideas. An example of this type of response might be, "Bug . . . uh . . . hard-shell . . . what do you call it . . . beetle."

(2) WERNICKE'S APHASIA. Wernicke's aphasia can be produced by lesions in the superior temporal gyrus back to the end of the sylvan fissure. Language is typically more complex and fluent but contains paraphasias at either the phonemic, semantic, or neologistic level. Language is also rather empty and can be devoid of meaning. On the Rorschach, we might expect longer responses, without pronounced word-finding difficulties. The responses may have a poverty of thought content, as well as peculiar, queer, and neologistic verbalizations. Wernicke's aphasia is notorious for marked comprehension problems, making it likely that the subject will have difficulty understanding the instructions to the task.

Other aphasiac syndromes include conduction, trancortical sensory, transcortical motor, anomic, and global aphasia. Each presents with either fluent or nonfluent language output and some variety of paraphasias. Rorschach responses may reflect pronounced word-finding problems, along with varying degrees of deviant verbalizations.

Aphasia can truly be considered a disorder of language, as opposed to psychotic thinking. Strub and Black (1977) distinguished aphasic from psychotic language by both historical data and qualitative features.

Regarding history, age of onset typically differs markedly between psychosis and aphasia, with acute onset of aphasia occurring more often in the elderly following strokes. A longer or prodromal history of language deterioration in a younger person argues in favor of a schizophrenia. Qualitatively, paraphasias, even of the neologistic type, tend to be more symbolic in schizophrenia (and other functional psychoses) and more random and nonsymbolic in aphasia.[7] Word-finding difficulties are typically not expected among psychotic individuals. Conversely, confabulatory speech is not expected in aphasia but may certainly occur in other forms of "functional" psychosis and neuropathology (as in dementia, for example).

IMPAIRMENTS IN VISUOSPATIAL FUNCTIONS. Perceptual organizational abilities are differentiated between the left and right hemispheres and can influence Rorschach responses. The left hemisphere is superior in identifying and interpreting parts or fine details, while the right is specialized for processing the gestalt and integrating parts into wholes. Hall et al. (1968) examined the impact of lesions in the right versus left hemisphere on a number of Rorschach variables, including combinatory thinking, form level, perplexity, and rejection of cards. The left hemisphere patients were characterized by high scores on perplexity and card rejection and a tendency to attend to the outline of the blot, while ignoring any other attributes of the card. Right hemisphere patients, by contrast, scored low on both card rejection and perplexity. However, their thinking was characterized by inappropriate elaboration of details and bizarre fabulized combinations.

Perry and Potterat speculated that damage to the posterior area of the left temporal lobe would interfere with an individual's ability to detect and process small details on the Rorschach. Such individuals would tend to produce an abundance of whole (W) responses, even on Cards IX and X, which are more difficult to make into whole responses. One would expect that the form quality of many of these whole responses would be poor because the subject would likely sacrifice the precision of accurate detail, necessary for F+ responses, for the press of achieving a whole response. One might also speculate about the presence of DW responses (the CONFAB score in the Comprehensive System), as subjects would quickly overgeneralize from a part to the whole.

Right hemispheric damage typically results in difficulties forming an integrated whole response, referred to as constructional aparaxia. On the Rorschach, these individuals would likely be able to perceive indi-

---

7. Interestingly, Gerson, Benson, and Frazier (1977) found that neologisms in general were more common among aphasic subjects than those with schizophrenia.

vidual details but be unable to form a gestalt necessary for a whole response. This is essentially what Kestenbaum-Daniels and her colleagues found in their study comparing Rorschach TDI scores of subjects with right-sided cortical damage to those with schizophrenia and mania (Kestenbaum-Daniels et al., 1988). Twenty-three patients with unilateral right hemisphere cortical damage, status post cerebral vascular accidents, were compared to similar numbers of schizophrenic and bipolar manic patients on the TDI. With corrections for number of responses, there were no significant differences in total TDI scores for the three groups; however, there were distinct qualitative differences between the groups. Using a principal components analysis, the researchers consolidated all TDI scoring categories into five factors, which included (1) combinatory thinking (flippant thinking, incongruous combinations, playful confabulations); (2) fragmented thinking (excessive qualification, concrete thinking, vagueness, fragmentation, confusion); (3) idiosyncratic thinking (peculiar, queer, absurd, neologisms, incoherence); (4) associative looseness (clanging, perseverations, inappropriate distance, looseness, fabulized combinations); and (5) arbitrary thinking (autistic logic, fluid thinking, confusion). Patients with right-sided damage demonstrated significantly more fragmented thinking than did the other patients. When these subjects gave more than one response per card, they were typically fragments of a whole response instead of separate responses. For example, a subject may look at Card V and state, "I see wings . . . antennae . . . and legs" but not intend for these to form an integrated whole. Rorschach (1921) labeled this type of response a "Do" or "oligophrenic" response, by which he meant a response was given to a detail that was ordinarily seen by most subjects as part of a whole—for example, seeing a crab's claw but seeing the whole crab, too.

Consistent with previous TDI research, schizophrenic subjects scored significantly higher on the Idiosyncratic Verbalization factor, whereas the manic group exhibited significantly greater scores on the Combinatory factor. Both manic and schizophrenic groups gave significantly more responses scored at the .75 level of severity than the brain-damaged group, and the schizophrenic group gave more 1.0 level responses than the other two groups. All three had roughly equivalent numbers of .25 level responses.

COMPLEX PROBLEM-SOLVING FUNCTIONS. Implicated in a range of tasks, the frontal lobes have remained somewhat enigmatic, leading neuroscientists to search for a unified theory of frontal lobe function. Other than knowing that the frontal lobes play a crucial role in the formation of complex behavior, the precise functions of the frontal cortex have eluded investigators. The frontal cortex has been assumed to be important for abstract thinking, planning, utilizing feedback to modify behavior, inhibiting action tendencies, and working memory. Kimberg, D'Esposito, and Farah (1997) reviewed various theories of frontal lobe function and favored the "working memory" theory. They concluded that all tasks sensitive to frontal lobe damage can be linked together by their dependence on working memory. Executing complex behaviors is dependent on memories of past experience. According to Kimberg et al., working memory is a form of functional short-term memory, analogous to a mental scratch pad. The prefrontal cortex expands the temporal perspectives of working memory, thus allowing it to integrate newer and more complex behavior (Fuster, 1980). Thus, the frontal lobes are critical for memory functioning.

According to Perry and Potterat (1997), frontal lobe impairment interferes with the efficient organization, storage, and retrieval of information, all of which are necessary for successful memory functioning. Thus problems in encoding and retrieval may result in perseverative tendencies. Bilder and Goldberg (1987) suggested that all types of perseveration involve impairments in frontal cortex-mediated executive functioning, which results in a greater frequency of perseverations in thought, speech, and action. In general, frontal patients do not utilize (or assimilate into working memory?) feedback to use as cue for modifying their behavior.

Perry et al.'s (1996) scale for assessing paraphasias included three types of perseverative errors in Rorschach responses. The first type, called "phonemic perseveration" is scored for a repetition of a phonemic or morphemic quality of a previous response. The second form, called "stuck-in-set perseveration" involves the compulsive use of a strategy from a previous response. The third type is the "thematic perseveration," scored when a theme or content from a previous response reappears. Making further links to the neuropsychological literature, Perry et al. reported that stuck-in-set perseverations are most characteristic of frontal lobe pathology, whereas thematic perseverations are more common in aphasic and Alzheimer patients (Sandson and Albert, 1984).

EMOTIONAL REACTIONS AND CORTICAL IMPAIRMENT. Patients with unilateral hemispheric damage manifest contrasting emotional reactions to their brain impairment and to their productions on different tasks. Patients with damage to the left hemisphere demonstrate "catastrophic" reactions characterized by heightened anxiety and depression. While taking the Rorschach, these subjects may display disorganizing anxiety or agitation. They may be extremely sensitive to the difficulties they have attending to relevant details, making sense of the cards, and communicating their responses to the examiner. As Hall et al. found, left hemisphere patients tend to express more perplexity regarding their responses and to reject cards more often.

Right-sided subjects demonstrate the opposite emotional reaction. They react to taking the Rorschach the same way they react to their deficits, with denial and indifference. Unlike patients with left hemisphere damage, they tend to be oblivious to their difficulties and unflappable in the face of their distortions, fragmentation, and even their expressed confusion. Another characteristic reaction sometimes observed in right-sided patients is their relative disinhibition and use of sarcasm. These individuals may actually respond in ways similar to hypomanic patients, with flippant and inappropriate comments.

Thought Disorder Scores and Cortical Impairment

As can be seen from this review, a number of specific scores from the TDI and Comprehensive System appear to reflect different kinds of cognitive deficits found in brain-damaged individuals. Table 16-1 summarizes some of the scores that are most relevant to the differential assessment of disordered thinking in neurologically impaired patients. As can be seen, the majority of the scores fall in the mild to moderate categories.

Table 16-1 Thought Disorder Scores Associated with Cortical Impairment

Thought Disorder Score (C.S.)	Severity Level (TDI)	Clinical Manifestation
Excessive Qualification	0.25	Perplexity
Vagueness	0.25	Perplexity
Confusion	0.50	Impotence, Perplexity
Peculiar Responses (DV1)	0.25	Paraphasias
Word-Finding Difficulty	0.25	Paraphasias
Queer Responses (DV2)	0.50	Paraphasias
Neologisms (DV2)	1.00	Paraphasias
Concreteness	0.25	Stimulus-bounded
Perseveration (PSV)	0.25	Rigidity
Fragmentation	0.50	Integrative failure
DW (CONFAB)	0.75	Integrative failure
Loss of Distance	0.25	Catastrophic reaction
Flippant Response	0.25	Denial, Indifference

CHAPTER

17

CREATIVITY OR
DISORDERED THINKING?

There is a frequently cited, but no less compelling, anecdote that is germane to the subject of this chapter. The story tells of a professional conversation between C. G. Jung and James Joyce about the nature of Joyce's daughter's mental illness. Joyce, increasingly distraught over his 21-year-old daughter's apparent descent into schizophrenia, was, in the early 1930s, urged by his patrons to bring his daughter, Lucia, to meet with the eminent Swiss psychiatrist. Joyce, perhaps in desperation, insisted that Lucia's poetry contained the strands of a new form of literature. Following his examination, Jung, the twentieth doctor to be consulted, told Joyce that Lucia was suffering from dementia praecox and that her poems were "random."

> "How do you know, Dr. Jung?" Joyce asked. Jung replied that her thinking and speech were so deviant and distorted that he could conclude that she was suffering from this particular form of madness. Joyce protested that in his own writing, he purposefully stretched the English language, distorted words, fused thoughts and images. "What is the difference?" he asked. Jung replied that Joyce and his daughter were like two people going to the bottom of a river, but whereas Joyce dove into the deep water, his daughter fell into it. Jung later wrote, "The ordinary patient cannot help himself talking and thinking in such a way, while Joyce willed it and moreover developed it with all his creative forces" [Johnston and Holzman, 1979, p. 16, quoting Ellmann, 1959, p. 692].

What distinguishes the idiosyncratic speech and peculiar ideas of the creative mind from those of the thought disordered one? Disentangling creative or artistic thought from that which is disturbed and pathological has interested philosophers and scientists for centuries. Although Jung provided a useful organizing concept for making the distinction, diagnosticians need to rely on more specific empirical and conceptual signs to help them differentiate the two.

In this chapter, I present some information regarding pertinent theories of creativity and introduce concepts that should prove helpful in understanding creative processes on the Rorschach. Next, I review how some have conceptualized creativity on the inkblot test. Finally, I turn to the specific case example of Linus Pauling, whose Rorschach presents a number of complex issues regarding the distinction between creative and pathological processes.

THEORIES OF CREATIVITY

Sublimation and Regression in the Service of the Ego

In his psychoanalytic study of Leonardo da Vinci, Freud (1910) concluded that da Vinci's artistic talent and creativity were, in part, a product of "his extraordinary capacity for sublimating the primitive instincts" (p. 136). Freud wrote about the regressive shift which occurred in da Vinci's psychic equilibrium in his fifties, that it yielded access to "deeper layers" of his mind and acted "to the benefit of his art" (p. 134). In other words, Freud implied that da Vinci's sublimation of his erotic impulses acted in the service of his artistic talent.

Ernst Kris (1952) introduced the term "regression in the service of the ego" to build upon Freud's concept of sublimation and to place it squarely within the realm of the ego. Interested in creativity, art, and humor, Kris proposed that the ego of a healthy individual can relax its grip on the rules of secondary-process thinking in a deliberate and controlled manner. In doing so, primary-process thinking can be used at the discretion of the healthy ego for the purpose of a controlled and reversible regression in the service of creative or artistic expression. In discussing the contributions of Kris, Holt (1977) wrote, "A person who is not asleep and dreaming may therefore fragment and recombine ideas and images in ways that flout the demands of reality on either of two bases: because he cannot help it, due to a temporary or permanent impairment, or because he wants to, for fun or for creative purposes" (p. 379).

The concept of regression in the service of the ego formed the original basis for understanding the mental substratum of creativity. Since

Kris's seminal contribution, others have attempted to conceptualize the specific psychological underpinnings of creativity. As described in chapter 4, Holt attempted to operationalize the concept of "adaptive regression" in his Rorschach scoring system for primary process thinking. Holt wanted to measure the balance of primary-process material that was admitted into consciousness along with the accompanying control or defense mechanisms that brought the former into the service of the ego.

From his extensive study of schizophrenic cognition, Arieti (1964) introduced the term "tertiary process" to describe how creative processes reflect the special combination of primary and secondary processes. Instead of rejecting primitive ideas as illogical, the creative mind plays with and intentionally integrates these with higher level logic in a synergistic process that allows a novel synthesis to emerge. More specifically, Arieti pointed out that the creative act involves perceiving relationships between two seemingly dissimilar entities or engaging in a kind of creative "combinatory play." This capacity to perceive commonalities or identities between ostensibly unrelated things is a property of the primary process.[1] The creative act emerges from the linking of this primary process-based perceptual identity with a secondary process based conceptual understanding.

As described in chapter 11, Rothenberg (1971, 1976) introduced the term "Janusian process" (after the Roman god, Janus, whose faces simultaneously look in opposite directions), to describe the cognitive process that lies at the heart of creative breakthroughs. Rothenberg indicated that Janusian thinking has superficial similarities to the "thinking in opposites" and to the paralyzing ambivalence attributed to schizophrenia. However, in creative endeavors, conceiving of opposites is a conscious, ego-directed act that transcends conventional logic and results in a creative leap. Rothenberg's concept of "homospatial process" described the simultaneous placing of two discrete entities in the same perceptual-cognitive space. Koestler (1964) used the term "bisociation" to describe a similar concept in which previously unrelated dimensions of experience are superimposed to form a creative synthesis. In both concepts, separate images or objects are condensed, leading to the articulation of a new entity. According to Rothenberg, homospatial process is a primary factor in metaphor creation. He gave the example of a poetic image of a horse and rider, in which the components of each interact in a poetic manner that does not simply result in the image of a centaur or other combination of horse and human (i.e., an incongruous combination). In many ways, Rothenberg's concept

---

1. Freud (1900) indicated that no contradictions exist in the primary process realm of experience.

comes close to capturing the creative use of condensation, the adaptive counterpart to the Rorschach contamination response, which is typically regarded as an ominous harbinger of psychotic thinking.

Creativity and Mental Illness

The link between creativity and madness has intrigued people for a millennium. Plato referred to poetic inspiration as "divine madness" (Jowett, 1924), while Aristotle said that "no great genius was without a mixture of insanity" (Langsdorf, 1900). In the field of psychiatry, Lombroso (1895) wrote extensively at the turn of the century about the link between creativity and mental illness.

Freudian theory led generations of researchers to relate the mechanisms of primary process functioning to schizophrenic regression on the one hand and artistic creations on the other. Because the same mechanisms that were observed in the mental functioning of schizophrenic patients were found in dreams, humor, and art, researchers reasoned that there must be a close relationship between the two. At the very least, creative geniuses were expected to be eccentric and, at worst, insane.

Surrealistic painter Salvador Dali had a great deal to say about the relationship between psychopathology and creativity. Referring to himself as a "paranoiac," Dali believed that he possessed a special capacity to recognize double images because he felt that his disturbed mind was hypersensitive to hidden appearances that were real or imagined. A master of creative condensation, Dali called his technique the "paranoiac-critical method," which he defined as a "spontaneous method of irrational knowledge based on the interpretative-critical association of delirious phenomena" (Dali, 1930, in Arnason, 1977). In his book *La Femme Visible*, Dali wrote, "I believe the moment is at hand when, by a paranoiac and active advance of the mind, it will be possible (simultaneously with automatism and other passive states) to systematize confusion and thus to help discredit completely the world of reality" (p. 359).

Given his self-proclaimed paranoia, the nightmarish images in his paintings, and his peculiar prose, could Dali be considered insane? Eccentric probably, but it is doubtful that he suffered from a psychotic condition. Arieti (1976) does not believe that he was truly paranoid in the legal or clinical case. Instead, Arieti's interpretation was that Dali had a heightened sensitivity to the primary process. Dali actively sought to create in his art a specific documentation of Freud's theories which he applied to himself. He began a painting with the first image that came to his mind and then went from one association to the next, superimposing images of persecution and megalomania, like a true paranoiac. It becomes clearer that Dali expressed his contempt for conventional and formalist art by actively and intentionally diving into the depths of madness and primary process.

Andreasen and her colleagues began to examine the relationship between creativity and mental illness (Andreasen and Canter, 1974; Andreasen and Powers, 1975; Andreasen, 1980). Initially expecting to find a closer relationship between creativity and schizophrenia, Andreasen and Canter were surprised to find a strong family history of affective illness in their sample of creative writers. Furthermore, they found that 66% of a sample of creative writers reported having experienced an episode of affective illness. More than half of their sample reportedly met diagnostic criteria for cyclothymia. In a later study, Andreasen (1987) reported that an even higher percentage (80%) of a sample of creative writers had experienced some form of affective illness.

In terms of the underlying cognitive mechanisms, Andreasen and Powers (1975) investigated the conceptual styles among groups of manics, schizophrenics, and creative writers. In their study, which did not control for intellectual or educational levels, Andreasen and Powers discovered that the creative writers resembled the manic group in their performance on an object-sorting test. Like the manic subjects, the writers scored high on measures of conceptual overinclusiveness, in that both groups tended to broaden, blur, and shift conceptual boundaries. Furthermore, like the manic group, the creative writers were energetic, productive, and intellectually adroit. Jamison's (1993) findings, presented in chapter 14, are quite consistent with this. Recall that Jamison found that both creative and hypomanic thinking are characterized by fluency, rapidity, and flexibility. Jamison also concluded that, for both groups, a greater speed of thinking leads to a greater quantity of thoughts and associations which may produce some unique ideas and associations.

The creative writers and manics in Andreasen and Power's study were equally overinclusive in their conceptual spans and significantly different from the schizophrenic subjects who tended to be both conceptually underinclusive and idiosyncratic in their thinking. However, the writers could be distinguished from the manic subjects by the quality of their overinclusiveness. Whereas the manics demonstrated conceptual overinclusiveness and idiosyncratic thinking, the creative writers demonstrated overinclusiveness and ideational richness. Thus, whereas creative individuals may demonstrate unusual associations that are rich and literary, manics tend to have difficulty maintaining a focus and filtering out distractions that render their associations bizarre and idiosyncratic.

A different point of view was presented by Rothenberg (1983, 1990) who criticized the methodology in the studies of Andreasen and Jamison linking creativity to affective illness. Although he acknowledged that disappointment and elation are frequent consequences of creative endeavors, Rothenberg did not believe that mood fluctuations intrinsically reflect or result from underlying affective illness. Instead, he believed that creativity stems from a more complex array of factors. Likewise, he believed that it is erroneous to view creativity as a product of primary process. The similarities are there for sure; however, according to Rothenberg, the underlying psychological dynamics are quite different. He agreed that, although some creative geniuses may cross the line between creativity and psychosis, imagination and creativity involve special cognitive abilities, talents, and motivations to transcend one's experience in order to bring forth new ideas and creations.

CREATIVITY AND THE RORSCHACH

Among his 28 clinical examples, Rorschach included the case of an "imaginative individual." In addition to noting that this subject gave accurately perceived and original responses, Rorschach twice indicated that there were no confabulations in her record. Instead, he noted that she demonstrated an excellent capacity for creative synthesis as evidenced by a wealth of associations and combinations. Interestingly, he hinted that this capacity for creative synthesis was also related to the subject's tendency toward moodiness. "[T]he factors making for combination (synthesis) become so powerful in the moody spells which sometimes appear that they lead to the evolution of 'forebodings' and like experiences" (p. 139). Examples of a few of this woman's responses illustrate the richly combinative and lively nature of her associations.

Card III.	Two jilted suitors who are meeting each other; they hold bouquets in their hands. W M+ H
Card VII.	Two women's heads with rococo hairdress pointing upwards. D F+ Hd
Card VIII.	A bear climbing a tree-stump. D F+ Ad
	A fairy tale motif stylized. W FC+ Style
	A fire at the bottom. D CF+ Fire
	A buried treasure. D F+ obj. Orig.
	The root of the tree under which the treasure is buried. D F+ Pl.
	The animals guarding the treasure. D F+ A [p. 138].

Rorschach's scoring was crude by current standards, and we would, no doubt, score some of these responses a bit differently. For example, her response to Card VIII approaches a mild fabulized combination, and the fabulizing quality of several of her other responses borders on overspecificity. In general, however, the responses that drift toward overspecificity retain their good form and are not preposterous.

Aside from associating well-integrated combination responses with "good endowment and intelligence" (p. 424), Rapaport et al. (1968) had little to say about creativity on the Rorschach. Schafer (1954) took up this subject later as he linked the concept of regression in the service of the ego to creativity. Although he also did not address specific Rorschach indices of creativity, Schafer spoke of the creative process as a shift in level of functioning that requires a relaxation of the defensive organization that bars unconscious material from preconscious and conscious awareness. He described creative regression as an active process "of taking imaginative liberties and not an altogether passive process of being overwhelmed by alien forces" (p. 81).

An interesting departure from the traditional ego psychological approach to the issue of creativity on the Rorschach is contained in the work of Schachtel (1966). Unlike Rapaport, who held that normal subjects felt that they must give responses that are completely acceptable to conventional logic, Schachtel believed that the very nature of the Rorschach Test invites "the play of imagination and fantasy" (p. 26). For Rapaport, strict adherence to the dictates of "conventional logic" was the sine qua non of a good Rorschach response; for Schachtel it represented a straitjacket. What is merely acceptable to everyday logic leaves, in Schachtel's view, little room for everything that is creative and capable of penetrating beneath the surface of conventionality. He referred to the Card VIII response given by Rorschach's imaginative subject as an example of an image that would be deemed pathological (perhaps by Rapaport, he thought) only if one assumed that the subject understood the test instructions to mean that she was to give completely realistic and conventionally logical responses. Schachtel indicated that an imaginative or artistic person certainly will not understand the instructions in such a way.

In addressing the role of imagination on the Rorschach, Schachtel stated, "Imagination does not form new images out of nothing; it transforms, recombines, varies known images" (p. 65). Thus, like others, he linked imaginative activity to the recombining of ideas or images in novel ways. Schachtel also referred to Werner's (1948) concept of "physiognomic perception" as an integral part of the creative response process. Werner considered this a more primitive type of perception found in primitive societies, psychopathology, and children. Schachtel felt that physiognomic perception should not be relegated solely to the realm of primitivity or immaturity, but that it also related to art and poetry. Developing from an individual's sensitivity to the expressive meaning of the human face, physiognomic perception can enliven our experience of phenomena such as landscapes, objects, and works of art with animistic qualities. Schachtel felt that perceiving nonhuman objects as warm, cold, inviting, eternal, gentle, ominous, and so forth, enriched one's experience and deepened the sense of reality. He wrote, "Unless we are able to perceive the 'character' of a landscape in a physiognomic way, it remains a closed book to us, it does not speak to us, we remain unrelated rather than open to it" (p. 69). Schachtel indicated that physiognomic perceptions on the Rorschach were pathological only if they were absurd, incompatible with the contours of the inkblots, occurred too frequently together with Dds, were perseverative, or were taken as real by the subject.

A number of studies have compared the Rorschach performances of creative individuals to those of noncreative normals and psychiatric controls. Hersch (1962) analyzed creative processes from a developmental perspective. Based on Werner's comparative developmental theory (1957), which, among other things, held that a person's capacity for creativity depended on a dynamic balance between regressive and progressive forces, Hersch proposed that creative people would demonstrate greater cognitive flexibility in terms of having access to developmentally mature and primitive levels of experience. Hersch hypothesized that creative individuals would demonstrate both mature and primitive responses on the Rorschach. Additionally, Hersch wondered whether the regressive experiences of the "creators," as they emerged on the Rorschach, would differ from the primitive responses of schizophrenic patients.

Narrowing his focus to only those variables that best reflected Werner's developmental concepts of maturity (differentiation, articulation, and integration) and primitivity (diffuseness and syncretism), Hersch compared six response categories among three groups of adult male subjects (each with an N of 20): creators (in this case, eminent artists), noncreative normals, and schizophrenics. The following Rorschach variables were considered to reflect developmental maturity: (1) Human Movement Responses (M), indicating the capacities to evaluate cognitively, to delay one's motoric responses, and to differentiate self from environment; (2) Integrative Responses (I), essentially the appropriate integration of two or more accurately perceived blot elements into an organized and articulated whole; and (3) Form Dominant Responses (FD), indicative of both articulation and differentiation. Hersch defined developmental primitivity by the following response categories: Form Subordinate Responses (FS), reflecting greater diffuseness and less differentiation; Physiognomic Responses (PR), described as a fabulized enlivenment of the inkblot; and Primitive Thought Responses (PT).

Werner (1957) defined "physiognomic perception" as a primitive cognitive process in which the subject fuses his or her own motoric or affective impressions with the sensory stimulation of the blot. Because Werner felt that this mode of perception reflected an undifferentiated relationship between the self and the external environment, Hersch considered physiognomic Rorschach responses to be more developmentally primitive. Hersch's final type of primitive response (PT) included a general category that included contaminations, fabulized combinations, and confabulations. He felt that each of these reflected varying degrees of diffuse or syncretic functioning.

Hersch found that the artists gave more Ms (human movement responses), FDs (form dominant responses), PRs (physiognomic responses), and PT (primitive thought) responses than the noncreative normals, suggesting that they were capable of blending developmentally mature with more primitive experiences. There were no differences between the two groups in frequency of I (integrative responses) or FS responses (form subordinate responses). Compared to the schizophrenic subjects, the artists gave more Ms, Is, and FDs, as well as PRs. Neither FS nor PT was significantly different in the two groups. Hersch concluded that his findings supported the hypothesis that cognitive functioning in creative people is characterized by greater availability of both relatively mature and primitive processes. The primitive responses of the creative individuals occurred in the context of good Ms and more highly organized and form-dominated responses. Hersch postulated that the physiognomic responses of creative people reflect their ability to fuse self-affective experience with environmental stimuli but to then pull back and reflect on this experience, objectifying it and distinguishing between what is inside and outside. Schizophrenic individuals, on the other hand, may fuse subject and object and lose their ability to reflect and maintain appropriate reality testing.

It is interesting to note that, in terms of primitivity, the schizophrenic and creative subjects differed only in the frequency of physiognomic responses, and not in the number of traditional thought disorder signs. However, if one looks at Hersch's data, one finds that both groups had comparatively low levels of measured thought disorder (median for each group was one response per record). This seems unusually low for a sample of schizophrenic subjects.

Rawls and Slack (1968) found that a group of artists had a greater number of Ws, cut-off Ws, and a richer variety of M and H responses. These subjects seemed to prefer complexity and demonstrated a greater tolerance for ambiguity. They also gave more sexual and abstract content than comparison groups. Dudek (1968) compared 41 artists, operationally defined as "good" or talented, to 19 similarly defined unsuccessful artists and 22 high M nonartist controls. The groups did not differ in their production of M responses, leading Dudek to conclude that M is related to creativity but not to talent, motivation, or the potential to use creativity. What distinguished the two groups of artists from each other and from the control group, however, was the extent of primary process content in their records. Seventy-two percent of the artists, as opposed to 36% of the controls, showed evidence of primary process thinking on their Rorschachs. The successful artists demonstrated more primary process material, richer associations, and more spontaneous affectively-tinged comments than both the unsuccessful artists and the nonartist controls. Eighty percent of the successful artists gave responses containing primary process material, whereas less than 16% of the unsuccessful group gave a substantial number of these responses. Dudek added that those "bad," that is, unsuccessful, artists who did give more primary process responses were independently rated as having the greatest potential of becoming good, that is, successful.

Successful artists gave responses that reflected primitive sexual or aggressive content and bizarre elaboration. Confabulatory responses with good form level occurred frequently in the records of the successful artists. Dudek reported that the tone of these embellished and combinatory responses was generally positive and constructive, a finding that was supported by De Sluttitel and Sorribas (1972) who found creative combinatory responses with positive content in the records of artists. Some examples of these responses are given below.

Card II, given by a highly talented sculptor whose work hangs in several outstanding modern museums of art: "Suggests to me fire and water. The central part like the calyx of a flower which is quite cool, yet it is surrounded by fire which mixes in through this mistlike form and emerges as fire on the upper side too. But this mixture of fire and water fuses well in that they merge."

Card IX, given by a talented painter: "A yearning sort of feeling; birth, something attempted to move through this very small channel and being closed in upon by many forms. Some of it has managed to get through and then to find some sort of haven or peace in that upper area. The feeling of something attempting to be born. Feeling of the process of birth in the first stages. The pastel form might be a child still in his mother's womb" [p. 545].

In any context, such responses would surely be scored as confabulations, formless M's, and overly abstract symbolizations, suggesting a potential, if not actual, psychotic regression.

Dudek and Chamberland-Bouhaduna (1982) compared the extent of primary process Rorschach manifestations between two groups of artists, one renowned and the other students. Using Holt's PRIPRO system, the researchers found no difference between the two groups in the total amount of primary process content (Levels 1 and 2). The mature artists, however, gave more primary process content per response and more responses characterized by Holt's contradiction of reality score (Ctr-R 1&2). Recall that this score included responses in which subjects attempt to deliberately mold the inkblot into what they want it to be, as exemplified by the response, "I'm going to make this one colorful, full of rich purple hues, even though it is really just grey." Contradictions in reality can also include unlikely or inappropriate combinations of images and actions, much like the type of incongruous combinations responses, in which animals or people are performing inappropriate activities. At the same time, the renowned artists also showed more efficient and adaptive defenses (Defense Efficiency), a higher F+%, and an overall greater capacity for regression in the service of the ego (Adaptive Regression).

Other researchers have demonstrated that creative, intelligent people may produce very original, elaborate, and unorthodox responses that may be mistaken for psychotic thinking (Barrett, 1957; Gallagher and Crowder, 1957; Selig, 1958; Gallucci, 1989). Both Selig and Gallucci found a high incidence of what appeared to be disturbed thinking in the records of highly intelligent subjects. Gallucci administered the Rorschach to 72 adolescents with IQs greater than 135 and found that these subjects tended to give a high number of DVs, DRs, Dds, and X-responses. More impressively, 72% of these adolescents, who did not differ from a normal control group on psychiatric symptom checklists, were positive on the SCZI. The results seem to suggest that highly intelligent subjects may encode and process information in unusual ways, and that divergent responses may often appear to be less in line with conventional reality.

Franklin and Cornell (1997) extended this paradigm by comparing the Rorschachs of 43 girls who gained early admission to college (mean age = 14) to 19 similarly-aged gifted high school girls. The accelerated admission girls had significantly higher average SCZIs and DEPIs than the comparison group. To put this in context, 34% of the accelerated subjects had a SCZI of 4 or higher versus only 10% of the comparison group. Keep in mind that none of Exner's normative sample of youngsters between the ages of 12 and 16 (N=585) had a SCZI of 4 or greater! Furthermore X+% was low and X–% high in both groups. Forty-two percent of the accelerated group, versus 16% of the comparison subjects, gave M– responses. Nevertheless, despite these ominous findings, both groups had fairly low WSUM 6 totals, and only one subject from the combined sample had more than one Level 2 special score. Franklin and Cornell suggested that the low incidence of Level 2 scores may differentiate these creative and intelligent subjects from those suffering from psychopathology.

What makes these findings all the more important is that the researchers found that the SCZI correlated positively with a number of measures of social and emotional maturity in their index group. They were independently rated as more emotionally mature, socially competent, flexible, independent, and optimistic. The unconventional nature of their approach to the Rorschach was best typified by the response of one young subject who began the test by announcing, "I could say a bat, but everyone sees a bat, so I won't" (p. 195).

Based on the above findings, we would not be surprised to find primary process content, formal signs of thought disorder, and lower form level in the records of creative individuals. However, we would also not expect to find evidence of more severe indices of disordered thinking. Thought disordered responses, when they were given, would be milder and occur in the context containment and control, benign or creative thematic material, and possibly some good Ms.

THE RORSCHACH OF LINUS PAULING

Studying the Rorschach responses of one scientific luminary allows us to examine whether these characteristics are accurate when applied to a single case. The figure is Linus Pauling, heralded as one of the most distinguished scientists of the past century (Goertzel and Goertzel, 1995). An exceptionally intelligent and creative thinker, Pauling won two Nobel Prizes for his extraordinary contributions. Linus agreed to be a subject in two Rorschach studies concerning personality characteristics among scientists (Roe, 1952; Eiduson, 1962). His original Rorschach became part of the public record when it was published in a recent chapter which used his Rorschach to gain insight into his personality makeup (Gacono, DeCato, and Goertzel, 1997).

Before commenting on the issues of creativity versus thought disorder in Pauling's Rorschach, it is important to acknowledge several sources of error inherent in the analysis of his protocol. To begin with, Pauling took the Rorschach under experimental, as opposed to clinical, conditions, which may well have affected his response productivity and threshold for giving unusual responses. We have no way of knowing whether Pauling would have produced this same type of record under clinical conditions. It is not even clear what instructions he was given for taking the Rorschach. In other words, the context of the testing situation and instructions given may have affected his willingness or reluctance to respond openly and spontaneously. Additionally, Pauling gave an inordinate number of responses (65), which should ratchet down, slightly, our sensitivity and readiness to interpret pathology in this very dilated record. Furthermore, all efforts to interpret Pauling's Rorschach are hampered by a poor inquiry and questionable verbatim transcription, making valid scoring extremely difficult. Scoring deviant types of verbalization requires a verbatim record and careful inquiry in order to evaluate the extent and nature of the pathological thought processes involved.

Structural Data

Gacono et al. scored Pauling's lengthy protocol according to the Comprehensive System. Table 17-1 summarizes the structural data pertaining to the scoring of thought disorder. Pauling's form level percentages were uniformly low (X + % = 31; F + % = 35; X − % = 25) as measured by the Comprehensive System, suggesting at the very least a marked propensity to view the world in an idiosyncratic manner and, at worst, a tendency toward distortion of reality. However, these low form level percentages are not inconsistent with some of the findings reviewed above. Furthermore, the fact that Pauling's SCZI was 3 and that 38% of his responses contained unusual and even bizarre-sounding responses with accompanying thought disorder scores should also come as no surprise.

If the presence of scorable signs of thought disorder in his record is not surprising, then what would distinguish Pauling's Rorschach from that given by a psychotic individual? Do we find the features, reported in the literature, that distinguish creativity from craziness? Likewise, is there anything about Pauling's Rorschach that does not fit with what we might have predicted?

I believe there are aspects of Pauling's Rorschach that run contrary to empirically based expectations about creative processes, that raise further questions about how to make sense of his complex Rorschach. For example, one is hard pressed to find evidence supporting the kind of "relatively mature processes" (Hersch, 1962), or ego strength, that enables a creative person to regress in an adaptive manner. A qualitative analysis of Pauling's thought disordered responses suggests that, on the average, his primary process content and formal variables exceeded his capacity to control and adaptively contain this material. Despite ample evidence of his intellectual prowess and vast fund of literary and scientific knowledge, the bizarre nature of many of his responses does not seem to be counterbalanced by successful containing or contextualizing efforts. Instead, there is a great deal of intellectualizing that is not supported by adequate form or convincing rationale. Everything we have learned in this chapter suggests that creative individuals are distinguished by their abilities to play with primitive ideas and unconventional forms of logic while simultaneously demonstrating a number of critical ego strengths.

Regarding additional discontinuities, unlike Hersch's artists, Pauling's Rorschach lacks evidence of other indications of ego strength such as good Ms and form-dominated responses. Of his seven Ms, only one was given

Table 17-1 Summary of CS Critical Special Scores Indices for
Pauling's Rorschach

Thought Disorder Measure	Score
SCZI	3
SUM6	27
WSUM6	90
Percent responses with critical special scores	42%
Percent Level 1 special scores	67%
Percent Level 2 special scores	33%
Percent Deviant Verbalizations (DV & DR)	52%
Percent Inappropriate Combinations (INCOM, FABCOM, CONTAM)	37%
Percent Inappropriate Logic (ALOG)	11%
X + %	31%
F + %	35%
X – %	25%
M–	2

From Gacono et al. (1997).

with good form level, while two were minus and four unusual. Furthermore, Pauling gave 20 shading and color responses, only four of which were form-dominated. The majority were dominated by either color or shading, with form a secondary determinant. Finally, unlike the intelligent, creative subjects in Franklin and Cornell's study (1997), whose critical special scores were almost without exception Level 1 in severity, 33% of Pauling's critical special scores were Level 2. And what is more, according to Gacono's scoring, Pauling's record contains four ALOGs. While some may feel that these ALOGs were overscored (Levy and Holzman, personal communication, September 3, 1998), I believe that Pauling gave at least one response with a marked tendency toward autistic logic. One example of scorable idiosyncratic logic was his response to Card II below (with scoring from PRIPRO, TDI, and Comprehensive System):

II. 8) This reminds me of blood and the black of ink, carbon and the structure of graphite.
PRIPRO: Ag2R; VP2; Au lg1; Fa; Cx–I–; R–min (DD = 3.0; DE = –1.0)
TDI: Autistic logic-tend (.50);
CS: Wv+ C.C'Fu Bl, Art, Id 4.5 ALOG

E: (Rpts Ss response)
S: Structure, because I was thinking of carbon and I always think of structure. The straight lines in the little central figure are puzzling, because the general impression is curvature.

Although Pauling's creativity and intelligence may provide some explanation for his strikingly unusual Rorschach, these factors do not account for everything. DeCato's blind interpretation of Pauling's Rorschach (Gacono et al., 1997) highlighted the degree to which Pauling was given to "intermittent disruptions in reality testing" and "unrealistic and distorted thinking" (p. 424). Biographical knowledge of Pauling's life would not support the conclusion that he suffered from an underlying psychotic illness; however, factors other than psychosis, latent or manifest, may help explain how his Rorschach could be riddled with deviant thinking without evidence of sufficient moderating elements.[2]

There is considerable evidence from biographical sources (Goertzel, Goertzel, and Goertzel, 1980; Goertzel and Goertzel, 1995) that Pauling was an extremely narcissistic individual, who tended to overvalue his personal worth and seek approval from others for his accomplishments. A gifted and charismatic speaker, Pauling apparently loved to espouse his scientific and political views in front of admiring audiences. Interestingly, many of his Rorschach responses had an exhibitionistic quality, as if he were delighting in displaying his wit, intelligence, and unconventionality. At the same time, he did not appear particularly invested in explaining himself to the examiner (who, unfortunately, did not ask enough about his responses). Consider, for example, the following response to Card IV, in which Pauling seemed to exhibit his scientific knowledge in a self-absorbed manner:

IV. 23) A little group of very small dots that remind me of the spots on a Laue photograph that makes me think of a 2-dimensional lattice, of course a great number of ideas go through my head as a result of that.

PRIPRO: VP2; FV; Cx-I+; R-time (DD = 2.0; DE = 1.0)

TDI: Peculiar (.25);

CS: Ddo Fu Sc PER, DR2

E: (Rpts Ss response)
S: Laue was the one who got the Nobel prize for discovering X-ray diffraction by crystals.

---

2. I am indebted to Debbie Levy, Ph.D. and Phil Holzman, Ph.D. for their suggestions about applying the TDI to Pauling's Rorschach. It should be noted that Levy and Holzman scored Pauling's Rorschach and came up with a more conservative total TDI score (1.6) than I did (9.18). Their experience scoring the records of floridly psychotic subjects has surely given them a very critical eye and somewhat higher threshold for scoring thought disordered verbalizations on the Rorschach than the average clinician gen-

In addition to the scientific method of carefully testing hypotheses, Pauling utilized another approach to problem solving. This alternative strategy was characterized by his tendency to adopt quickly and fervently a stance that was not adequately supported by empirical evidence. At best, this strategy reflected his intuitive genius; at worst, it reflected his tendency to jump to biased conclusions while ignoring contradictory evidence. Pauling's rashness spawned an arrogant and iconoclastic attitude that led him to rebel against scientific and political authorities who did not subscribe to his vision of the truth. A number of his Rorschach responses seem to reflect this self-indulgent, solipsistic quality, reflecting his tendency to bend reality to fit his predilections. For example, Pauling's Card II response ("This reminds me of blood and the black of ink, carbon and the structure of graphite") is, at a minimum, not a very differentiated response; and most would agree that it reflects difficulties with affect integration and regulation. However, when the response was inquired into, Pauling responded "Structure, because I was thinking of carbon and I always think of structure." Scored as an ALOG (and more conservatively as a tendency toward Autistic logic on the TDI), this response reflects not simply his unconventional and perhaps strained reasoning, but also his tendency to perceive the world in an egocentric manner. He justified his response, not on the basis of aspects of external reality per se, but because he was simply thinking of it.

In a response on Card IV, Pauling saw a "carcass of an animal spread open." He went on to say, "I seem to see a cleaver, not in the picture but the act of cleaving is suggested to me. I must have seen a butcher cleave one open" (p. 439). Here again, we see a similar lack of objectivity, as Pauling based his response not on empirical data in the card but on a whim, something entirely subjective and not easily shared or validated by others. Thus, as suggested in chapter 15, narcissistic individuals may give thought-disordered responses because they either enjoy flouting reality or indulging themselves by shaping their perception of the external world or "the truth" into that which they wish it to be. However, Pauling's inclination towards self-indulgent subjectivism and idiosyncratic thinking was undergirded by his brilliance, which also enabled him spontaneously to create original ideas by using his intuition.

Although in some cases adaptive, Pauling's tendency to perceive the world according to his own inclinations may have also run him afoul of the scientific community in his impassioned support for a theory that was

---

erally possesses. In this regard, it is also interesting to note how Gacano, using the Comprehensive System, scored the record more liberally for thought disorder signs. The issue of thresholds is a critical one that can make it difficult to replicate findings from one research group to another.

not grounded in empirical evidence. I am speaking here of his commitment to the belief that megadoses of Vitamin C could prevent and treat a wide array of diseases. Not only did he extend his inferences beyond his area of expertise, but he also selectively sought out evidence to support his theory and minimized or viciously attacked findings that contradicted his beliefs. The Goertzels described his narcissistic rage against a colleague, Arthur Robinson, who released data that might have raised public doubts about Vitamin C. According to their report, Pauling

> demanded that Robinson immediately leave the building and not return for at least a year. He ordered Robinson to turn over all his research data, projects, and equipment to Pauling, and insisted that since the institute was named after him he was entitled to 100 percent of the research funds, leaving nothing for Robinson's research. Pauling was livid with rage when Robinson refused to give in to these demands. Claiming that Robinson's research was defective, he threatened to have the mice killed in order to prevent continuation of the experiment [Goertzel et al., 1980, p. 379].

Furthermore, Pauling's tendency to form rapid conclusions may have cost him in his pursuit of other scientific discoveries. According to the Goertzels, his rapid, highly individualized approach to problem solving was productive in many cases, but in others it led to major blunders. For example, they cite his work in the area of DNA, in which he "rushed into print with a paper that incorporated errors so basic that they should have been caught by any student who had mastered Pauling's introductory chemistry text" (Goertzel et al., 1980, p. 372).

These biographical vignettes may reflect his combined tendencies to develop ideas on the basis of inspired intuition, to rush to judgment, to cling tenaciously to conclusions that were not grounded in thoroughly researched observations, and to mount irrational attacks against those who did not adhere to his version of the truth. In the cases of both his DNA and Vitamin C research, Pauling may have formulated his conclusions in a rash and faulty manner, much like the style of reasoning he exhibited in some of his Rorschach responses. In fact, one might wonder whether his ALOG tendencies reflected this propensity to jump to conclusions that at times turned out to be ingenious and at other times biased, seemingly irrational, and not grounded in scientific fact.

In the end, we are left with an enigma. Pauling, the creative genius, produced a Rorschach with notable signs of thought disorder and insufficient signs of a directing ego or a capacity for adaptive regression. As I indicated earlier, I am by no means suggesting that Pauling was latently thought disordered; however, simply concluding that his idiosyncratic Rorschach is the product of "creativity" is not acceptable either. Thus, we are left with the stew of human complexity that does not lend itself well to unidimensional conclusions. Pauling was most likely a Janusian thinker, who was rather egocentric in the way he formulated his ideas. That this two-time Nobel Prize winner was capable of brilliance and creativity cannot be disputed. However, when he felt narcissistically threatened, his thinking could become idiosyncratic, irrational, and not well grounded in reality. Pauling may certainly not have characteristically "fallen" into the river of primary process experience, but at least his Rorschach suggests that he may not have always successfully "dived" into the depths either.

CHAPTER
18

FINAL THOUGHTS

Hermann Rorschach probably never intended for his inkblots to be used as a primary method for measuring, much less for diagnosing or studying, disordered thinking. He developed the Rorschach as a test of perceptual functioning, from which various aspects of behavior and personality structure could be inferred. However, in addition to its broad utility as a test of personality functioning and internal representation, the Rorschach has proven to be an enormously useful instrument for detecting disorders of thinking and for helping us conceptualize the different processes that underlie them.

As detailed in the chapters of this book, the Rorschach assessment of thought disorder has evolved through a series of approaches, each based on varying degrees of empirical and theoretical scaffolding. A variety of formal systems have been devised, and researchers have attempted to extend the boundaries of Rorschach thought disorder scoring to the understanding of object relations, transference phenomena, psychological development, differential diagnosis, and creativity. Three general approaches to using the Rorschach to assess disordered thinking can be identified: (1) a Global Sign approach, (2) a Differential Diagnostic Sign approach, and (3) a Conceptual approach. Each represents a more complex, comprehensive, and differentiated approach than the previous one, and each subsumes the strategies of the former.

GLOBAL SIGN APPROACH. Based on typical test signs, or scores, the Global Sign Approach is essentially binary and descriptive. It is binary in the sense that it focuses primarily on the presence or absence of thought disorder. Generally "thought disorder" is recognized as a static

346

entity that exists in an all or nothing form. Little attention is paid to the conditions under which thinking becomes disturbed. This approach is also descriptive in the sense that the presence of "thought disorder signs" simply implies to the diagnostician that the "subject may suffer from a thought disorder." The more signs, the greater the likelihood. Little if any attention is paid to the differential meaning or diagnostic implications of different thought disorder scores. Instead, reference is made to global descriptors such as "disorganized thinking" or "strained reasoning." Used in its most elementary, cookbook manner, the Comprehensive System lends itself to such a binary and descriptive approach.

DIFFERENTIAL DIAGNOSTIC SIGN APPROACH. Like the global sign approach, the Differential Diagnostic Sign Approach focuses on the quantitative measurement of thought disorder but goes a step further and emphasizes the qualitative differences in "thought disorder profiles" between different types of diagnostic entities, usually psychotic disorders. Represented primarily by the work of the TDI research group, the differential diagnostic sign approach is rooted in a nomothetic tradition that searches for markers that distinguish different diagnostic groups from one another. The contributions of this tradition are clear; disordered thinking is recognized both as existing along a continuum of severity and as manifesting itself differently in different clinical syndromes. Despite these contributions, clinicians are often left wondering what the scores themselves mean in terms of an individual patient's psychological functioning. Making conceptual sense of the different scores in terms of their psychological, as opposed to diagnostic, implications is typically beyond the scope of this tradition.

CONCEPTUAL APPROACH. Best represented by the contributions of Holt, Weiner, Athey, and Blatt, the Conceptual Approach is characterized by efforts to flesh out the meaning of thought disorder signs for an individual's adaptation. Unlike the differential sign approach, the mission of the conceptual approach is not differential diagnosis, although identifying differences between diagnostic groups is clearly of interest. Instead, conceptual approaches seek to broaden the understanding of intrapsychic and interpersonal implications of different types of thought disordered responses. The search for a deeper meaning and a broader understanding of what these responses suggest to us about how a person might think about herself, relate to others, or perceive his therapist is what interests clinicians the most. This is essentially the approach I found most lacking in the literature and the approach I wanted to emphasize in this book.

My interest in this third approach begs the question, "What is so important about an approach that emphasizes the conceptual understanding of different thought disorder scores?" After all, the approach I describe is less firmly rooted in a strict empirical tradition and, as such, remains open to critics who ask "where's the proof?" Furthermore, implicit in a conceptual approach is the expenditure of more time and effort—costly commodities that are hard to afford nowadays. In our current professional climate with its zeitgeist of fast and furious clinical work, where all of us are pressured to do less with each patient we see, an approach that emphasizes careful and in-depth understanding of an individual's thought processes might seem anachronistic. Yet it is precisely for this reason that an approach that values careful diagnostic assessment of psychological functioning and seeks to understand subtlety of meaning is critically important. Broadly speaking, the erosion of meaning and appreciation of complexity in the field of psychodiagnostic assessment is a grave threat not only to the profession but to the dignity and worth of the people we serve.

The conceptual approach is important because it reflects the inherent value of thorough diagnostic understanding. Nowhere is this value more eloquently articulated than in the wisdom of Paul Pruyser (1984), who tenaciously defended the traditional approach to diagnostic assessment cultivated by psychologists at the Menninger Clinic over many decades of work. Pruyser's words ring even more true today than at the time at which he wrote them.

> In the helping professions and especially in medicine, thoroughness is a value—a virtue—to be emulated; thoroughness, not from fear of malpractice suits or from ambition to get the institution's top job, but from the humanistic conviction that the patient is entitled to the best, and that anything shoddy is an offense to the patient's and physician's own dignity [Pruyser, 1984, p. 14].

Regarding the inherent complexity of human psychological functioning, Pruyser wrote, "The more we acknowledge that human problems of health and illness are typically complex, the more thoroughness and comprehensiveness should be our diagnostic reasoning" (p. 14). Pruyser also addressed the inherent pleasure that many of us derive in achieving an in-depth understanding of another human being:

> Within the limits of the professional and the patient's rights, no stone should be left unturned to foster the patient's (and doctor's) understanding of the ailment, the condition, or the problem. The patient is worth the effort, and diligence and zest in one's work, now experienced as a collaborative task, are the physician's professional *joie de vivre* [p. 14].

Careful understanding of the meaning of thought disorder scores is important also because of what the scores might tell us about the organizing principles of an individual's personality. Here I am reminded of Rapaport's rather abstruse, yet perspicacious, words that every aspect of behavior, "bears the imprint of the organization of the behaving personality, and permits—if felicitously chosen—of reconstruction of the specific organization principles of that personality" (Rapaport, 1950, p. 339).

These words describe a philosophy of inference making that underscores the essence of careful diagnostic work. Just as one cell contains the genetic blueprint that makes for a unique individual, one segment of behavior may similarly have generalizable significance and contain some broad organizing principles about how that person lives his or her life. But how do we label and understand the segment of behavior we choose? In terms of studying disturbances in thinking, do we simply label these as "thought disorder" and conclude that the person is "thought disordered" or "disorganized" in his thinking? If so, where do we take this static inference; what do we do with it; how do we "play" with it and enlarge it so that we get beyond the reified and monolithic concept of "thought disorder" to make broader and deeper inferences about the "organizing principles" of that individual's personality?

Say we're looking at the presence of FABCOMs in a record. Notice the difference, for example, if instead of labeling the behavior in question as "thought disorder," "strained reasoning," or even "combinatory thinking," we call it, instead, "the propensity to combine ideas and situations unrealistically or the tendency to base causality on contiguity and coincidence"; we are then in a better position to look at how this behavioral inclination might manifest itself in a variety of situations. For example, we can think about this individual's tendency to blur boundaries between different events, thoughts, people, and affect states, as the person relates things that typically do not go together. We might also wonder how this tendency would manifest itself in an intimate relationship, like psychotherapy. From here, we would naturally ask about transference implications.

The conceptual understanding of psychological implications of thought disorder scoring is consistent with the holistic approach to psychodiagnosis. In discussing implications for neuropsychology, Allen, Lewis, Peebles, and Pruyser (1986) advocated taking a holistic approach to understanding the relationship between mind and body. These authors reviewed the various philosophical underpinnings of different traditions in the neurosciences. They argued against the position of Reductionistic Monism, whereby the complex relationship between mind and body is reduced to either all of one or the other. In particular, they criticized neuropsychological interpretations that excluded the realm of mental functioning and avoided dealing with conceptual difficulties in the relationship between brain and mind by focusing only on the observable relationship between brain and behavior. According to Allen et al. (1986):

> [T]he neuropsychologist's task is to go beyond the assessment of organic contributions to impairment and to specify as far as possible the manner in which neuropsychological and psychological considerations are intertwined for a given patient. Perforce, we often employ the language of interactionism, while aiming for the best holistic synthesis [p. 17].

The implications for the assessment and interpretation of disordered thinking are evident. Whether one takes a global or a differential diagnostic sign approach, or whether one views disorders of thinking as neurocognitive anomalies in associative semantic and working memory (Spitzer, 1997) or temporal lobe pathology (Nestor et al., 1998), effective clinical psychodiagnostic assessment begs for the translation of static conclusions into action implications for how the individual may experience the world and live his or her life.

The shift from relying on static scores or test signs to "breathing" meaningful life into them can be compared to Schafer's concept of "action language" (1976). Objecting to the language of impersonal forces and structures of psychoanalytic metapsychology, Schafer proposed a new language for psychoanalysis, in which every psychological process, event, experience, response, or other item of behavior should be conceived as an action. Schafer believed that actions should not be explained in terms of causes, but in terms of reasons. Unlike causes, which rely on some force or circumstance that precedes the action, reasons refer to personal meanings of the action. Harty (1986) applied Schafer's concepts to psychological testing reports and argued that the overly abstract, experience-distant language of impersonal forces and structures is unnecessary and inappropriate when trying to understand what patients are doing.

Although the focus in this book has been a narrow one, examining the meaning of various types of disordered thinking, I am a strong advocate for understanding the significance of any aspect of testing-derived behavior in the larger context of the testing battery. Looking for a convergence of signs from different tests and behavioral manifestations between patient and examiner is the sine qua non of competent psychodiagnostic work. Furthermore, we should never be content in making the conclusion that a patient's thinking is disordered, or even that the disorder is characterized primarily by one type or another. An individual's thinking is rarely disturbed across the board, in every setting and situation. Psychodiagnosticians can provide invaluable service by specifying not only whether the patient's thinking is disturbed, how disturbed it is, or even the meaning of the particular form of disturbance, but ultimately the conditions under which the patient's thinking regresses.

In essence, the finding that the patient has a "thought disorder" should not be viewed as the endpoint of a search but as a springboard for a set of new questions, each more refined than the other, regarding the nature of the thought disturbance, how severe it is, when it is most likely to occur, what it might reveal about the patient's ego functioning, self-experience, and object relations, and how the patient reacts to these slippages in language or reasoning. This last question is particularly important if one remembers Harrow and Quinlin's concept of "impaired perspective," or the capacity to discern whether or not one is making sense and can be understood by the listener. Clearly the ability to maintain this critical perspective has significant prognostic implications. In regard to one's ability to take distance from one's responses, will a person's comments about and reaction to his or her thought disordered responses give us clues about creative potential, whether they are willingly "diving" or "falling" into the river of primary process?

Finally, we should venture to ask whether patients' disordered thinking might serve them in some way. If we take a holistic approach which assumes that behavior has meaning for the individual and can be used for adaptive and defensive purposes, then all behavior, including disorders in thinking, might aid us in our search for meaning and a deeper understanding of the puzzle of the personality.

Problems in the Rorschach Assessment and Interpretation of Disordered Thinking

The foregoing recommendations notwithstanding, what is the cost and what are the problems in attempting to make such a careful analysis of the meaning and implications of an individual's disordered Rorschach responses? I think there are a number that are worth mentioning here.

Specificity of Diagnosis and Meaning

First, there is the issue of specificity. I am not talking simply about the old issue of whether disordered thinking is specific to a particular clinical syndrome, but the issue of whether specific thought disorder signs always have specific differential diagnostic significance or specific psychological meanings. Although there are broad guidelines for associating certain types of scores with certain diagnoses or meaningful interpretations, there is clearly no isomorphic relationship that exists between scoring type and implication. Consider, for example, that different people can produce confabulations or combinatory responses for different reasons. Diagnostically, they may be bipolar, borderline, traumatized, or suffer from some combination of the above. Likewise, the meaning of these processes may differ from one person to the next. On the other hand, one individual may produce a variety of thought disorder signs/scores for essentially the *same* reason. For example, consider the acutely psychotic individual who produces a record so full of idiosyncratic and bizarre ideas and verbiage that it becomes almost impossible to score, much less tease out the significance of different types of thought disturbances. The following response to Card II was given by such an acutely psychotic patient.

> This reminds me of a rocket ship for some reason. This is the gas here. This is the nose of the cone. These two remind me of outer space. I used to see these horses with wings flying through the air, and things like that remind me of outer space. I want to read books on Greek mythology and things like that. Now this reminds me of blood, I must be honest. And this right here would be the name of the company that built the space ship. That's about all. (INQ—Outline the rocket ship?) OK, here are the sides, this is the cone, here's the nose. These two symbols remind me of outer space, because they are so dangling, like they are just floating in the air. (INQ—What would those two things be?) Just the sky . . . (INQ—You saw the gas?) Oh, yeah, my first impression was gas and my second was blood. (INQ—What made it look like gas?) I don't know, it kind of just doesn't have any specific design. Gas is something you can't see and when you see something like this it reminds me of gas in a way, because it looks intangible. I can't really apply the symbolism to anything except blood or gas.

Where does one begin with such a response? There is evidence of confabulatory thinking in the form of absurd overspecificity ("and right here would probably be the name of the company that built the space ship"); combinative thinking ("horses with wings flying through the air"); autistic logic ("These two symbols remind me of outer space, *because* they are so dangling, like they are just floating in the air"); peculiar verbalization ("the nose of the cone" and "it reminds me of gas in a way, because it looks intangible"); idiosyncratic image symbolism ("These two symbols remind me of outer space"); and frank looseness ("I want to read books on Greek mythology and things like that"). What we have in this extended response is the Rorschach equivalent of someone mixing the various colors on a pallet together to form black. The distinctive character of each individual color is lost in the blackness of the mixture. Likewise, it seems almost futile to try to tease apart the implications and meanings of the six varieties of disordered thinking in this one response. Specific clues about the nature of the underlying illness type seem to have been largely obscured by the florid nature of the psychotic process. The most economical interpretation is that the acuity of psychotic disorganization has left the patient massively confused, unable to reason clearly, to conceptualize at appropriate levels of abstraction and objectivity, to bound his ideas adequately, and to step back and observe the severity of his impairment to communicate his ideas.

Scoring Threshold and Time Requirements

Although it is possible with practice for research teams to establish satisfactory interrater reliability in their scoring of thought disordered responses, this presents a potential problem for the average clinician attempting to do such scoring. First, it is time consuming to learn the intricacies of using scoring systems like the TDI or PRIPRO. Not only does it take time and practice to master the scoring, but applying these methods to individual records can be enormously time consuming. Few clinicians have the luxury of time to do this on a regular basis. Furthermore, even if a clinician has the time to both learn the techniques and apply them to his or her work, then there is the problem of scoring thresholds. In a critique of thought disorder scoring on the Rorschach, Frank (1994) pointed out that scorers differ in their tolerance of deviant thinking. What may strike one clinician as highly idiosyncratic may be assessed differently by another clinician. The developers of the TDI recommend that individuals who intend to use the instrument for research (and, I would argue, to achieve clinical mastery as well) calibrate their scoring to the threshold of the McLean Hospital research group by attending an intensive scoring workshop that they sponsor.

Empirical Studies

There are a number of areas that call for further empirical study both for heuristic purposes and to help with designing treatment interventions for patients with disorders in thinking. First, it would be useful to have more controlled studies addressing the question of how thought disorder appears differently in the Rorschach records of OCD patients; patients with borderline disorders, with and without a history of trauma; and traumatized patients, with and without comorbid borderline disorders. Furthermore, we should know more about the manifestations of disordered thinking in nonclinical subjects and devise scoring techniques sensitive to these more subtle emergences of deviant thinking.

Two promising areas of research should also be pursued, both of which have the potential to make more refined thought disorder scoring available to a wider range of clinicians. The TDI is probably the most sensitive and well researched of all current Rorschach systems for assessing disordered thought. However, the TDI was developed, and is currently used, with the Rapaport method of administering the Rorschach. Because the Rapaport method is used by a relatively small enclave of individuals nowadays, the vast majority of clinicians who use the Comprehensive System have been left either unaware of the TDI or aware of but unable to apply the TDI to their clinical Rorschachs. Developing a way of adapting the TDI for use with the Comprehensive System would have a great deal of practical value for those interested in the kind of diagnostic practice described in this book. Similarly, finding ways to simplify Holt's PRIPRO, especially his control and defense measures, so that they also could be used with the Comprehensive System would be of use to the clinician seeking to distinguish adaptive from maladaptive regression in his or her subjects' disordered responses.

If there is one particular area that has gotten short shrift in this book, it may have been the area of deviant or idiosyncratic verbalizations. Much has been said about the manifold implications of confabulatory, combinatory, contaminatory, and paleological thinking but less attention was devoted to understanding the subtleties of idiosyncratic verbalization response. When I contemplated writing a chapter addressing the nuances of peculiar and queer verbalizations, I soon realized how this aspect of "thought disorder" occupies a borderland between psychiatry, linguistics, and neuropsychology. Each field may attempt to lay claim to an exclusive understanding of the nature of deviant forms of verbalization, whether based in psychological, linguistic, or neurocognitive terminology. One useful effort to synthesize these areas when focusing on verbalization is the work of Perry et al. (1996), who proposed a system for classifying linguistic and perseveration errors on the Rorschach.

CONCLUSION

Before closing with a personal statement, I want to acknowledge for a last time the seminal contributions to this area in the field of psychodiagnostic testing.

Hermann Rorschach introduced the idea that the nature of thought organization could be assessed by using the inkblots. Rapaport, Gill, and Schafer elevated this idea and developed an approach to categorizing and explaining the psychological rationale of Rorschach manifestations of disordered thinking. Holt applied psychoanalytic theory to Rapaport's structural scaffolding, further systematized it, and conceptualized manifestations of thought disorder on the Rorschach as not simply signs of ego weaknesses but as harbingers of possible creative regression as well. Stauffacher and Watkins, and later Schuldberg and Boster, took Rapaport's rich clinical categories of Rorschach thought disorder and made them both more quantifiable and conceptually understandable. Weiner and Exner operationalized and simplified Rapaport's categories and packaged them in a more user-friendly form. Johnston and Holzman took Stauffacher and Watkin's Delta Index and added methodological sophistication and empirical rigor to identify qualitative differences in the thought disorder profiles of patients suffering from different types of psychotic syndromes. Athey, Blatt, and Ritzler broadened static categories of thought disorder and imbued them with clinically meaningful implications. Finally, Leichtman added a much needed developmental perspective to our understanding of thought disordered responses on the Rorschach. Each of these figures contributed something unique to the unraveling of the tangles of disordered thinking and helped us understand how the Rorschach may offer valuable clues to making sense of what at first appears to be nonsense.

Although I do not advocate eclecticism for its own sake, I do believe it is important for students and clinicians alike to be familiar with the work of each of these individuals. In today's pressured professional and academic climates, however, some may ask, what is lost by not knowing about Rapaport's definition of confabulation, Holt's concept of adaptive regression, Weiner's clarity in defining the varieties of impairments in reasoning, Athey's creative endeavor to relate Rorschach thought disorder scores to transference paradigms, and, finally, the TDI research on differential diagnosis? I believe much is lost, because it has been my experience that integrating these concepts enriches significantly our diagnostic work by helping our patients feel understood, by answering the complex questions that our referring colleagues pose to us, and, last but not least, to paraphrase Pruyser, by contributing to our professional joie de vivre.

REFERENCES

Abraham, P. P., Lewis, M. G., Lepisto, B. L. & Nahabedian, C. (1993), Rudimentary origins of obsessive-compulsive disorder reflected in Rorschach records of adolescents. *British Journal of Projective Psychology*, 38:2–8.

Achkova, M. (1976), Neurotic-like and psychopathic-like forms of schizophrenia in children and teenagers (in Bulgarian). *Nevrologia, Psikhiatria i Neurokhirurgia (Sofia)*, 15:326–332.

Aita, J., Reitan, R. & Ruth, J. (1947), Rorschach's test as a diagnostic aid in brain injury. *American Journal of Psychiatry*, 103:770–779.

Akiskal, H. S. & Puzantian, V. R. (1979). Psychotic forms of depression and mania. *Psychiatric Clinics of North America*, 2:419–440.

———— (1981), Subaffective disorders: Dysthymic, cyclothymic and bipolar II disorders in the "borderline" realm. *Psychiatric Clinics of North America*, 4:25–46.

———— Chen, S. E., Davis, G. G., Puzantian, V. R., Kashgarian, M. & Bolinger, J. M. (1985), Borderline: An adjective in search of a noun. *Journal of Clinical Psychiatry*, 46:41–48.

Alexander, M. P. (1997), Aphasia: Clinical and anatomic aspects. In: *Behavioral Neurology and Neuropsychology*, ed. T. E. Feinberg & M. J. Farah. New York: McGraw-Hill, pp. 133–149.

Allen, J., Lewis, L., Peebles, M. J. & Pruyser, P. W. (1986), Neuropsychological assessment in a psychoanalytic setting: The mind-body problem in clinical practice. *Bulletin of the Menninger Clinic*, 50:5–21.

Allison, J. (1962), Adaptive regression and intense religious experiences. *Journal of Nervous and Mental Disease*, 145:452–463.

———— Blatt, S. J. & Zimet, C. N. (1968), *The Interpretation of Psychological Tests*. New York: Harper & Row.

American Heritage Dictionary of the English Language (1981), Boston: Houghton Mifflin.

American Psychiatric Association (1994), *Diagnostic and Statistical Manual of Mental Disorders*, 4th ed. Washington, DC: Author.

Ames, L. B., Learned, J., Metraux, R. W. & Walker, R. N. (1952), *Child Rorschach Responses*. New York: Paul B. Hoeber.

Andreasen, N. C. (1976), Do depressed patients show thought disorder? *Journal of Nervous and Mental Disease*, 163:186–192.

———— (1978), *The Scale for the Assessment of Thought, Language, and Communication (TLC)*. Iowa City: University of Iowa Press.

———— (1979a), Thought, language, and communication disorders, I: Clinical assessment, definition of terms, and evaluation of their reliability. *Archives of General Psychiatry*, 36:1315–1321.

———— (1979b), Thought, language, and communication disorders, II: Diagnostic significance. *Archives of General Psychiatry*, 36:1325–1330.

———— (1980), Mania and creativity. In: *Mania: An Evolving Concept*, ed. R. H. Belmaker & H. M. Van Praag. New York: Spectrum, pp. 377–386.

———— (1982), Negative symptoms in schizophrenia. *Archives of General Psychiatry*, 39:784–788.

———— (1984), *Scale for the Assessment of Positive Symptoms (SAPS)*. Iowa City: University of Iowa Press.

———— (1986), Scale for the assessment of thought , language, and communication (TLC). *Schizophrenia Bulletin*, 12:473–482.

———— (1987), Creativity and mental illness: Prevalence rates in writers and their first-degree relatives. *American Journal of Psychiatry*, 144:1288–1292.

———— & Akiskal, H. S. (1983), The specificity of Bleulerian and Schneiderian symptoms: A critical reevaluation. *Psychiatric Clinics of North America*, 6:41–53.

———— & Canter, A. (1974), The creative writer: Psychiatric symptoms and family history. *Comprehensive Psychiatry*, 4:123–131.

———— & Grove, W. M. (1986), Thought, language, and communication in schizophrenia: Diagnosis and prognosis. *Schizophrenia Bulletin*, 12:348–359.

———— Hoffman, R. E. & Grove, W. M. (1985), Mapping abnormalities in language and cognition. In: *Controversies in Schizophrenia*, ed. M. Alpert. New York: Guilford Press, pp. 199–226.

———— & Pfohl, B. (1976), Linguistic analysis of speech in affective disorders. *Archives of General Psychiatry*, 33:1361–1367.

———— & Powers, P. S. (1974), Overinclusive thinking in mania and schizophrenia. *British Journal of Psychiatry*, 125:452–456.

———— & ———— (1975), Creativity and psychosis: An examination of conceptual style. *Archives of General Psychiatry*, 32:70–73.

———— Tsuang, M. T. & Canter, A. (1974), The significance of conceptual style. *Archives of General Psychiatry*, 32:70–73.

Angst, J., Felder, W. & Lohmeyer, B. (1980), Course of schizoaffective psychoses: Results of a follow-up study. *Schizophrenia Bulletin*, 6:579–585.

Appelbaum, S. A. (1975), *A Rorschach Test System for Understanding Personality*. Unpublished manuscript, The Menninger Clinic, Topeka, KS.

Arboleda, C. & Holzman, P. S. (1985), Thought disorder in children at risk for psychosis. *Archives of General Psychiatry*, 42:1004–1013.

Arieti, S. (1955), *Interpretation of Schizophrenia*. New York: Brunner.

———— (1964), The rise of creativity: From primary to tertiary process. *Contemporary Psychoanalysis*, 1:51–68.

———— (1967), *The Intrapsychic Self: Feeling and Cognition in Health and Mental Illness*. New York: Basic Books.

———— (1974), *Interpretation of Schizophrenia*, 2nd ed. New York: Basic Books.

———— (1976), *Creativity: The Magic Synthesis*. New York: Basic Books.

Arlow, J. A. & Brenner, C. (1964), *Psychoanalytic Concepts and the Structural Theory*. New York: International Universities Press.

Armstrong, J. (1991), The psychological organization of multiple personality disordered patients as revealed in psychological testing. *Psychiatric Clinics of North America*, 14:533–546.

——— (1994a), Reflections on multiple personality disorder as a developmentally complex adaptation. *The Psychoanalytic Study of the Child*, 49:349–370. New Haven, CT: Yale University Press.

——— (1994b), Disordered thinking, disordered reality: Issues and insights from dissociative and traumatized patients. Presented at Thought Disorder Conference, The Menninger Clinic, Topeka, KS.

——— & Lowenstein, R. J. (1990), Characteristics of patients with multiple personality and dissociative disorders on psychological testing. *Journal of Nervous and Mental Diseases*, 178:448–454.

——— Silberg, J. L. & Parente, F. J. (1986), Patterns of thought disorder on psychological testing: Implications for adolescent psychopathology. *Journal of Nervous and Mental Disease*, 174:448–456.

Arnason, H. H. (1977), *The History of Modern Art: Paintings, Sculpture, and Architecture*. New York: Harry N. Abrams, p. 359.

Arndt, S., Alliger, R. J. & Andreasen, N. C. (1991), The distinction of positive and negative symptoms: The failure of a two-dimensional model. *British Journal of Psychiatry*, 158:317–320.

Arnold, F. & Saunders, E. (1989), Reframing borderline disorder: Etiology, conceptualization, and treatment. Presented at the Harvard Medical School, Cambridge.

Arnow, D. & Cooper, S. (1988), Toward a Rorschach psychology of the self. In: *Primitive Mental States and the Rorschach*, ed. H. D. Lerner & P. M. Lerner. New York: International Universities Press, pp. 53–70.

Aronow, E., Reznikoff, M. & Moreland, K. (1994), *The Rorschach Technique: Perceptual Basics, Content Interpretations, and Applications*. Boston: Allyn and Bacon.

Astrup, K. & Noreik, K. (1966), *Functional Psychosis: Diagnosis and Prognosis Models*. Springfield, IL: Thomas.

Athey, G. I. (1974), Schizophrenia thought organization, object relations, and the Rorschach test. *Bulletin of the Menninger Clinic*, 38:406–429.

——— (1986), Rorschach thought organization and transference enactment in the patient-examiner relationship. In: *Assessing Object Relations Phenomena*, ed. M. Kissen. Madison, CT: International Universities Press, pp. 19–50.

——— Colson, D. & Kleiger, J. H. (1992), *Manual for Scoring Thought Disorder on the Rorschach*. Unpublished 5th draft, The Menninger Clinic, Topeka, KS.

——— ——— & ——— (1993), *Manual for Scoring Thought Disorder on the Rorschach*. Unpublished manuscript, The Menninger Clinic, Topeka, KS.

——— Fleischer, J. & Coyne, L. (1980), Rorschach object representation as influenced by thought and affect organization. In: *Borderline Phenomena and the Rorschach Test*, ed. J. Kwawer, H. Lerner, P. Lerner & A. Sugarman. New York: International Universities Press, pp. 275–298.

Bachrach, H. (1968), Adaptive regression, empathy, and psychotherapy. *Psychotherapy: Theory, Practice, and Research*, 5:203–209.

Balint, M. (1942), Contributions to reality testing. *British Journal of Medical Psychology*, 19:201–214.

Barrett, H. O. (1957), An intensive study of 32 gifted children. *Personnel and Guidance Journal*, 36:192–194.

Beck, A. T. (1963), Thinking and depression: I. Idiosyncratic content and cognitive distortions. *Archives of General Psychiatry*, 9:36–45.

———— (1964), Thinking and depression: II. Theory and therapy. *Archives of General Psychiatry*, 10:561–571.

———— (1967), *Depression: Clinical, Experimental and Theoretical Aspects.* New York: Harper & Row.

———— (1971), Cognition, affect, and psychopathology. *Archives of General Psychiatry*, 24:495–500.

Beck, S. J. (1933), Configurational tendencies in Rorschach responses. *American Journal of Psychology*, 45:433–443.

———— (1938), Personality structure in schizophrenia: A Rorschach investigation in 81 patients and 64 controls. *Nervous and Mental Disorders Monograph*, 63:ix-88.

———— (1949), *Rorschach's Test, Vol. 1: Basic Processes,* 2nd ed. New York: Grune & Stratton.

———— Rabin, A. I., Thiesen, W. G., Molish, H. & Theftford, W. N. (1950), The normal personality as projected on the Rorschach. *Journal of Psychology*, 30:241–298.

———— Leavitt, E. E. & Molish, H. B. (1961), *Rorschach's Test Vol. 1: Basic Processes,* 3rd ed. New York: Grune & Stratton.

Becker, W. C. (1956), A genetic approach to the interpretation and evaluation of the process-reactive distinction in schizophrenia. *Journal of Abnormal and Social Psychology*, 53:229–236.

Bellak, L. (1949), A multiple-factor psychosomatic theory of schizophrenia. *Psychiatric Quarterly*, 23:730–750.

———— (1969), Research on ego function patterns. In: *The Schizophrenic Syndrome*, ed. L. Bellak & L. Lober. New York: Grune & Stratton.

Belmaker, R. H. & Van Praag, H. M., eds. (1980), *Mania: An Evolving Concept.* New York: Spectrum.

Benfari, R. C. & Calogeras, R. C. (1968), Levels of cognition and conscience typologies. *Journal of Projective Techniques and Personality Assessment*, 32:466–474.

Benjamin, J. D. (1944), A method for distinguishing and evaluating formal thinking disorders in schizophrenia. In: *Language and Thought in Schizophrenia*, ed. J. S. Kasinin. New York: Norton, pp. 65–90.

Beres, D. (1956), Ego deviation and the concept of schizophrenia. *The Psychoanalytic Study of the Child*, 11:164–235. New York: International Universities Press.

Berg, J. L., Packer, A. & Nunno, V. J. (1993), A Rorschach analysis: Parallel disturbance in thought and in self/object representation. *Journal of Personality Assessment*, 61:311–323.

Berg, M. (1984), Borderline psychopathology as displayed on psychological tests. *Journal of Personality Assessment*, 47:120–133.

Bergen, J. R. (1965), Pitch perception, imagery, and regression in the service of the ego. *Journal of Research in Music Education,* 13:15–32.

Berlyne, N. (1972), Confabulation. *British Journal of Psychiatry,* 120:31–39.

Bilder, R., & Goldberg, E. (1987), Motor perseverations in schizophrenia. *Archives of Clinical Neuropsychology,* 2:195–214.

Birnie, W. A. & Littman, S. K. (1978), Obsessionality and schizophrenia. *Canadian Psychiatric Association Journal,* 23:77–81.

Blatt, S. J. (1990), The Rorschach: A test of perception on an evaluation of representation. *Journal of Personality Assessment,* 55:394–416.

——— Allison, J. & Feirstein, A. (1969), The capacity to cope with cognitive complexity. *Journal of Personality,* 37:269–288.

——— & Ritzler, B. A. (1974), Thought disorder and boundary disturbances in psychosis. *Journal of Consulting and Clinical Psychology,* 42:370–381.

——— & Wild, C. (1976), *Schizophrenia: A Developmental Analysis.* New York: Academic Press.

——— Tuber, S. B. & Auerbach, J .S. (1990), Representation of interpersonal interactions on the Rorschach and level of psychopathology. *Journal of Personality Assessment,* 54:711–728.

Bleuler, E. (1911), *Dementia Praecox or the Group of Schizophrenias,* trans. J. Zinkin. New York: International Universities Press, 1950.

Bohm, E. (1958), *Rorschach Test Diagnosis.* New York: Grune & Stratton.

Braff, D. L. & Beck, A. T. (1974), Thinking disorder in depression. *Archives of General Psychiatry,* 31:456–459.

——— & Geyer, M. A. (1990), Sensorimotor gating and schizophrenia: Human and animal model studies. *Archives of General Psychiatry,* 47:181–188.

——— & Saccuzzo, D. P. (1981), Information processing dysfunction in paranois schizophrenia: A two-factor deficit. *American Journal of Psychiatry,* 138:1051–1056.

——— Grillon, C. & Geyer, M. A. (1992), Gating and habituation of the startle reflex in schizophrenic patients. *Archives of General Psychiatry,* 49:206–215.

——— Saccuzzo, D. P. & Geyer, M. A. (1991), Information processing dysfunctions in schizophrenia: Studies of visual backward masking, sensorimotor gating and habituation. In: *Handbook of Schizophrenia, Vol. 5: Neuropsychology, Psychophysiology, and Information Processing,* ed. S. Steinhauer, J. H. Gruzelier et al. Amsterdam: Elsevier, pp. 303–334.

Breuer, J. & Freud, S. (1893/1895), Studies on hysteria. *Standard Edition,* 2:1–311. London: Hogarth Press, 1955.

Briere, J. (1997), *Psychological Assessment of Adult Posttraumatic States.* Washington, DC: American Psychological Association.

Bumke, O. (1906), Die psychischen Zwanger-scheinungen (The manifestations of psychic compulsion). *Allgemeine Zeitschrift fur Psychiatrie und Psychische-Gerichtliche Medizine,* 63:138–148.

Buros, O. K. (1965), *The Sixth Mental Measurements Yearbook.* New York: Gryphon Press.

Burstein, A. G. & Loucks, S. (1989), *Rorschach Test: Scoring and Interpretation.* New York: Hemisphere Publishing.

Butcher, J. N., Graham, J. R., Williams, C. L. & Ben-Porath, Y. (1989), *Development and Use of the MMPI-2 Content Scales.* Minneapolis: University of Minnesota Press.

Butler, R. W., Jenkins, M. A., Geyer, A. A. & Braff, D. L. (1991), Wisconsin Card Sorting deficits and diminished sensorimotor gating in a discrete subgroup of schizophrenic patients. In: *Schizophrenia Research: Advances in Neuropsychiatry and Psychopharmacology, Vol. 1,* ed. C. A. Tamminga, S. C. Schultz et al. New York: Raven Press, pp. 163–168.

Bychowski, G. (1952), The problem of latent psychosis. *Journal of the American Psychoanalytic Association,* 1:484–503.

Cameron, N. (1938), Reasoning, regression and communication in schizophrenics. *Psychological Monographs,* 50:1–340.

———— (1939), Deterioration and regression in schizophrenic thinking. *Journal of Abnormal and Social Psychology,* 34:265–270.

Cancero, R. (1969), Clinical prediction of outcome in schizophrenia. *Comprehensive Psychiatry,* 10:349–354.

Carlson, E. B. & Armstrong, J. (1995), The diagnosis and assessment of dissociative disorders. In: *Dissociation: Clinical and Theoretical Perspectives,* ed. S. J. Lynn & J. L. Rhue. New York: Guilford Press, pp. 159–174.

Carpenter, J. T., Coleman, M. J., Waternaux, C., Perry, J., Wong, H., O'Brian, C. & Holzman, P. S. (1993). The Thought Disorder Index: Short for assessments. *Psychological Assessment,* 5:75–80.

Carpenter, W. T., Strauss, J. S. & Muleh, S. (1973), Are there pathognomic symptoms in schizophrenia? An empiric investigation of Schneider's first-rank symptoms. *Archives of General Psychiatry,* 28:847–852.

Carr, A. (1984), Content interpretation re: Salley and Teillings' "Dissociated rage attacks in a Vietnam veteran: A Rorschach study." *Journal of Personality Assessment,* 48:420–421.

———— & Goldstein, E. (1981), Approaches to the therapy of borderline condition by use of psychology tests. *Journal of Personality Assessment,* 45:563–574.

———— ———— Hunt, H. F. & Kernberg. O. F. (1979), Psychological tests and borderline patients. *Journal of Personality Assessment,* 43:582–590.

Carroll, B. J., Greden, J. F. & Feinberg, T. E. (1981), Neuroendocrine evaluation of depression in borderline patients. *Psychiatric Clinics of North America,* 4:89–99.

Carsky, M. & Bloomgarden, J. W. (1981), Subtyping in the borderline realm by means of Rorschach analysis. *Psychiatric Clinics of North America,* 4:101–116.

Carter, M. L. (1986), The assessment of thought deficit in psychotic unipolar depression and chronic paranoid schizophrenia. *Journal of Nervous and Mental Disease,* 174:336–341.

Cauwels, J. M. (1992), *Imbroglio: Rising to the Challenges of Borderline Personality Disorder.* New York: Norton.

Cerney, M. (1990), The Rorschach and traumatic loss: Can the presence of traumatic loss be detected from the Rorschach? *Journal of Personality Assessment,* 55:781–789.

Chaika, E. O. (1990), *Understanding Psychotic Speech: Beyond Freud and Chomisky.* Springfield: Thomas.

Chapman, L. & Chapman, J. P. (1973), *Disordered Thought in Schizophrenia.* New York: Appleton-Century-Croft.

——— & ——— (1988), The genesis of delusions. In: *Delusional Beliefs*, ed. T. Oltmanns & B. Maher. New York: Wiley.

——— ——— & Miller, E. N. (1982), Reliabilities and intercorrelations of eight measures of proneness to psychosis. *Journal of Consulting and Clinical Psychology*, 50:187–195.

——— ——— & Raulin, M. L. (1978), Body-image aberration in schizophrenia. *Journal of Abnormal Psychology*, 87:399–407.

——— Edell, W. S. & Chapman, J. P. (1980), Physical anhedonia, perceptual aberration and psychosis proneness. *Schizophrenia Bulletin*, 6:639–653.

Chopra, H. D. & Beatson, J. A. (1986), Psychotic symptoms in borderline personality disorder. *American Journal of Psychiatry*, 143:1605–1607.

Christensen, A. L. (1985), Acute cerebral disorders and the Rorschach test. Presented at Eighth European Conference. *International Neuropsychological Society*, June 12–15.

Claude, H., Vidart, L. & Longeut, Y. (1941), Le journal d'un schizoide: Réflexions sur les rapports de la psychasthénie, la schizoidie et la schizophrénie (The diary of a schizoid: Reflections on the relationship among psychasthenia, schizoidism, and schizophrenia). *Encéphale*, 2:323–338.

Clayton, P. J., Rodin, L. & Winokur, G. (1968), Family history studies: III. Schizoaffective disorder, clinical and genetic factors including a one to two year follow-up. *Comprehensive Psychiatry*, 9:31–79.

Cohen, J. H. (1960), An investigation of the relationship between adaptive regression, dogmatism, and creativity using the Rorschach and dogmatism scale. Unpublished doctoral dissertation, Michigan State University.

Coleman, M. J., Carpenter, J. T., Waternaux, C., Levy, D. L., Shenton, M. E., Perry, J., Medoff, D., Wong, H., Monoach, D., Meyer, P., O'Brian, C., Valentino, C., Robinson, D., Smith, M., Makowski, D. & Holzman, P. S. (1993), The thought disorder index: A reliability study. *Psychological Assessment*, 5:336–342.

——— Levy, D. L. & Lenzenweger, M. F. (1996), Thought disorder, perceptual aberrations, and schizotypy. *Journal of Abnormal Psychology*, 105:469–473.

Coonerty, S. (1986), An exploration of separation individuation in the borderline personality disorder. *Journal of Personality Assessment*, 50:501–511.

Cooper, S. (1983), An object relations view of borderline defenses: A Rorschach analysis. Unpublished manuscript.

Coursey, R. D. (1984), The dynamics of obsessive-compulsive disorder. In: *New Findings in Obsessive-Compulsive Disorder*, ed. T. R. Insel. Washington, DC: American Psychiatric Press, pp. 104–121.

Croughan, J. L., Welner, A. & Robins, E. (1974), The group of schizoaffective and related psychoses: Critique, record, follow-up, and family studies: II. Record studies. *Archives of General Psychiatry*, 31:632–637.

Crow, T. J. (1980), Molecular pathology of schizophrenia: More than one dozen procedures. *British Medical Journal*, 280:66–68.

Dali, S. (1930), *La Femme Visible (The Visible Woman)*. Paris: Editions Surréalistes.

DeCato, C. M. (1993), Piotrowski's enduring contributions to the Rorschach: A review of Perceptanalysis. *Journal of Personality Assessment*, 61:584–595.

Deese, J. (1978), Thought into speech. *American Science*, 66:314–321.

―――― (1980), Pauses, prosody, and the demands of production in language. In: *Temporal Variables in Speech: Studies in Honor of Frieda Goldman-Eisler*, ed. H. W. Dechert & M. Raupach. The Hague: Mouton, pp. 69–84.

De Sluttitel, S. I. & Sorribas, E. (1972), The Rorschach Test in a research of artists. Unpublished manuscript.

Deutsch, H. (1942), Some forms of emotional disturbance and their relationships to schizophrenia. *Psychoanalytic Quarterly*, 11:301–321.

Donnelly, E. F., Waldman, I. N., Murphy, D. L., Wyatt, R. J. & Goodwinn, F. K. (1980), Primary affective disorder: Thought disorder in depression. *Journal of Abnormal Psychology*, 89:315–319.

Dorken, H. & Kral, V. A. (1952), The psychological differentiation of organic brain lesions and their localization by means of the Rorschach test. *American Journal of Psychiatry*, 108:764–770.

Dudek, S. (1968), Regression and creativity: A comparison of the Rorschach records of successful vs. unsuccessful painters and writers. *Journal of Nervous and Mental Disease*, 147:535–546.

―――― & Chamberland-Bouhaduna, G. (1982), Primary process in creative persons. *Journal of Personality Assessment*, 46:239–247.

Eckblad, M. & Chapman, L. J. (1983), Magical ideation as an indicator of schizotypy. *Journal of Consulting and Clinical Psychology*, 51:215–225.

Edell, W. (1987), Role of structure in disordered therapy in borderline and schizophrenia disorders. *Journal of Personality Assessment*, 51:23–41.

Eggers, C. (1969), Zwang und jugendliche psychosen. (Compulsions and juvenile psychoses.) *Praxis der Kinderpsychologie und Kinderpsychiatrie*, 118:202–208.

Eiduson, B. (1962), *Scientists: Their Psychological World*. New York: Basic Books.

Ellmann, R. (1959), *James Joyce*. New York: Oxford University Press.

Evans, R. B. & Marmorston, J. (1963), Psychological test signs of brain damage in cerebral thrombosis. *Psychological Reports*, 12:915–930.

―――― & ―――― (1964), Rorschach signs of brain damage in cerebral thrombosis. *Perceptual Motor Skills*, 18:977–988.

Exner, J. E. (1969), *The Rorschach Systems*. New York: Grune & Stratton.

―――― (1974), *The Rorschach, Vol. 1*. New York: Wiley.

―――― (1978), *The Rorschach, Vol. 2*. New York: Wiley.

―――― (1981), The response process and diagnostic efficiency. 10th International Rorschach Congress, Washington, DC.

―――― (1984), The Schizophrenia Index. *Alumni Newsletter*. Bayville, NY: Rorschach Workshops.

―――― (1986a), *The Rorschach, Vol. 1*, 2nd ed. New York: Wiley.

―――― (1986b), Some Rorschach data comparing schizophrenics with borderline and schizotypal personality disorders. *Journal of Personality Assessment*, 50:455–471.

―――― (1990), *Rorschach Workbook for the Comprehensive System*, 3rd ed. Asheville, NC: Rorschach Workshops.

—— (1991), *The Rorschach, Vol. 2*, 2nd ed. New York: Wiley.

—— (1993), *The Rorschach, Vol. 1*, 3rd ed. New York: Wiley.

—— & Weiner, I. B. (1982), *The Rorschach, Vol. 3*. New York: Wiley.

—— & —— (1995), *The Rorschach, Vol. 3*, 2nd ed. New York: Wiley.

—— —— & Schuyler, S. (1976), *A Rorschach Workbook for the Comprehensive System*. Bayville, NY: Rorschach Workshops.

—— Collogan, S. C., Hillman, L. B., Ritzler, B. A., Sciara, A. D. & Viglione, D. J. (1995), *A Rorschach Workbook for the Comprehensive System*, 4th ed. Ashville, NC: Rorschach Workshops.

Farris, M. (1988), Differential diagnoses for borderline and narcissistic personality disorders. In: *Primitive Mental States and the Rorschach*, ed. H. D. Lerner & P. M. Lerner. Madison, CT: International Universities Press, pp. 299–338.

Fear, C. F. & Healy, D. (1997), Probabilistic reasoning in obsessive-compulsive and delusional disorders. *Psychological Medicine*, 27:199–208.

Federn, P. (1952), *Ego Psychology and the Psychoses*. New York: Basic Books.

Feirstein, A. (1967), Personality correlates of tolerance for unrealistic experiences. *Journal of Consulting Psychology*, 31:387–395.

Fenton, W. S. & McGlashan, T. H. (1986), The prognostic significance of obsessive-compulsive symptoms in schizophrenia. *American Journal of Psychiatry*, 143:437–441.

Fish, F. J. (1962), *Schizophrenia*. Bristol: John Wright & Sons.

Fisher, S. (1955), Some observations suggested by the Rorschach test concerning the "ambulatory schizophrenic." *Psychiatric Quarterly Supplement*, 29:81–89.

—— & Cleveland, S. E. (1958), *Body Image and Personality*. New York: Van Nostrand.

Ford, M. (1946), Application of the Rorschach test to young children. *University of Minnesota, The Institute of Child Welfare Monograph Series*, 23. Minneapolis: University of Minnesota Press.

Forer, B. R. (1950), The latency of latent schizophrenia. *Journal of Projective Techniques*, 14:297–302.

Frances, A., Clarkin, J., Gilmore, M., Hurt, S. & Brown, R. (1984), Reliability of criteria for borderline personality disorder: A comparison of DSM-III and the Diagnostic Interview for Borderline Patients. *American Journal of Psychiatry*, 141:1080–1083.

Frank, G. (1994), On the assessment of thought disorder from the Rorschach. *Psychological Reports*, 75:375–383.

Franklin, K. W. & Cornell, D. G. (1997), Rorschach interpretation with high-ability adolescent females: psychopathology on creative thinking? *Journal of Personality Assessment*, 68:184–196.

Freeman, A. M., Kaplan, H. I. & Saddock, B. J. (1976), *Comprehensive Textbook of Psychiatry, Vol. 2*. Baltimore: Williams & Wilkins.

Freud, A. (1937), *The Ego and the Mechanisms of Defense*. New York: International Universities Press.

Freud, S. (1895), Project for a scientific psychology. *Standard Edition*, 1:283–397. London: Hogarth Press, 1966.

—— (1900), The interpretation of dreams. *Standard Edition*, 4 & 5. London: Hogarth Press, 1953.

—— (1905), Jokes and their relation to the unconscious. *Standard Edition*, 8:9–236. London: Hogarth Press, 1960.

—— (1908), Character and anal erotism. *Standard Edition*, 9:167–175. London: Hogarth Press, 1959.

—— (1910), Leonardo da Vinci and a memory of his childhood. *Standard Edition*, 11:63–137. London: Hogarth Press, 1957.

—— (1911), Psycho-analytic notes on an autobiographical account of a case of paranoia (dementia paranoides). *Standard Edition*, 12:1–82. London: Hogarth Press, 1958.

—— (1923), The ego and the id. *Standard Edition*, 19:12–66. London: Hogarth Press, 1961.

Friedman, H. (1952), Perceptual regression in schizophrenia: An hypothesis suggested by the use of the Rorschach test. *Journal of Genetic Psychology*, 87:63–98.

—— (1953), Perceptual regression in schizophrenia: An hypothesis suggested by the use of the Rorschach test. *Journal of Projective Techniques*, 17:171–185.

Frith, C. D. (1992), *The Cognitive Neuropsychology of Schizophrenia*. Hillsdale, NJ: Lawrence Erlbaum Associates.

Fuster, J. M. (1980), *The Prefrontal Cortex*. New York: Raven.

Gacono, C. B., DeCato, C. M. & Goertzel, T. G. (1997), Vitamin C or pure C: The Rorschach of Linus Pauling. In: *Contemporary Rorschach Interpretation*, ed. J. R. Meloy, M. W. Acklin, C. B. Gacono, J. F. Murray & C. A. Peterson. Mahwah, NJ: Lawrence Erlbaum Associates, pp. 421–451.

Gallagher, J. J. & Crowder, T. (1957), The adjustment of gifted children in the regular classroom. *Exceptional Children*, 23:306–319.

Gallucci, N. T. (1989), Personality assessment with children of superior intelligence: Divergence vs. psychopathology. *Journal of Personality Assessment*, 53:749–760.

Gartner, J., Hurt, S. & Gartner, A. (1989), Psychological test signs of borderline personality disorder: A review of the empirical literature. *Journal of Personality Assessment*, 53:423–441.

Gerson, S. N., Benson, D. F. & Frazier, S. H. (1977), Diagnosis: Schizophrenia versus posterior aphasia. *American Journal of Psychiatry*, 134:966–969.

Glasner, S. (1966), Benign paralogical thinking. *Archives of General Psychiatry*, 14:94–99.

Goertzel, T. & Goertzel, B. (1995), *Linus Pauling: A Life in Science and Politics*. New York: Basic Books.

—— Goertzel, M. G. & Goertzel, V. (1980), Linus Pauling: The scientist as crusader. *The Antioch Review*, 38:371–382.

Goldberg, L. R. (1965), Diagnosticians vs. diagnostic signs: The diagnosis of psychosis vs. neurosis from the MMPI. *Psychological Monographs*, 79:1–29.

Goldberger, L. (1961), Reactions to perceptual isolation and Rorschach manifestations of the primary process. *Journal of Projective Techniques*, 25:287–302.

Goldfried, M. R., Stricker, G. & Weiner, I. B. (1971), *Rorschach Handbook of Clinical and Research Application*. Englewood Cliffs, NJ: Prentice-Hall.

Goldman-Rakic, P. S. (1992), Working memory and the mind. *Scientific American*, Special Issue:111–117.

Goldstein, K. (1939), The significance of special mental tests for diagnosis and prognosis in schizophrenia. *American Journal of Psychiatry*, 96:575–588.

———— & Scheerer, M. (1941), Abstract and concrete behavior: An experimental study with special tests. *Psychological Monographs*, 53:1–151.

Goodglass, H. & Kaplan, E. (1983), *The Assessment of Aphasia and Related Disorders*, 2nd ed. Philadelphia: Lea & Febiger.

Goodwin, J., Cheeves, K. & Connell, V. (1990), Borderline and other severe symptoms in adult survivors of incestuous abuse. *Psychiatric Annals*, 20: 22–32.

Gordon, A. (1926), Obsessions in their relation to psychoses. *American Journal of Psychiatry*, 5:647–659.

Gorham, D. R. (1956), Use of the proverbs test for differentiating schizophrenics from normals. *Journal of Consulting Psychology*, 20:435–440.

Grala, C. (1980), The concept of splitting and its manifestations on the Rorschach test. *Bulletin of the Menninger Clinic*, 44:253–271.

Gray, J. J. (1969), The effect of productivity on primary process and creativity. *Journal of Projective Techniques and Personality Assessment*, 33:213–218.

Grinker, R. R. (1979), Diagnosis of borderlines: A discussion. *Schizophrenia Bulletin*, 5:47–52.

———— & Holzman, P. E. (1973), Schizophrenic pathology in young adults. *Archives of General Psychiatry*, 28:168–175.

———— Werble, B. & Drye, R. C. (1968), *The Borderline Syndrome*. New York: Basic Books.

Guirdham, A. (1935), The effects of experimental drive arousal on response to subliminal stimulation. Unpublished doctoral dissertation, New York University.

Gunderson, J. G. (1977), Characteristics of borderline. In: *Borderline Personality Disorders: The Concept, the Syndrome, the Patient*, ed. P. Hartocollis. New York: International Universities Press, pp. 173–192.

———— (1984), *Borderline Personality Disorder*. Washington: American Psychiatric Press.

———— & Kolb, J. (1978), Discriminating features of borderline patients. *American Journal of Psychiatry*, 135:792–796.

———— & Phillips, K. A. (1991), A current view of the interface between borderline personality disorder and depression. *American Journal of Psychiatry*, 148:967–975.

———— & Singer, M. T. (1975), Defining borderline patients: An overview. *American Journal of Psychiatry*, 132:1–10.

———— Kolb, J. E. & Austin, V. (1981), The diagnostic interview for borderline patients. *American Journal of Psychiatry*, 138:896–903.

Gur, R. E., Mozley, P. D., Resnick, S. M., Levick, S. & Gur, R. C. (1991), Relations among clinical scales in schizophrenia. *American Journal of Psychiatry*, 148:472–478.

Guttman, L. (1968), A general nonmetric technique for finding the smallest coordinate space for a configuration of points. *Psychometrika*, 33:469–506.

Haimo, S. F. & Holzman, P. S. (1979), Thought disorder in schizophrenics and normal controls: Social class and race differences. *Journal of Consulting and Clinical Psychology*, 47:963–967.

Hall, C. S. & Lindzey, G. (1957), *Theories of Personality*. New York: Wiley.

—— Hall, G. C. & Lavoie, P. (1968), Ideation in patients with unilateral or bilateral midline brain lesions. *Journal of Abnormal Psychology*, 73:526–531.

Hanfmann, E. & Kasanin, J. S. (1942), Conceptual thinking in schizophrenia. *Nervous and Mental Disorders Monograph Series*, 67:vii–115.

Harris, O. (1993), The prevalence of thought disorder in personality-disordered outpatients. *Journal of Personality Assessment*, 61:112–120.

Harrow, M. & Grossman, L. S. (1984), Outcome in schizoaffective disorders: A critical review and reevaluation of the literature. *Schizophrenia Bulletin*, 10:87–108.

—— & Quinlan, D. (1977), Is disordered thinking unique to schizophrenia? *Archives of General Psychiatry*, 34:15–21.

—— & —— (1985), *Disordered Thinking and Schizophrenic Psychopathology*. New York: Garden Press.

—— Grossman, L. S., Silverstein, M. L. & Meltzer, H. Y. (1980), Are manic patients thought disordered? *Scientific Proceedings of the American Psychiatric Association*. Washington, DC: American Psychiatric Association.

—— —— —— & —— (1982), Thought pathology in manic and schizophrenic patients. *Archives of General Psychiatry*, 39:665–671.

Hartman, W., Clark, M., Morgan, M., Dunn, V., Fine, A., Perry, G. & Winsch, D. (1990), Rorschach structure of a hospitalized sample of Vietnam veterans with PTSD. *Journal of Personality Assessment*, 54:149–159.

Hartmann, H. (1953), The metapsychology of schizophrenia. *The Psychoanalytic Study of the Child*, 8:177–198. New York: International Universities Press.

—— Kris, E. & Loewenstein, R. M. (1946), Comments on the formation of psychic structure. In *Psychological Monographs: No. 14. Papers on Psychoanalytic Psychology*. New York: International Universities Press, pp. 27–55.

Harty, M. K. (1986), Action language in the psychological test report. *Bulletin of the Menninger Clinic*, 50:456–463.

Harvey, P. D. & Neale, J. (1983), The specificity of thought disorder to schizophrenia: Research methods in their historical perspective. *Progress in Experimental Methods of Personality Research*, 12:153–180.

Heinrichs, T. F. (1964), Objective configural rules for discriminating MMPI profiles in a psychiatric population. *Journal of Clinical Psychology*, 20:157–159.

Herman, J. L. (1992), *Trauma and Recovery*. New York: Basic Books.

—— Perry, J. & van der Kolk, B. (1986), Childhood trauma in borderline personality disorder. *American Journal of Psychiatry*, 146:490–495.

Hersch, C. (1962), The cognitive functioning of the creative person: A developmental analysis. *Journal of Projective Techniques*, 26:193–200.

Hertz, M. R. (1938), Scoring the Rorschach ink-blot test. *Journal of Genetic Psychology*, 52:15–64.

—— (1942), The scoring of the Rorschach ink-blot method as developed by the Brush Foundation. *Rorschach Research Exchange*, 6:16–27.

—— (1977), The organization activity. In: *Rorschach Psychology*, 2nd ed., ed. M. A. Rickers-Ovsiankina. New York: Krieger, pp. 29–82.

—— (1986), Rorschachbound: A 50-year memoir. *Journal of Personality Assessment*, 50:396–416.

———— & Loehrke, L. M. (1954), The application of the Piotrowski and Hughes signs of organic defect to a group of patients suffering from post-traumatic encephalopathy. *Journal of Projective Techniques*, 18:183–196.

———— & Paolino, A. F. (1960), Rorschach indices of perceptual and conceptual disorganization. *Journal of Projective Techniques*, 24:370–388.

Hilsenroth, M. & Handler, L. (1995), A survey of graduate students' experiences, interests, and attitudes about learning the Rorschach. *Journal of Personality Assessment*, 64:243–257.

———— Fowler, J. C. & Pawader, J. R. (1998), The Rorschach Schizophrenia Index (SCZI): An examination of reliability, validity, and diagnostic efficiency. *Journal of Personality Assessment*, 70:514–534.

Hoch, P. & Polatin, P. (1949), Pseudoneurotic forms of schizophrenia. *Psychiatric Quarterly*, 33:248–276.

Hoffman, R. E., Stopek, S. & Andreasen, N. C. (1986), A comparative study of manic vs. schizophrenic speech disorganization. *Archives of General Psychiatry*, 43:831–838.

Holt, R. R. (1956), Gauging primary and secondary process in Rorschach responses. *Journal of Projective Techniques*, 20:14–25.

———— (1966), Measuring libidinal and aggressive motives and their controls by means of the Rorschach test. In: *Nebraska Symposium on Motivation*, ed. D. Levine. Lincoln: University of Nebraska Press.

———— (1967), The development of primary process: A structural view. In: *Motives and Thought: Psychoanalytic Essays in Honor of David Rapaport, Psychological Issues*, 5:345–383.

———— (1970), *Manual for the Scoring of Primary Process Manifestations and Their Controls in Rorschach Responses*. New York: Research Center for Mental Health.

———— (1977), A method for assessing primary process manifestations and their control in Rorschach responses. In: *Rorschach Psychology*, 2nd ed., ed. M. A. Rickers-Ovsiankina. New York: Krieger, pp. 375–420.

———— (1989), *Freud Reappraised: A Fresh Look at Psychoanalytic Theory*. New York: Guilford Press.

———— & Havel, J. (1960), A method for assessing primary and secondary process in the Rorschach. In: *Rorschach Psychology*, ed. M. A. Rickers-Ovsiankina. New York: Wiley, pp. 263–318.

———— Rapaport, D., Gill, M. & Schafer, R., eds. (1968), *Diagnostic Psychological Testing*, revised ed. New York: International Universities Press.

Holzman, P. S. (1978), Cognitive impairment and cognitive stability: Towards a theory of thought disorder. In: *Cognitive Defects in the Development of Mental Illness*, ed. G. Serban. New York: Brunner/Mazel, pp. 361–376.

———— Shenton, M. E. & Solovay, M. R. (1986), Quality of thought disorder in differential diagnosis. *Schizophrenia Bulletin*, 12:360–371.

Huber, G. & Gross, G. (1989), The concept of basic symptoms in schizophrenic and schizoaffective psychoses. *Recent Progress in Medicine*, 80:646–652.

Hughlings-Jackson, J. (1931), *Selected Writings*, ed. J. Taylor. London: Hodder & Stoughton.

Hunt, K. C. & Appel, K. E. (1936–1937), Prognosis in the psychoses lying midway between schizophrenia and manic-depressive psychoses. *American Journal of Psychiatry,* 93:313–329.

Hunter, R. & MacAlpine, I. (1963), *Three Hundred Years of Psychiatry.* London: University Press.

Hurt, S. W., Holzman, P. S. & Davis, J. M. (1983), Thought disorder. *Archives of General Psychiatry,* 40:1281–1285.

Hwang, M. Y. & Hollander, E. (1993), Schizo-obsessive disorders. *Psychiatric Annals,* 23:396–400.

Hymowitz, P., Hunt, H. F., Carr, A. C., Hurl, S. & Spear, W. E. (1983), The WAIS and Rorschach in diagnosing borderline personality. *Journal of Personality Assessment,* 47:588–596.

Ianzito, B. M., Cadoret, R. J. & Pugh, D. D. (1974), Thought disorder in depression. *American Journal of Psychiatry,* 131:703–707.

Insel, T. R. & Akiskal, H. S. (1986), Obsessive-compulsive disorder with psychotic features: A phenomenologic analysis. *American Journal of Psychiatry,* 143:1527–1533.

Ipp, H. (1986), Object relations of feminine boys: A Rorschach assessment. Unpublished doctoral dissertation, New York University.

Isaacs, S. (1948), The nature and function of phantasy. *International Journal of Psycho-Analysis,* 29:73–97.

Jaffee, L. S. (1990), The empirical foundations of psychoanalytic approaches to psychological testing. *Journal of Personality Assessment,* 55:746–755.

Jamison, K. R. (1993), *Touched with Fire.* New York: Free Press.

Jampala, V. C., Taylor, M. A. & Abrams, R. (1989), The diagnostic implications of formal thought disorder in mania and schizophrenia: A reassessment. *American Journal Psychiatry,* 146:459–463.

Janoff, I. (1951), The relation between Rorschach form quality measures and children's behavior. Unpublished doctoral dissertation, Yale University Library.

Janowsky, D. S., Leff, M. & Epstein, R. S. (1970), Playing the manic game. *Archives of General Psychiatry,* 22:252–261.

Jenike, M. A., Baer, L. & Carey, R. J. (1986), Co-existent obsessive-compulsive disorder and schizotypal personality disorder: A poor prognosis indicator (letter). *Archives of General Psychiatry,* 43:296.

Johnston, M. H. (1975), Thought disorder in schizophrenics and their relatives. Unpublished doctoral dissertation, University of Chicago.

——— & Holzman, P. S. (1979), *Assessing Schizophrenic Thinking.* San Francisco: Jossey-Bass.

Jonas, J. M. & Pope, H. G. (1984), Psychosis in borderline personality disorder. *Psychiatric Developments,* 4:295–308

Jones, J. E. (1975), Transactional style deviance in families of disturbed adolescents. Unpublished dissertation, University of California, Los Angeles.

Jortner, S. (1966), An investigation of certain cognitive aspects of schizophrenia. *Journal of Projective Techniques and Personality Assessment,* 30:559–568.

Joseph, R. (1986), Confabulation and delusional denial: Frontal lobe and lateralized influences. *Journal of Clinical Psychology,* 42:507–520.

Jowett, B., ed. & trans. (1924), Phaedrus. In: *The Dialogues.* Oxford: Oxford University Press.

Judd, L. L., McAdams, L., Budnick, B. & Braff, D. L. (1992), Sensory gating deficits in schizophrenia: New results. *American Journal of Psychiatry*, 149:488–493.

Kasanin, J. (1933), The acute schizoaffective psychoses. *American Journal of Psychiatry*, 13:97–126.

Kaser-Boyd, N. (1993), Rorschachs of women who commit homicide. *Journal of Personality Assessment*, 60:458–470.

Kay, S. R. (1986), Thought deficit in psychotic depression and chronic paranoid schizophrenia: Methodological and conceptual issues. *Journal of Nervous and Mental Disease*, 174:342–347.

Kernberg, O. F. (1966), Structural derivatives of objective relationships. *International Journal of Psycho-Analysis*, 47:236–295.

———— (1967), Borderline personality organization. *Journal of the American Psychoanalytic Association*, 15:641–685.

———— (1980), *Internal World and External Reality*. New York: Jason Aronson.

Kestenbaum-Daniels, E., Shenton, M. E., Holzman, P. S., Benowitz, L. I., Coleman, M., Levin, S. & Levine, D. (1988), Patterns of thought disorder associated with right cortical damage, schizophrenia, and mania. *American Journal of Psychiatry*, 145:944–949.

Kety, S. S., Rosenthal, D., Wender, P. H. & Schulsinger, F. (1968), Mental illness in the biological and adoptive families of adopted schizophrenia. In: *The Transmission of Schizophrenics*, ed. D. Rosenthal & S. S. Kety. Oxford: Pergamon Press, pp. 345–362.

Khadivi, A., Wetzler, S. & Wilson, A. (1997), Manic indices on the Rorschach. *Journal of Personality Assessment*, 69:365–375.

Kimberg, D. Y., D'Esposito, M. & Farah, M. J. (1997), Frontal lobes: Cognitive neuro-psychological aspects. In: *Behavioral Neurology and Neuropsychology*, ed. T. E. Feinberg & M. J. Farah. New York: McGraw-Hill, pp. 409–425.

Kirkwood, J. (1960), *There Must Be a Pony!* New York: Dell Publishing.

Kleiger, J. H. (1992a), A conceptual critique of the EA : es comparison in the Comprehensive Rorschach System. *Psychological Assessment*, 4:288–296.

———— (1992b), A response to Exner's comments on "A conceptual critique of the EA : es comparison in the Comprehensive Rorschach System." *Psychological Assessment*, 4:301–302.

———— (1997), Rorschach shading responses: From a printer's error to an integrated psychoanalytic paradigm. *Journal of Personality Assessment*, 69:342–364.

———— & Peebles-Kleiger, M. J. (1993), Toward a conceptual understanding of the deviant response in the Comprehensive Rorschach System. *Journal of Personality Assessment*, 60:74–90.

Klein, D. (1930), The importance of symbol-formation in the development of the ego. In: *Contributions to Psycho-analysis, 1921–1945*. London: Hogarth Press, 1968, pp. 236–250.

———— (1975), Psychopharmacology and the borderline patient. In: *Borderline States in Psychiatry*, ed. J. Mack. New York: Grune & Stratton.

———— (1977), Psychopharmacological treatment and delineation of borderline disorders. In: *Borderline Personality Disorders: The Concept, the Syndrome, the Patient*, ed. P. Hartocollis. New York: International Universities Press, pp. 365–384.

Klopfer, B. & Kelley, D. M. (1942), *The Rorschach Technique: A Manual for a Projective Method of Personality Diagnosis*. Yonkers-on-Hudson, New York: World Book Company.

—— & Margulies, H. (1941), Rorschach reactions in early childhood. *Rorschach Research Exchange*, 5:1–23.

—— Spiegelman, M. & Fox, J. (1956), The interpretation of children's records. In: *Developments in the Rorschach Technique, Vol. 2* ed. B. Klopfer. New York: Harcourt, Brace & World, pp. 22–44.

—— Ainsworth, M., Klopfer, W. & Holt, R. (1954), *Developments in the Rorschach Technique, Vol. 1*. New York: Harcourt, Brace & World.

Knight, R. A. & Blaney, P. H. (1977), The interrater reliability of the psychotic inpatient profile. *Journal of Clinical Psychology*, 33:647–653.

—— Elliot, D. S., Roff, J. D. & Watson, C. G. (1986), Concurrent and predictive validity of components of disordered thinking in schizophrenia. *Schizophrenia Bulletin*, 12:427–446.

Knight, R. P. (1953), Borderline states. *Bulletin of the Menninger Clinic*, 17:1–12.

Koenigsberg, H. (1982), A comparison of hospitalized and nonhospitalized borderline conditions in an outpatient setting. *Archives of General Psychiatry*, 139:1292–1297.

Koestler, A. (1964), *The Act of Creation*. New York: Macmillan.

Kohut, H. & Wolf, E. (1978), The disorders of the self and their treatment: An outline. *International Journal of Psychoanalysis*, 59:413–425.

Koistinen, P. (1995), *Thought Disorder and the Rorschach*. Oulu: Oulun Yliopistd.

Korchin, S. J. (1960), Form perception and ego functioning. In: *Rorschach Psychology*, ed. M. Rickers-Ovsiankina. New York: Wiley, pp. 109–129.

Korsakoff, S. S. (1890), Eine psychische storung combinirt mit multipler neuritis (A psychic disturbance combined with polyneuritis). *Allgemeine Zeitschrift fur Psychischgerichtliche Medizin und Psychiatrie*, 46:475–485.

—— (1892), Erinnerungstreuschungen (pseudoreminicenzen) bei polyneuritischen psychose (memory disturbances [pseudo-reminiscences] in polyneurotic psychoses). *Allgemeine Zeitschrift fur Psychischgerichtliche Medizin und Psychiatrie*, 47:390–410.

Kowitt, M. (1985), Rorschach content interpretation in posttraumatic stress disorder: A reply to Carr. *Journal of Personality Assessment*, 49:21–24.

Kraepelin, E. (1896), *Dementia Praecox and Paraphrenia*, trans. R. M. Barclay. Chicago: Chicago Medical Books, 1919.

—— (1921), *Manic-Depressive Insanity and Paranoia*. Edinburgh: E. & S. Livingston.

Kringlen, E. (1965), Obsessional neurotics: A long term follow-up. *British Journal of Psychiatry*, 111:709–722.

Kris, E. (1952), *Psychoanalytic Explorations in Art*. New York: International Universities Press.

Kroll, J., Sines, L., Martin, K., Lari, S., Pyle, R. & Zander, J. (1981), Borderline personality disorder: A constrict validity of the concept. *Archives of General Psychiatry*, 38:1021–1026.

Kwawer, J. (1980), Primitive interpersonal modes, borderline phenomena, and Rorschach content. In: *Borderline Phenomena and the Rorschach Test*, ed. J. Kwawer, H. Lerner, P. Lerner & A. Sugarman. New York: International Universities Press, pp. 89–106.

———— Lerner, H., Lerner, P. & Sugarman, A., eds. (1980a), *Borderline Phenomena and the Rorschach Test*. New York: International Universities Press.

Langsdorf, C. (1900), *Tranquility of Mind*. New York: G. P. Putnam's Sons.

Lanin-Kettering, I. & Harrow, M. (1985), The thought behind the words: A view of schizophrenic speech and thinking disorders. *Schizophrenia Bulletin*, 11:1–7.

Larson, D. G. (1974), The Borderline Syndrome in the Rorschach: A Comparison with Acute and Chronic Schizophrenics. Thesis, University of California, Psychology Department, Berkeley, CA.

Lazar, Z. L. & Schwartz, F. (1982), The contaminated Rorschach response: Formal features. *Journal of Clinical Psychology*, 38:415–419.

Lebowitz, A. (1963), Patterns of perceptual and motor organization. *Journal of Projective Techniques*, 27:302–308.

Leichtman, M. (1988), When does the Rorschach become the Rorschach? Stages in the mastery of the test. In: *Primitive Mental States and the Rorschach*, ed. H. D. Lerner & P. M. Lerner. Madison, CT: International Universities Press, pp. 559–600.

———— (1996), *The Rorschach: A Developmental Perspective*. Hillsdale, NJ: The Analytic Press.

Lerner, H. & Lerner, P. (1982), A comparative study of defensive structure in neurotic, borderline, and schizophrenic patients. *Psychoanalysis and Contemporary Thought*, 5:77–115.

———— & ———— (1986), Contributions of object relations theory towards a general psychoanalytic theory of thinking. *Psychoanalysis and Contemporary Thought*, 9:469–513.

———— & ———— eds. (1988), *Primitive Mental States and the Rorschach*. Madison, CT: International Universities Press.

———— & St. Peter, S. (1984), Patterns of object relations in neurotic, borderline, and schizophrenic patients. *Psychiatry*, 47:77–92.

———— Sugarman, A. & Barbour, C. G. (1985), Patterns of ego boundary disturbance in neurotic, borderline, and schizophrenic patients. *Psychoanalytic Psychology*, 2:47–66.

Lerner, P. (1988), Rorschach measures of depression, the false self, and projective identification with narcissistic personality disorders. In: *Primitive Mental States and the Rorschach*, ed. H. D Lerner & P. M Lerner. Madison, CT: International Universities Press, pp. 71–94.

———— (1990), The clinical inference process and the role of theory. *Journal of Personality Assessment*, 55:426–431.

———— (1991), *Psychoanalytic Theory and the Rorschach*. Hillsdale, NJ: The Analytic Press.

———— (1996), Rorschach assessment of cognitive impairment from an object relations perspective. *Bulletin of the Menninger Clinic*, 60:351–365.

———— (1998), *Psychoanalytic Perspectives on the Rorschach*. Hillsdale, NJ: The Analytic Press.

———— & Lerner, H. (1980), Rorschach assessment of premature defenses in borderline personality structure. In: *Borderline Phenomena and the Rorschach Test*, ed. J. Kwawer, H. Lerner, P. Lerner & A. Sugarman. New York: International Universities Press, pp. 257–274.

———— & Lewandowski, A. (1975), The measurement of primary process manifestations: A review. In: *Handbook of Rorschach Scales*, ed. P. Lerner. New York: International Universities Press, pp. 181–214.

Levey, D. M. & Beck, S. J. (1934), The Rorschach test in manic-depressive psychosis. *Research Publication of the Association for Nervous and Mental Disorders*, 4:31–42.

Levin, P. (1993), Assessing post-traumatic stress disorder with the Rorschach projective technique. In: *International Handbook of Traumatic Stress Syndromes*, ed. J. P. Wilson & B. Raphael. New York: Plenum, pp. 189–200.

———— & Reis, B. (1996), The use of the Rorschach in assessing trauma. In: *Assessing Psychological Trauma and PTSD*, ed. J. Wilson, & T. Keane. New York: Guilford Press, pp. 529–543.

Levitt, E. E. (1989), *The Clinical Application of MMPI Special Scales*. Hillsdale, NJ: Lawrence Erlbaum Associates.

Levy-Bruhl, L. (1910), *Les Fonctions Mentales dans les Sociétés Inférieures (The Mental Functions of Primitive Societies)*. Paris: Alcan.

Lewine, R. J. & Sommers, A. A. (1985), Clinical definition of negative symptoms as a reflection of theory and methodology. In: *Controversies in Schizophrenia: Changes and Constancies: Proceedings of the 74th Annual Meeting of the American Psychopathological Association, New York, March 1–3*, ed. A. Murray et al. New York: Guilford Press, pp. 267–277.

Lezak, M. (1976), *Neuropsychological Assessment*. New York: Oxford University Press.

Lidz, T., Cornelison, A., Terry, D. & Fleck, S. (1958), The transmission of irrationality. In: *Schizophrenia and the Family*, ed. T. Lidz, S. Fleck, A. Cornelison et al. New York: International Universities Press, pp. 171–187.

Lipkin, K. M., Dyrud, J. & Meyer, G. G. (1970), The many faces of mania: Therapeutic trial of lithium carbonate. *Archives of General Psychiatry*, 22:262–267.

Loehrke, L. M. (1952), An evaluation of the Rorschach method for the study of brain injury. Unpublished doctoral dissertation, Western Reserve University Library.

Lombroso, C. (1895), *The Man of Genius*. New York: Charles Scribner's Sons.

Loranger, A. W., Oldham, J. M. & Tulis, E. H. (1982), Familial transmission of DSM-III borderline personality disorder. *Archives of General Psychiatry*, 39:795–799.

Lorr, M. & Vestre, N. (1969), The Psychotic Inpatient Profile: A nurse's observation scale. *Journal of Clinical Psychology*, 25:137–140.

Lovitt, R. & Lefkof, G. (1985), Understanding multiple personality disorder with the comprehensive Rorschach system. *Journal of Personality Assessment*, 59:289–294.

Maher, B. A. (1974), Delusional thinking and perceptual disorder. *Journal of Individual Psychology*, 30:98–113.

———— (1988), Anomalous experience and delusional thinking: The logic of explanations. In: *Delusional Beliefs*, ed. T. F. Ottmanns & B. A. Maher. New York: John Wiley & Sons, pp. 15–33.

———— & Ross, J. S. (1984), Delusions. In: *Comprehensive Handbook on Psychopathology*, ed. H. E. Adams & P. B. Sutker. New York: Plenum Press, pp. 383–409.

Mahler, M., Pine, F. & Bergman, A. (1975), *The Psychological Birth of the Human Infant*. New York: Basic Books.

Makowski, D., Waternaux, C., Lajonchere, C. M., Dicker, R., Smoke, N., Kopelwiez, H., Minn, D., Mendell, N. R. & Levy, D. L. (1997), Thought disorder in adolescent-onset schizophrenia. *Schizophrenia Research*, 23:147–166.

Manschreck, T. C. (1979), The assessment of paranoid features. *Comprehensive Psychiatry*, 20:370–377.

———— (1995), Pathogenesis of delusion. *The Psychiatric Clinics of North America*, 18:213–229.

Marengo, J. T., Harrow, M., Lanin-Kettering, I. & Wilson, A. (1986), Evaluating bizarre-idiosyncratic thinking: A comprehensive index of positive thought disorder. *Schizophrenia Bulletin*, 12:497–509.

———— & Harrow, M. (1985), Thought disorder: A function of schizophrenia, mania, or psychosis? *Journal of Nervous and Mental Disease*, 173:35–41.

Maupin, E. W. (1965), Individual differences in response to a Zen meditation exercise. *Journal of Consulting Psychology*, 29:139–145.

Mayman, M. (1960), Measuring introversiveness on the Rorschach. Unpublished manuscript, Menninger Foundation, Topeka, KS.

———— (1964), Form quality of Rorschach responses. Unpublished manuscript, Menninger Foundation, Topeka, KS.

———— (1977), A multidimensional view of the Rorschach movement response. In: *Rorschach Psychology*, ed. M. Rickers-Ovsiankina. Huntington, NY: Krieger, pp. 229–250.

———— (1982), *Rorschach Training Manual*. Unpublished manuscript, The Menninger Clinic, Topeka, KS.

McConaghy, N. & Clancy, M. (1968), Familial relationships of allusive thinking in university students and their parents. *British Journal of Psychiatry*, 114:1079–1087.

McCully, R. S. (1962), Certain theoretical considerations in relation to borderline schizophrenia and the Rorschach. *Journal of Projective Techniques*, 26:404–418.

McGhie, A. & Chapman, J. (1961), Disorders of attention and perception in early schizophrenia. *British Journal of Medical Psychology*, 34:103–116.

McMahon, J. (1964), The relationship between "over-inclusion" and primary process thought in a normal and schizophrenic population. Unpublished doctoral dissertation, New York University.

Meehl, P. E. (1962), Schizotaxia, schizotypy, schizophrenia. *American Psychologist*, 17:827–838.

—— & Dahlstrom, W. G. (1960), Objective configural rules for discriminating psychotic from neurotic MMPI profiles. *Journal of Consulting Psychology*, 24:375–387.

Meissner, W. W. (1981), The schizophrenic and paranoid process. *Schizophrenia Bulletin*, 7:611–631.

Meloy, J. R. (1984), Thought organization and primary process in the parents of schizophrenics. *British Journal of Medical Psychology*, 57:279–281.

—— (1986), On the relationship between primary process and thought disorder. *Journal of the American Academy of Psychoanalysis*, 14:47–56.

—— & Singer, J. (1991), A psychoanalytic view of the Rorschach Comprehensive System "special scores." *Journal of Personality Assessment*, 56:202–217.

Mercer, M. & Wright, S. C. (1950), Diagnostic testing in a case of latent schizophrenia. *Journal of Projective Techniques*, 14:287–296.

Mignard, M. (1913), De l'obsession: Émotive ou délire d'influence (On obsession: Emotional or delusion of influence). *Annales Médecine Psychologique* (Paris), 71:333–343.

Morrison, J. R. & Flanagan, T. A. (1978), Diagnostic errors in psychiatry. *Comprehensive Psychiatry*, 19:109–117.

Mortimer, A. M., Lund, C. E. & McKenna, P. J. (1990), The positive-negative dichotomy in schizophrenia. *British Journal of Psychiatry*, 157:41–49.

Moscovitch, M. (1989), Confabulation and the frontal system: Strategic versus associative retrieval in neuropsychological theories of memory. In: *Varieties of Memory and Consciousness: Essays in Honour of Endel Tulving*, ed. H. L. Roediger & F. I. Craik. Hillsdale, NJ: Lawrence Erlbaum Associates, pp. 133–160.

Muller, C. (1953), Der ubergong von zwangsnekrose in schizophrenie im licht der katumnese (Transformation of compulsive neurosis into schizophrenia in light of the case history). *Schweiz. Arch. Neurol. Psychiatr.*, 72:218–225.

Murray, J. & Russ, S. W. (1981), Adaptive regression and types of cognitive flexibility. *Journal of Personality Assessment*, 45:59–65.

Myers, T. & Kushner, E. N. (1970), *Sensory tolerance as a function of primary process defense demand and defense effectiveness.* Unpublished manuscript, Bethesda, MD: Naval Research Institute.

Nathaniel-James, D. A. & Frith, C. D. (1996), Confabulation in schizophrenia: Evidence of a new form. *Psychological Medicine*, 26:391–399.

Neiger, A. G., Slemon, A. G. & Quirk, D. (1962), The performance of chronic schizophrenic patients on Piotrowski's Rorschach sign list for organic CNS pathology. *Journal of Projective Techniques*, 26:419–428.

Nestor, P. G., Shenton, M. E., McCarley, R. W., Haimson, J., Smith, R. S. & O'Donnell, B. F. (1993), Neuropsychological correlates of MRI temporal lobe abnormalities in schizophrenia. *American Journal of Psychiatry*, 150:1849–1855.

—— —— Wible, C., Hokama, H., O'Donnell, B. F., Law, S. & McCarley, R. W. (1998), A neuropsychological analysis of schizophrenic thought disorder. *Schizophrenia Research*, 29:217–225.

Nigg, J. T., Lohr, N. E., Westen, D., Gold, L. J. & Silk, K. R. (1992), Malevolent object representations in borderline personality disorder and major depression. *Journal of Abnormal Psychology*, 101:61–67.

Nims, J. P. (1959), Logical reasoning in schizophrenia: The von Domarus Principle. Unpublished doctoral dissertation, University of Southern California, Los Angeles.

Nuechterlein, K. H. & Dawson, M. E. (1984), Information processing and attentional functioning in the developmental course of schizophrenic disorders. *Schizophrenia Bulletin*, 10:160–203.

—— Edell, W. S., Norris, M. & Dawson, M. E. (1986), Attentional vulnerability indicators, thought disorder, and negative symptoms. *Schizophrenia Bulletin*, 12:408–426.

O'Connell, M., Cooper, S., Perry, C. & Hoke, L. (1989), The relationship between thought disorder and psychotic symptoms in borderline personality disorder. *Journal of Nervous and Mental Disease*, 177:273–278.

Patrick, J. & Wolfe, B. (1983), Rorschach presentation of borderline personality disorder: Primary process manifestations. *Journal of Clinical Psychology*, 39:442–447.

Payne, R. W., Mattusek, P. & George, E. I. (1959), An experimental study of schizophrenic thought disorder. *Journal of Mental Science*, 105:627–652.

Peebles, M. J. (1986), Low intelligence and intrapsychic defenses. *Bulletin of the Menninger Clinic*, 50:33–49.

Perris, C. (1966), A study of bipolar (manic depressive) and unipolar recurrent depressive psychoses. *Acta Psychiatrica Scandenavica*, 42 (suppl. 194):1–189.

Perry, J. C. & Klerman, G. L. (1980), Clinical features of the borderline personality disorder. *American Journal of Psychiatry*, 137:165–173.

Perry, W. & Braff, D. L. (1994), Information-processing deficits and thought disorder in schizophrenia. *American Journal of Psychiatry*, 151:363–367.

—— & Potterat, E. (1997), Beyond personality assessment: The use of the Rorschach as a neuropsychological instrument in patients with amnestic disorders. In: *Contemporary Rorschach Interpretation*, ed. J. R. Meloy, M. W. Acklin, C. B. Gacono, J. F. Murray & C. A. Peterson. Mahwah, NJ: Lawrence Erlbaum Associates, pp. 557–575.

—— —— Auslander, L., Kaplan, E. & Jeste, D. (1996), A neuropsychological approach to the Rorschach in patients with dementia of the alzheimer type. *Assessment*, 3:351–363.

—— Viglione, D. & Braff, D. (1992), The Ego Impairment Index and schizophrenia: A validation study. *Journal of Personality Assessment*, 59:165–175.

—— —— (1991), The Ego Impairment Index as a predictor of outcome in melancholic depressed patients treated with tricyclic antidepressants. *Journal of Personality Assessment*, 56:487–501.

Peterfreund, E. (1978), Some critical comments on psychoanalytic conceptualizations of infancy. *International Journal of Psycho-Analysis*, 59:427–441.

Peterson, A. O. D. (1954), A comparative study of Rorschach scoring methods in evaluating personality changes resulting from psychotherapy. *Journal of Clinical Psychology*, 10:190–192.

Phillips, L., Kaden, S. & Waldman, M. (1959), Rorschach indices of developmental level. *Journal of Genetic Psychology*, 94:267–285.

———— & Smith, J. G. (1953), Rorschach Interpretation: Advanced technique. New York: Grune & Stratton.

Piaget, J. (1959), *The Language and Thought of the Child*. London: Routledge & Kegan Paul.

Pine, F. (1990), *Drive, Ego, Object, and Self: A Synthesis for Clinical Work*. New York: Basic Books.

———— & Holt, R. R. (1960), Creativity and primary processs: A study of adaptive aggression. *Journal of Abnormal and Social Psychology*, 61:370–379.

Piotrowski, Z. A. (1937), The Rorschach ink-blot method in organic disturbances of the central nervous system. *Journal of Nervous and Mental Disease*, 86:525–537.

———— (1957), *Perceptanalysis*. New York: Macmillan.

———— & Berg, J. (1955), Verification of the Rorschach Alpha diagnostic formula for underactive schizophrenics. *American Journal of Psychiatry*, 112:443–450.

———— & Lewis, N. D. (1950), An experimental Rorschach diagnostic aid for some forms of schizophrenia. *American Journal of Psychiatry*, 107:360–366.

Pious, W. (1950), Obsessive-compulsive symptoms in an incipient schizophrenic. *Psychoanalytic Quarterly*, 19:327–339.

Piran, N. (1988), Borderline phenomena in anorexia and bulimia. In: *Primitive Mental States and the Rorschach*, ed. H. D. Lerner & P. M. Lerner. New York: International Universities Press, pp. 363–376.

Pogue-Geile, M. F. & Harrow, M. (1984), Negative and positive experience in schizophrenia and depression: A follow-up study. *Schizophrenia Bulletin*, 10:371–387.

Pope, B. & Jensen, A. R. (1957), The Rorschach as an index of pathological thinking. *Journal of Projective Techniques*, 21:54–62.

Pope, H. G. & Lipinski, J. F. (1978), Diagnosis in schizophrenia and manic-depressive illness: A reassessment of the specificity of "schizophrenic" symptoms in light of current research. *Archives of General Psychiatry*, 35:811–828.

———— Jonas, J. M., Hudson, J. I., Cohen, B. M. & Gunderson, J. (1983), The validity of DSM-III borderline personality disorder: A phenomenologic, family history, treatment, and long-term follow-up study. *Archives of General Psychiatry*, 40:23–30.

———— ———— ———— ———— & Tohen, M. (1985), An empirical study of psychosis in borderline personality disorder. *American Journal of Psychiatry*, 142:1285–1290.

Powers, W. T. & Hamlin, R. M. (1955), Relationship between diagnostic category and deviant verbalizations on the Rorschach. *Journal of Consulting Psychology*, 19:120–124.

Pruyser, P. W. (1984), The diagnostic process: Touchstone of medicine's values. In: *Diagnostic Understanding and Treatment Planning*, ed. F. Shectman & W. H. Smith. New York: Wiley, pp. 5–17.

Putnam, F. (1997), *Dissociation in Children and Adolescents*. New York: Guilford Press.

Quinlan, D., Harrow, M., Tucker, G. & Carlson, K. (1972), Varieties of "disordered" thinking on the Rorschach findings in schizophrenic and nonschizophrenic patients. *Journal of Abnormal Psychology*, 79:49–53.

────── ────── ────── & ────── (1973), *Manual for Assessment of Deviant Responses on the Rorschach*. ASIS/NAPS #02211. New York: Microfiche Publications.

────── Schultz, K. D., Davies, R. K. & Harrow, M. (1978), Overinclusion and transactional thinking on the Object Sorting Test of schizophrenic and nonschizophrenic patients. *Journal of Personality Assessment*, 42:401–408.

Rabkin, J. (1967), Psychoanalytic assessment of change in organization of thought after psychotherapy. Unpublished doctoral dissertation, New York University.

Raine, A. (1991), The SPQ: A scale for the assessment of schizotypal personality based on DSM-III-R criteria. *Schizophrenia Bulletin*, 17:555–564.

Rapaport, D., Gill, M. & Schafer, R. (1968), *Diagnostic Psychological Testing*, revised ed., ed. R. R. Holt. New York: International Universities Press.

────── ed. (1951), *Organization and Pathology in Thought*. New York: Columbia University Press.

────── (1950), The theoretical implications of diagnostic testing procedures. In: *The Collected Papers of David Rapaport*, ed. M. M. Gill. New York: Basic Books, pp. 334–356.

Rasmussen, S. A. & Tsuang, M. (1986), Clinical characteristics and family history in DSM-III obsessive-compulsive disorder. *American Journal of Psychiatry*, 143:317–322.

Rattenbery, F. R., Silverstein, M. L., DeWolfe, A. S., Kaufman, C. F. & Harrow, M. (1983), Associative disturbance in schizophrenia, schizoaffective disorder and major affective disorders: Comparison between hospital and one year follow-up. *Journal of Consulting and Clinical Psychology*, 51:621–623.

Rawls, J. R. & Slack, G. K. (1968), Artists vs. non-artists: Rorschach determinants and artistic creativity. *Journal of Projective Techniques and Personality Assessment*, 32:233–237.

Reed, G. F. (1985), *Obsessional Experience and Compulsive Behavior: A Cognitive-Structural Approach*. Orlando: Academic Press.

Regard, M. (1985), Diffuse cerebral damage and the Rorschach test. International Neuropsychological Society, Eighth European Conference, June 12–15, 1985 Copenhagen, Denmark.

Reitan, R. M. (1962), Psychological deficit. *Annual Review of Psychology*, 13:415–444.

Rickers-Ovsiankina, M. (1938), The Rorschach test as applied to normal and schizophrenic subjects. *British Journal of Medical Psychology*, 17:227–257.

Robinson, S., Winnik, H. Z. & Weiss, A. A. (1976), Obsessive psychosis: Justification for a separate clinical entity. *Israeli Annals of Psychiatry*, 14:39–48.

Roe, A. (1952), *The Making of a Scientist*. New York: Dodd, Mead.

Rogolsky, M. M. (1968), Artistic creativity and adaptive regression in third-grade children. *Journal of Projective Techniques and Personality Assessment*, 32:53–62.

Rorschach, H. (1921), *Psychodiagnostics*, 5th ed. Bern: Hans Huber, 1942.

Rosen, I. (1957), The clinical significance of obsessions in schizophrenia. *Journal of Mental Science*, 103:773–785.

Rosenthal, D., Wender, P. H., Kety, S. S., Schulsinger, F., Welner, J. & Oster-gaard, L. (1968), Schizophrenics' offspring reared in adoptive homes. In: *The Transmission of Schizophrenia*, ed. D. Rosenthal & S. S. Kety. Oxford: Pergamon Press, pp. 371–391.

Ross, W. D. & Ross, S. (1944), Some Rorschach ratings of clinical value. *Rorschach Research Exchange*, 8:1–9.

Rothenberg, A. (1969), The iceman changeth: Toward an empirical approach to creativity. *Journal of the American Psychoanalytic Association*, 17:549–607.

———— (1971), The process of Janusian thinking in creativity. *Archives of General Psychiatry*, 24:195–205.

———— (1976), The process of Janusian thinking in creativity. In: *The Creativity Question*, ed. A. Rothenberg & C. Hausman. Durham, NC: Duke University Press, pp. 305–327.

———— (1983), Psychopathology and creative cognition. *Archives of General Psychiatry*, 40:937–942.

———— (1990), *Creativity and Madness. New Findings, Old Stereotypes*. Baltimore: Johns Hopkins.

Ruchlis, H. & Oddo, R. (1990), *Clear Thinking: A Practical Introduction*. New York: Prometheus Books.

Rudin, G. (1953), Ein beitrag zur frage der zwangskran kheit (A contribution to the question of compulsive disease). *Archiv fur Psychiatrie und Nervenkrankheiten*, 191:14–54.

Russ, S. W. (1980), Primary process integration on the Rorschach and achievement in children. *Journal of Personality Assessment*, 44:338–344.

———— (1981), Primary process integration on the Rorschach and achievement in children: A follow-up study. *Journal of Personality Assessment*, 45:473–477.

———— (1982), Sex differences in primary process thinking and flexibility in problem solving in children. *Journal of Personality Assessment*, 46:569–577.

———— (1988), Primary process thinking, divergent thinking, and coping in children. *Journal of Personality Assessment*, 52:539–549.

———— & Grossman-McKee, A. (1990), Affective expression in children's fantasy play, primary process thinking on the Rorschach, and divergent thinking. *Journal of Personality Assessment*, 54:756–771.

Rust, J. (1987), The Rust Inventory of Schizotypal Cognitions (RISC). *Schizophrenia Bulletin*, 14:317–322.

Sadoun, R. (1957), Formes cliniques et diagnostiques des modes de début de la schizophrénie (Clinical and diagnostic types of the onset of schizophrenia). *Encéphale*, 46:1–7, 9–14.

Sandson, J. & Albert, M. L. (1984), Varieties of perseveration. *Neuropsychologia*, 22:715–732.

Saretsky, T. (1966), Effects of chlorpromazine on primary process thought manifestations. *Journal of Abnormal Psychology*, 71:247–252.

SAS Institute (1982), *SAS Users' Guide: Statistics.* Cary, NC: Author.

Saunders, E. A. (1991), Rorschach indicators of sexual abuse. *Bulletin of the Menninger Clinic,* 55:48–71.

Savard, R. J., Rey, A. C. & Post, R. M. (1980), Thinking in depression. *Archives of General Psychiatry,* 4:456–459.

Schachtel, E. (1966), *Experiental Foundations of the Rorschach Test.* New York: Basic Books.

Schafer, R. (1948), *The Clinical Application of Psychological Tests.* New York: International Universities Press.

—— (1954), *Psychoanalytic Interpretation in Rorschach Testing.* New York: Grune & Stratton.

—— (1976), *A New Language for Psychoanalysis.* New Haven, CT: Yale University Press.

Schmidt, H. O. & Fonda, C. P. (1954), Rorschach scores in the manic state. *Journal of Psychology,* 38:427–437.

Schneider, K. (1939), Begriffiche untersuchung uber den Zwang (Comprehensive examination of compulsion). *Allgemeine Zeitschrift der Psychiatrie und Ihre Grenze,* 112:17–24.

—— (1959), *Clinical Psychopathology,* trans. M. W. Hamilton. New York: Grune & Stratton.

Schuldberg, D. & Boster, J. S. (1985), Back to Topeka: Two types of distance in Rapaport original Rorschach thought disorder categories. *Journal of Abnormal Psychology,* 94:205–215.

Schwartz, F. & Lazar, Z. (1984), Contaminated thinking: A specimen of the primary process. *Psychoanalytic Psychology,* 4:319–334.

Scroppo, J. C., Drob, S. L., Weinberger, J. L. & Eagle, P. (1997), Identifying dissociative identity disorder: A self-report and projective study. *Journal of Abnormal Psychology,* 107:272–284.

Selig, K. (1958), The personality structure as revealed by the Rorschach technique of a group of children who test at or above 170 I.Q. on the 1937 revision of the Standford-Binet Scale: Volume I-V. *Dissertation Abstracts,* 19:3373–3374.

Shakow, D. (1950), Some psychological features of schizophrenia. In: *Feelings and Emotions,* ed. M. L. Reyment. New York: McGraw-Hill, pp. 383–390.

—— (1962), Segmental set: A theory of the formal psychological deficit in schizophrenia. *Archives of General Psychiatry,* 14:79–83.

Shapiro, D. (1954), Special problems in testing borderline patients. *Journal of Projective Techniques,* 18:387–394.

—— (1960), A perceptual understanding of the color response. In: *Rorschach Psychology,* 2nd ed., ed. M. A. Rickers-Ovsiankina. New York: Wiley, pp. 154–201.

—— (1965), *Neurotic Styles.* New York: Basic Books.

Shenton, M. E., Kikinis, R., Jolesz, F. A., Pollak, S. D., Lemay, M., Wible, C. G., Hokama, H., Martin, J., Metcalf, D., Coleman, M. & McCarley, R. W. (1992), Abnormalities of the left temporal lobe and thought disorder in schizophrenia. *New England Journal of Medicine,* 327:604–612.

—— Solovay, M. R. & Holzman, P. (1987), Comparative studies of thought disorders II schizoaffective disorder. *Archives of General Psychiatry,* 44:21–30.

———— ———— ———— Coleman, M. & Gale, H. J. (1989), Thought disorder in the relatives of psychotic patients. *Archives of General Psychiatry*, 46:897–901.

Shield, P., Harrow, M. & Tucker, G. (1974), Investigation of factors related to stimulus over inclusion. *Psychiatric Quarterly*, 48:1–8.

Siegel, E. L. (1953), Genetic parallels of perceptual structuralization in paranoid schizophrenia: An analysis by means of the Rorschach technique. *Journal of Projective Techniques*, 17:151–161.

Silberman, E. K., Weingartner, H. & Post, R.M. (1983), Thinking disorder in depression. *Archives of General Psychiatry*, 40:775–780.

Silverman, L. H. (1965), Regression in the service of the ego. *Journal of Projective Techniques and Personality Assessment*, 29:232–244.

———— (1966), A technique for the study of psychodynamic relationships: The effects of subliminally presented aggressive stimuli on the production of pathological thinking in a schizophrenic population. *Journal of Consulting Psychology*, 30:103–111.

———— & Candell, P. (1970), On the relationship between aggressive activation, symbiotic merging, intactness of body boundaries and manifest pathology in schizophrenics. *Journal of Nervous and Mental Disease*, 150:387–399.

———— & Goldweber, A. M. (1966), A further study of the effects of subliminal aggressive stimulation on thinking. *Journal of Nervous and Mental Disease*, 153:463–472.

———— & Spiro, R. (1967), Further investigation of the effects of subliminal aggressive stimulation on the ego functioning of schizophrenics. *Journal of Consulting Psychology*, 31:225–232.

———— Lapkin, B. & Rosenbaum, I.. (1962), Manifestations of primary process thinking in schizophrenia. *Journal of Projective Techniques*, 26:117–127.

Simpson, D. M. & Davis, G. C. (1985), Measuring thought disorder with clinical rating scales in schizophrenic and nonschizophrenic patients. *Psychiatric Research*, 15:313–318.

Singer, E. (1993), Transference and parataxic distortion. *Contemporary Psychoanalysis*, 29:418–440.

Singer, H. K. & Brabender, V. (1993), The use of the Rorschach to differentiate unipolar and bipolar disorders. *Journal of Personality Assessment*, 60:333–345.

Singer, M. T. (1973), Scoring Manual for Communication Deviances Seen in Individually Administered Rorschachs. Revision (mimeographed, pp. 1–100).

———— (1975), The borderline diagnosis and psychological tests: Review and research. In: *Borderline Personality Disorders: The Concept, the Syndrome, the Patient*, ed. P. Hartocollis. New York: International Universities Press, pp. 193–212.

———— (1977), The Rorschach as a transaction. In: *Rorschach Psychology*, ed. M. Rickers-Ovsiankina. Huntington, NY: Krieger, pp. 455–485.

———— & Larson, D. G. (1981), Borderline personality and the Rorschach test. *Archives of General Psychiatry*, 38:693–698.

———— & Wynne, L. C. (1966), Principles for scoring communication defects and deviances in parents of schizophrenics: Rorschach and TAT scoring manuals. *Psychiatry*, 29:260–288.

Skalweit, W. (1935), Der Rorschach-versuch als unterscheidungsmittel von konstitution und prozess (The Rorschach test as a means of differentiation between biological and constitution and disease process). *Zeitschrift fur die Gesamte Neurologie und Psychiatrie*, 152:605–610.

Skelton, M. O., Boik, R. J. & Madero, J. N. (1995), Thought disorder on the WAIS-R relative to the Rorschach: Assessing identity-disordered adolescents. *Journal of Personality Assessment*, 65:533–549.

Small, A., Teagro, L., Madero, J., Gross, H. & Ebert, M. (1982), A comparison of anorexia and schizophrenia on psychology therapy measures. *International Journal of Eating Disorders*, 2:17–36.

Smith, B. L. (1990), Potential space and the Rorschach: An application of object relations theory. *Journal of Personality Assessment*, 55:756–767.

Smith, K. (1980), Object relations concepts as applied to the borderline level of ego functioning. In: *Borderline Phenomena and the Rorschach Test*, ed. J. Kwawer, H. Lerner, P. Lerner & A. Sugarman. New York: International Universities Press, pp. 59–87.

Soloff, P. H. & Ulrich, R. F. (1981), Diagnostic interview of borderline patients: A replication study. *Archives of General Psychiatry*, 38:686–692.

Solovay, M. R., Shenton, M. E. & Holzman, P. S. (1987), Comparative studies of thought disorders. *Archives of General Psychiatry*, 44:13–20.

——— ——— Gasperetti, C., Coleman, M., Kestenbaum, E., Carpenter, T. & Holzman, P. S. (1986), Scoring Manual for the Thought Disorder Index. *Schizophrenia Bulletin*, 12:485–492.

Spitzer, M. (1997), A cognitive neuroscience view of schizophrenic thought disorder. *Schizophrenia Bulletin*, 23:29–50.

Spitzer, R. L., Endicott, J. & Robbins, E. (1977), *Research Diagnostic Criteria for a Selected Group of Functional Disorders*, 3rd ed. New York: Biometrics Research Division, New York Psychiatric Institute.

——— ——— ——— (1978), *Research Diagnostic Criteria for a Selected Group of Functional Disorders*. New York: Biometrics Research Division, New York Psychiatric Institute.

——— ——— & Gibbons, M. (1979), Crossing the border into borderline personality and borderline schizophenia: The development of criteria. *Archives of General Psychiatry*, 36:17–24.

Spohn, H. E., Coyne, L., Larson, J., Mittleman, F., Spray, J. & Hayes, K. (1986), Episodic and residual thought pathology in chronic schizophrenics: Effect of neuroleptics. *Schizophrenia Bulletin*, 12:394–407.

Sprock, J., Braff, D. L., Saccuzzo, D. P. & Atkinson, J. H. (1983), The relationship of depression and thought disorder in pain patients. *British Journal of Medical Psychology*, 56:351–360.

Steiner, M., Martin, S., Wallace, J. & Goldman, S. (1984), Distinguishing subtypes within the borderline domain: A combined psychoneuroendocrine approach. *Biological Psychiatry*, 19:907–911.

Stengel, E. (1931), Zur Kenntnis der beziehungen zwischen zwangsnevrose und paranoia (On the recognition of the relationships between compulsive neurosis and paranoia). *Archiv fur Psychiatrie und Nervenkrakheiten*, 95:8–23.

——— (1945), A study of some clinical aspects of the relationship between obsessional neurosis and psychotic reaction types. *Journal of Mental Sciences*, 41:166–187.

Stern, A. (1938), Psychoanalytic investigation and therapy in the borderline group of neuroses. *Psychoanalytic Quarterly*, 7:467–489.

Stern, D. N. (1985), *The Interpersonal World of the Infant*. New York: Basic Books.

Stern, E. (1930), Zwand und schizophrenie (Compulsion and schizophrenia). *Monatsschrift fur Psychiatrie und Neurologie*, 77:283–297.

Stone, H. K. & Dellis, N. P. (1960), An exploratory investigation into the levels of hypothesis. *Journal of Projective Techniques*, 24:333–340.

Stone, M. H. (1977), The borderline syndrome: Evolution of the term, genetic aspects, and prognoses. *American Journal of Psychotherapy*, 31:345–365.

—— (1978), Toward the detection of manic-depressive illness in psychoanalytic patients. *American Journal of Psychotherapy*, 32:427–439.

—— (1980), *The Borderline Syndromes: Constitution, Personality, and Adaptation*. New York: McGraw-Hill.

—— (1990), *Fate of Borderline Patients*. New York: Guilford Press.

—— Kuhn, E. & Flye, B. (1981), Psychiatrically ill relatives of borderline patients: A family study. *Psychiatric Quarterly*, 53:71–84.

Strub, R. L. & Black, F. W. (1977), *The Mental Status Examination in Neurology*. Philadelphia: F. A. Davis Company.

Stuart, J., Westen, D., Lohr, N. E., Silk, K. R., Becker, S., Vorus, N. & Benjamin, J. (1990), Object relations in borderlines, major depressives, and normals: Analysis of Rorschach human responses. *Journal of Personality Assessment*, 55:296–314.

Sugarman, A. (1986), An object relations understanding of borderline phenomena on the Rorschach. In: *Assessing Object Relations Phenomena*, ed. M. Kissen. Madison, CT: International Universities Press, pp. 77–88.

—— (1991), Where's the beef? Putting personality back into personality assessment. *Journal of Personality Assessment*, 56:130–144.

Sullivan, H. S. (1953), *The Interpersonal Theory of Psychiatry*. New York: Norton.

—— (1956), *Clinical Studies in Psychiatry*, ed. H. S. Gawel & M. Gibbon. New York: W. W. Norton.

Taulbee, E. S. & Sisson, B. D. (1957), Configural analysis of MMPI profiles of psychiatric groups. *Journal of Consulting Psychology*, 21:413–417.

Tausk, V. (1919), On the origin of the "influencing machine" in schizophrenia. *Psychoanalytic Quarterly*, 2:519–556, 1933.

Thiesen, J. W. (1952), A pattern analysis of structural characteristics of the Rorschach test in schizophrenia. *Journal of Consulting Psychology*, 16:365–370.

Tompkins, S. S. (1947), *The Thematic Apperception Test*. New York: Grune & Stratton.

Tsuang, M., Dempsey, G. & Rauscher, F. (1976), A study of atypical schizophrenia: Comparison with schizophrenia and affective disorder by sex, age of admission, precipitant, outcome, and family history. *Archives of General Psychiatry*, 33:1157–1160.

Urist, J. (1977), The Rorschach Test and the assessment of object relations. *Journal of Personality Assessment*, 41:3–9.

Van Der Does, A. J., Dingemans, P. M., Linzen, D. H., Nugter, M. A. & Scholte, W. F. (1993), Symptom dimensions and cognitive and social functions in recent onset schizophrenia. *Psychological Medicine*, 23:745–753.

van der Kolk, B. & Ducey, C. (1984), Clinical implications of the Rorschach in post-traumatic stress disorder. In: *Post-traumatic Stress Disorder: Psychological and Biological Sequelae*, ed. B. van der Kolk. Washington, DC: American Psychiatric Press, pp. 29–42.

——— & Ducey, C. (1989), The psychological processing of traumatic experience: Rorschach patterns in post-traumatic stress disorder. *Journal of Traumatic Stress*, 2:359–374.

Venables, P. H. (1960), The effect of auditory and visual stimulation on the skin potential responses of schizophrenics. *Brain*, 83:77–92.

——— Wilkins, S., Mitchell, D., Raine, A. & Bailes (1990), A scale for the measurement of schizotypy. *Personality and Individual Differences*, 11:481–495.

Vernon, P. (1933), The Rorschach Inkblot Test III. *British Journal of Medical Psychology*, 13:271–295.

Vigotsky, L. (1934), Thought in schizophrenia. *Archives of Neurology and Psychiatry*, 31:1063–1077.

von Domarus, E. (1944), The specific laws of logic in schizophrenia. In: *Language and Thought in Schizophrenia*, ed. J. S. Kasinin. New York: Norton, pp. 104–114.

Von Holt, H. W., Sengstake, C. B., Sonoda, B. & Draper, W. A. (1960), Orality, image fusion and concept formation. *Journal of Projective Techniques*, 24:194–198.

Waelder, R. (1949), Notes on prejudice. *Vassar Alumni Magazine* (May).

Wagner, E. (1998), TRAUT: A Rorschach index for screening thought disorder. *Journal of Clinical Psychology*, 54:719–762.

——— & Rinn, R. C. (1994), A proposed classification scheme for Rorschach autisms. *Perceptual and Motor Skills*, 77:1–2.

——— & Heise, M. (1974), A comparison of Rorschach protocols of three multiple personalities. *Journal of Personality Assessment*, 38:308–331.

Wahlberg, K. E. (1994), Vanhempien Kommunidaation merkitys lapsen ajatvshairioissa. *Acta Universitatis Ouluensis*, Series D, Medica 305.

Wallace, J. E. & Martin, S. (1988), Can psychological assessment address borderline phenomena? *Canadian Journal Psychiatry*, 33:344–349.

Watkins, J. G. & Stauffacher, J. C. (1952), An index of pathological thinking in the Rorschach. *Journal of Projective Techniques*, 16:276–286.

Wechsler, D. (1955), *Wechsler Adult Intelligence Scale Manual*. New York: Psychological Corporation.

Weiner, I. B. (1961), Three Rorschach scores indicative of schizophrenia. *Journal of Consulting Psychology*, 25:436–439.

——— (1962), Rorschach tempo as a schizophrenic indicator. *Perceptual and Motor Skills*, 18:484.

——— (1966), *Psychodiagnosis in Schizophrenia*. New York: Wiley.

——— (1972), Does psychodiagnosis have a future? *Journal of Personality Assessment*, 36:534–546.

——— (1977), Approaches to Rorschach validation. In: *Rorschach Psychology*, ed. M. A. Rickers-Ovsiankina. New York: Krieger, pp. 575–608.

——— (1986), Conceptual and empirical perspectives on the Rorschach assessment of psychopathology. *Journal of Personality Assessment*, 50:472–479.

Weinstein, E. A. (1996), Symbolic aspects of confabulation following brain injury: Influence of premorbid personality. *Bulletin of the Menninger Clinic*, 60:331–350.

——— Kahn, R. L. & Malitz, S. (1956), Confabulations as a social process. *Psychiatry*, 19:383–396.

Weiss, A. A., Robinson, S. & Winnick, H. Z. (1975), Obsessive psychosis: A cross validation study. *Israeli Annals of Psychiatry*, 13:137–141.

——— Robinson, S. & Winnick, H. Z. (1969), Obsessive psychosis: Psychodiagnostic findings. *Israeli Annals of Psychiatry*, 7:175–178.

Weiss, R. (1971), A study of some personality correlates of sensitivity to affective meaning. Unpublished doctoral dissertation, New York University.

Wender, P. (1977), The contribution of adoption studies to an understanding of the phenomenology and etiology of borderline schizophrenia. In: *Borderline Personality Disorders*, ed. P. Hartocollis. New York: International Universities Press, pp. 255–269.

——— Rosenthal, D. & Kety, S. S. (1968), The psychiatric assessment of adoptive parents of schizophrenics. In: *The Transmission of Schizophrenia*, ed. D. Rosenthal & S. S. Kety. Oxford: Pergamon Press, pp. 235–250.

Werner, H. (1948), *Comparative Psychology of Mental Development*. New York: Follett.

——— (1957), The concept of development from a comparative and organismic view. In: *The Concept of Development*, ed. D. B. Harris. Minneapolis: University of Minnesota Press, pp. 125–148.

——— & Kaplan, B. (1963), *Symbol Formation. An Organismic Approach to Language and the Expression of Thought*. New York: Wiley.

Westen, D., Lohr, N., Silk, K., Gold, L. & Kerber, K. (1990), Object relations and social cognition in borderlines, major depressives, and normals: A TAT analysis. *Psychological Assessment: A Journal of Consulting and Clinical Psychology*, 2:335–364.

——— Ludolph, P., Misle, B., Ruffins, S. & Block, J. (1990), Physical and sexual abuse in adolescents with borderline personality disorders. *American Journal of Orthopsychiatry*, 60:55–66.

Whitaker, L. (1973), *Whitaker Index of Schizophrenic Thinking: Manual*. Los Angeles: Western Psychological Services.

Widiger, T. A. (1982), Psychological tests and the borderline diagnosis. *Journal of Personality Assessment*, 46:227–238.

Wiggins, J. S. (1966), Substantive dimensions of self-report in the MMPI item pool. *Psychological Monographs*, 80:1–22.

Wilensky, H. (1959), Developmental scoring of Rorschachs of schizophrenics. Presented at the Annual Meeting of the Eastern Psychological Association, Atlantic City.

Williams, E. B. (1964), Deductive reasoning in schizophrenia. *Journal of Abnormal Social Psychology*, 69:47–61.

Wilson, A. (1985), Boundary disturbances in borderline and psychotic states. *Journal of Personality Assessment*, 49:346–355.

Wilson, S. (1994), Interpretive Guide to the Comprehensive Rorschach System. Laguna Beach, CA: Stuart Wilson, PhD.

Winnicott, D. (1961), Ego distortions in terms of true and false self. In: *The Maturational Processes and the Facilitating Environment*. Madison, CT: International Universities Press, 1965, pp. 140–152.

Winokur, G. (1973), Depression in menopause. *American Journal of Psychiatry*, 130:92–93.

—— (1991), *Mania and Depression. A Classification of Syndrome and Disease*. Baltimore: Johns Hopkins University Press.

—— Clayton, P. & Reich, T. (1969), *Manic Depressive Illness*. St. Louis: C.V. Mosby.

Wittenhorn, J. R. & Holzberg, J. D. (1951), The Rorschach and descriptive diagnosis. *Journal of Consulting Psychology*, 15:460–463.

Wolff, S. (1991), Schizoid personality in childhood and adult life: I. The vagaries of psychology labels. *British Journal of Psychiatry*, 159:615–620.

Wright, N. A. & Abbey, D. (1965), Perceptual deprivation tolerance and adequacy of defenses. *Perceptual & Motor Skills*, 20:35–38.

Wynne, L. C. (1967), Family transactions and schizophrenia: II. Conceptual considerations for a research strategy. In: *The Origins of Schizophrenia*, ed. J. Romano. Amsterdam: Excerpta Medica, pp. 165–178.

—— Singer, M. T. & Toohey, M. L. (1978), Communication disorders and the families of schizophrenics. In: *The Nature of Schizophrenia: New Approaches to Research and Treatment*, ed. L. Wynne, R. Cromwell & S. Matthysee. New York: Wiley, pp. 499–511.

—— —— Bartko, J. & Toohey, M. L. (1976), Schizophrenics and their families: Research on parental communication. In: *Developments in Psychiatric Research*, ed. J. M. Tanner. London: Hadden & Stoughton, pp. 254–286.

Yalom, I. (1992), *When Nietzsche Wept*. New York: Basic Books.

Yaryura-Tobias, J. & Neziroglu, F. (1997), *Obsessive Compulsive Disorder Spectrum: Pathogenesis, Diagnosis, and Treatment*. Washington, DC: American Psychiatric Press.

Zilboorg, G. (1941), Ambulatory schizophrenia. *Psychiatry*, 4:49–55.

Zillmer, E. & Perry, W. (1996), The neuropsychology of personality. *Assessment*, 3:205–263.

Zimet, C. N. & Fine, H. J. (1959), Perceptual differentiation and two dimensions of schizophrenia. *Journal of Nervous and Mental Disease*, 129:435–441.

Zucker, L. J. (1952), The psychology of latent schizophrenia. *American Journal of Psychotherapy*, 6:44–62.

INDEX